List of Online Cases

D0857919

THE
TEACHING
FILES Chest

THE TEACHING FILES Chest

C. Isabela S. Silva, MD, PhD
Research Associate, Department of Radiology
University of British Columbia
Vancouver, British Columbia, Canada

Nestor L. Müller, MD, PhD
Professor and Chairman, Department of Radiology
University of British Columbia
Head and Medical Director, Department of Radiology
Vancouver General Hospital
Vancouver, British Columbia, Canada

SAUNDERS

ELSEVIER

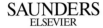

SAUNDERS
ELSEVIER

1600 John F. Kennedy Blvd.
Ste 1800
Philadelphia, PA 19103-2899

THE TEACHING FILES: CHEST   ISBN: 978-1-4160-6110-6

Notice

Knowledge and best practice in this field are constantly changing. As new research and experience broaden our knowledge, changes in practice, treatment, and drug therapy may become necessary or appropriate. Readers are advised to check the most current information provided (i) on procedures featured or (ii) by the manufacturer of each product to be administered, to verify the recommended dose or formula, the method and duration of administration, and contraindications. It is the responsibility of the practitioner, relying on his or her own experience and knowledge of the patient, to make diagnoses, to determine dosages and the best treatment for each individual patient, and to take all appropriate safety precautions. To the fullest extent of the law, neither the publisher nor the authors assume any liability for any injury and/or damage to persons or property arising out of or related to any use of the material contained in this book.

The Publisher

Library of Congress Cataloging-in-Publication Data
Silva, C. Isabela S.
    The teaching files. Chest/C. Isabela S. Silva, Nestor L. Muller. — 1st ed.
      p.;cm
    ISBN 978-1-4160-6110-6
    1. Chest—Diseases—Diagnosis. 2. Chest—Radiography. 3. Chest—Tomography. 4. Diagnosis, Radioscopic. 5. Diagnosis, Differential. I. Silva, C. Isabela S. II. Title.
      [DNLM: 1. Thoracic Diseases—diagnosis—Case Reports. 2. Diagnosis, Differential—Case Reports. 3. Diagnostic Imaging—methods—Case Reports.   WF 975 M958t 2010]
    RC941.M758 2010
    617.5'407572—dc22   2009032891

Acquisitions Editor: Rebecca Gaertner
Developmental Editor: Colleen McGonigal
Publishing Services Manager: Tina Rebane
Project Manager: Fran Gunning
Design Direction: Steve Stave

Printed in China

Last digit is the print number   9 8 7 6 5 4 3 2 1

To Alison and Phillip Müller and to Nicinha Silva

Preface

There are several ways to learn and teach chest radiology. The standard textbooks usually include a large number of disorders and the findings that are seen in each one of them. This format is particularly useful if the reader already knows what disorder the patient has and wants to learn more about it. However, in daily practice we are typically faced with a radiograph or CT image in a patient with an unknown condition and are asked to provide a specific diagnosis or a short differential diagnosis. Experienced chest radiologists usually have no difficulty providing the most likely differential diagnosis based on the pattern and distribution of findings and the clinical context. However, residents in training, respiratory physicians, and radiologists in general practice often have difficulty recognizing the main features that allow the expert to suggest a specific diagnosis. The aim of this book is to provide an overview of chest imaging based on key examples, or teaching files.

This teaching file book contains 200 cases that we consider key to learn and review the main concepts in chest radiology. They form the core teaching file of a chest radiologist with 25 years of experience in the field and one of the key learning and now teaching sources of a more junior chest radiologist.

This book is aimed at radiology residents, pulmonary physicians, and general radiologists with an interest in chest imaging. We believe that it provides a reasonably straightforward overview of the essential aspects of chest radiology, and we hope that it will succeed in making the subject enjoyable and gratifying to the reader.

C. Isabela S. Silva, MD, PhD
Nestor L. Müller, MD, PhD

Contents

THE TEACHING FILES Chest

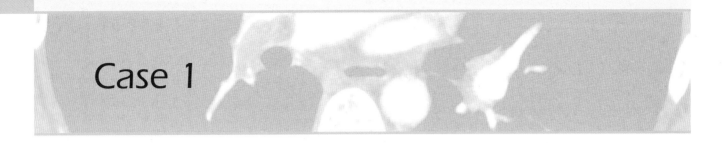

Case 1

DEMOGRAPHICS/CLINICAL HISTORY

A 30-year-old man with fever, undergoing radiography.

FINDINGS

Posteroanterior chest radiograph shows a focal area of consolidation in the right lower lung zone with obscuration of the right heart border (i.e., silhouette sign) that is consistent with right middle lobe pneumonia (Fig. 1). Posteroanterior chest radiograph of another patient shows a round, mass-like area of consolidation in the right middle lobe (Fig. 2).

DISCUSSION

Definition/Background

Consolidation on the chest radiograph and computed tomography (CT) is defined as a homogeneous increase in pulmonary parenchymal opacity that obscures the margins of vessels and airway walls. Air bronchograms may be present. Acute focal consolidation may result from pneumonia, aspiration, edema, hemorrhage, or pulmonary infarction.

Characteristic Clinical Features

Patients with pneumonia typically present with fever and cough, whereas those with pulmonary hemorrhage frequently present with hemoptysis. Pulmonary embolism resulting in infarction usually causes acute shortness of breath and pleuritic chest pain. Some patients may be asymptomatic or present with nonspecific symptoms.

Characteristic Radiologic Findings

The characteristic findings of acute focal consolidation consist of a focal (lobular, subsegmental, segmental, lobar, or round), fairly homogeneous area of increased opacity that obscures the underlying vessels.

Less Common Radiologic Manifestations

Air bronchograms are often present. Adjacent ground-glass opacities may be seen, particularly on CT. Hilar and mediastinal lymphadenopathy may be present in patients with focal consolidation due to pneumonia.

Differential Diagnosis
- Pneumonia
- Aspiration
- Hemorrhage
- Pulmonary edema
- Atelectasis

Discussion

The consolidation in pneumonia (i.e., bacterial, viral, or fungal) may be lobar (nonsegmental), round, or, more commonly, patchy and unilateral or bilateral. Focal consolidation due to aspiration typically involves a dependent lung region: the posterior segment of an upper or lower lobe or the superior segment of the lower lobe in the supine patient or the basal segments of a lower lobe in upright patients.

Segmental consolidation may be seen in pneumonia, distal to bronchial obstruction, and in association with acute pulmonary embolism. Spherical (round) areas of consolidation may occur in pneumonia, septic embolism, or occasionally in pulmonary hemorrhage.

Lung contusion results in focal consolidation that crosses normal anatomic boundaries. Focal right upper lobe pulmonary edema typically results from papillary muscle dysfunction after acute myocardial infarction. An important consideration in the differential diagnosis of focal consolidation is atelectasis. Atelectasis is typically associated with signs of volume loss, such as displacement of the adjacent interlobar fissure, hilum, or hemidiaphragm.

Diagnosis

Focal consolidation: acute causes

Suggested Readings

Gluecker T, Capasso P, Schnyder P, et al: Clinical and radiologic features of pulmonary edema. Radiographics 19:1507-1531, 1999.

Kim TH, Kim SJ, Ryu YH, et al: Differential CT features of infectious pneumonia versus bronchioloalveolar carcinoma (BAC) mimicking pneumonia. Eur Radiol 16:1763-1768, 2006.

Vilar J, Domingo ML, Soto C, Cogollos J: Radiology of bacterial pneumonia. Eur J Radiol 51:102-113, 1004.

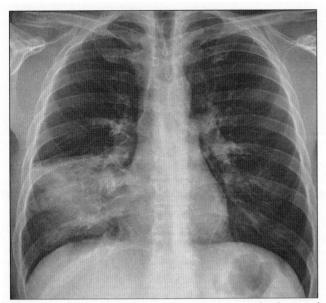

Figure 1. Posteroanterior chest radiograph shows a focal area of consolidation in the right lower lung zone with obscuration of the right heart border (i.e., silhouette sign) that is consistent with the diagnosis of right middle lobe pneumonia in a 30-year-old man with fever.

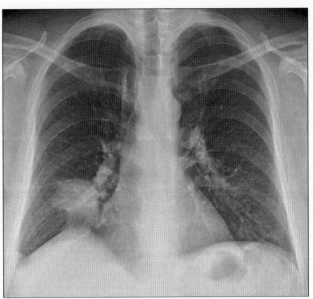

Figure 2. Round pneumonia was diagnosed in a 40-year-old man with fever and cough. Posteroanterior chest radiograph shows a round, mass-like area of consolidation in the right middle lobe.

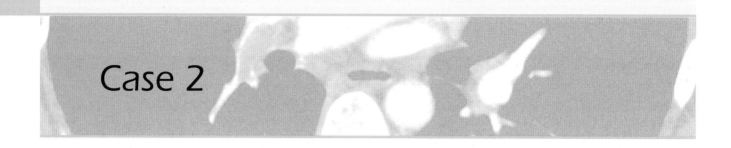

Case 2

DEMOGRAPHICS/CLINICAL HISTORY

A 53-year-old man who is asymptomatic but has an incidental radiographic finding, undergoing computed tomography (CT).

FINDINGS

CT shows a focal consolidation in the right upper lobe that is surrounded by minimal ground-glass opacity (Fig. 1). CT using soft tissue windows shows foci of fat attenuation within the consolidation that is consistent with lipoid pneumonia (Fig. 2). In another patient, CT shows a focal consolidation in the posterior basal segment of the left lower lobe (Fig. 3) and an artery originating from the descending thoracic aorta and extending into the consolidation consistent with intralobar sequestration (Fig. 4).

DISCUSSION

Definition/Background

Consolidation on the chest radiograph and CT is defined as a homogeneous increase in pulmonary parenchymal opacity that obscures the margins of vessels and airway walls. Air bronchograms may be present.

Characteristic Clinical Features

Patients are often asymptomatic or have nonspecific symptoms of cough or fever.

Characteristic Radiologic Findings

CT shows a fairly homogeneous area of increased opacity that obscures the underlying vessels and that may have well-defined or smoothly defined margins. An area of consolidation abutting a soft tissue structure typically obscures the margins of that structure (i.e., silhouette sign, which refers to the absence of the silhouette).

Less Common Radiologic Manifestations

Patients may have associated hilar or mediastinal lymphadenopathy. This is a nonspecific finding because the enlarged nodes may be reactive or contain tumor cells. A few patients may have ipsilateral pleural effusion.

Differential Diagnosis

- Obstructive pneumonitis distal to bronchial obstruction
- Lipoid pneumonia
- Intralobar sequestration
- Lung cancer (mainly adenocarcinoma)
- Pulmonary lymphoma (primary or secondary)

Discussion

Complete bronchial obstruction typically results in segmental or lobar areas of consolidation without air bronchograms. In most cases, there is associated volume loss (i.e., segmental, lobar, or, occasionally, entire lung atelectasis). The consolidation in extrinsic lipoid pneumonia usually contains areas of fat density evident on thin-section CT. Consolidation in intralobar sequestration typically affects the region of the posterior basal segment of the left lower lobe and is therefore in continuity with the diaphragm. Confirmation of the diagnosis can be made with contrast-enhanced CT, which shows the abnormal vessels originating from the descending aorta and supplying the intralobar sequestration. Pulmonary carcinoma or lymphoma should be suspected in patients with focal, round areas of ground-glass opacity or consolidation that progresses over several months.

Diagnosis

Focal consolidation: chronic causes

Suggested Readings

King LJ, Padley SP, Wotherspoon AC, et al: Pulmonary MALT lymphoma: Imaging findings in 24 cases. Eur Radiol 10:1932-1938, 2000.

Lee KS, Muller NL, Hale V, et al: Lipoid pneumonia: CT findings. J Comput Assist Tomogr 19:48-51, 1995.

Raz DJ, Kim JY, Jablons DM: Diagnosis and treatment of bronchioloalveolar carcinoma. Curr Opin Pulm Med 13:290-296, 2007.

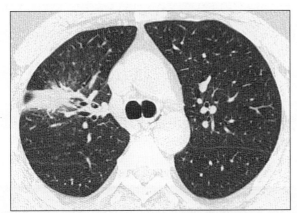

Figure 1. A 53-year-old man, asymptomatic, was diagnosed with lipoid pneumonia. CT shows focal consolidation in the right upper lobe surrounded by minimal ground-glass opacity.

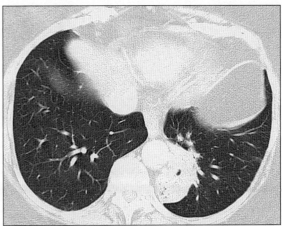

Figure 3. Intralobar sequestration was diagnosed in an 88-year-old woman. CT shows focal consolidation in the posterior basal segment of the left lower lobe.

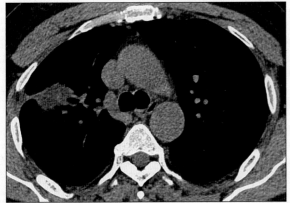

Figure 2. In the same patient, CT using soft tissue windows shows foci of fat attenuation within the consolidation that is consistent with lipoid pneumonia.

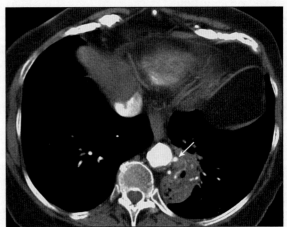

Figure 4. In the same patient, CT using soft tissue windows shows an artery originating from the descending thoracic aorta *(arrow)* and extending into the consolidation consistent with intralobar sequestration.

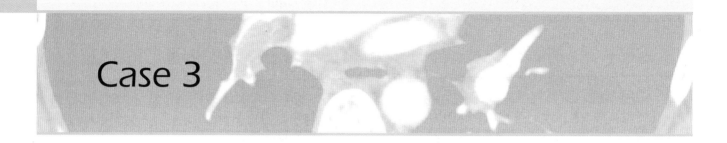

Case 3

DEMOGRAPHICS/CLINICAL HISTORY

A 44-year-old man with acute onset of fever and cough, undergoing radiography.

FINDINGS

Posteroanterior chest radiograph shows areas of consolidation in the right lung and bilateral hazy areas of increased opacity (Fig. 1). The culture was positive for *Streptococcus pneumoniae*. In a second patient, the posteroanterior chest radiograph shows consolidation in the right upper lobe and bilateral ground-glass opacity that are consistent with pulmonary hemorrhage (Fig. 2). In a third patient, the posteroanterior chest radiograph shows patchy consolidation in the left upper and lower lobes (Fig. 3). In a fourth patient, the chest radiograph shows multifocal consolidation involving mainly the dependent lung regions that are consistent with aspiration pneumonia (Fig. 4).

DISCUSSION

Definition/Background

Consolidation on the chest radiograph and computed tomography (CT) is defined as a homogeneous increase in pulmonary parenchymal opacity that obscures the margins of vessels and airway walls. Air bronchograms may be present.

Characteristic Clinical Features

Patients with pneumonia typically present with fever and cough, whereas those with pulmonary hemorrhage frequently present with hemoptysis. Pulmonary embolism resulting in infarction usually causes acute shortness of breath and pleuritic chest pain.

Characteristic Radiologic Findings

Patchy or confluent areas of increased opacity obscure the underlying vessels. Air bronchograms are seldom evident on the radiograph in patients with bronchopneumonia or pulmonary edema, but they are commonly seen on CT. Parenchymal consolidation also may result in poorly defined, 5- to 10-mm, nodular opacities known as air-space nodules. These nodular opacities have a centrilobular distribution and are more commonly seen on high-resolution CT scans than on radiographs.

Less Common Radiologic Manifestations

Hilar and mediastinal lymphadenopathy may be associated with bronchopneumonia. Pleural effusions may be present in patients with bronchopneumonia or pulmonary edema.

Differential Diagnosis
- Bronchopneumonia (bacterial, viral, fungal)
- Pneumonia
- Aspiration
- Pulmonary hemorrhage
- Pulmonary edema

Discussion

Acute multifocal consolidation is a common manifestation of bronchopneumonia. The areas of consolidation in aspiration pneumonia typically involve the dependent lung regions: the posterior segments of the upper and lower lobes and the superior segments of the lower lobes in the supine patient and the basal segments of the lower lobes in upright patients. Pulmonary hemorrhage may result in patchy or confluent, unilateral or bilateral ground-glass opacities or areas of consolidation. Multifocal or diffuse consolidation due to diffuse pulmonary hemorrhage is seen mainly in patients with vasculitis (e.g., Goodpasture syndrome, microscopic polyangiitis, Wegener granulomatosis). Multifocal consolidation due to hemorrhage is commonly seen in patients with blunt chest trauma (e.g., pulmonary contusion).

Diagnosis

Multifocal consolidation: acute causes

Suggested Readings

Gluecker T, Capasso P, Schnyder P, et al: Clinical and radiologic features of pulmonary edema. Radiographics 19:1507-1531, 1999.
Herold CJ, Sailer JG: Community-acquired and nosocomial pneumonia. Eur Radiol 14(Suppl 3):E2-E20, 2004.
Hiorns MP, Screaton NJ, Müller NL: Acute lung disease in the immunocompromised host. Radiol Clin North Am 39:1137-1151, vi, 2001.
Kjeldsberg KM, Oh K, Murray KA, Cannon G: Radiographic approach to multifocal consolidation. Semin Ultrasound CT MR 23:288-301, 2002.

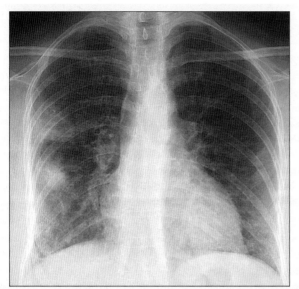

Figure 1. A 44-year-old man had acute onset of fever and cough. The posteroanterior chest radiograph shows areas of consolidation in the right lung and bilateral hazy areas of increased opacity. The culture was positive for *Streptococcus pneumoniae*.

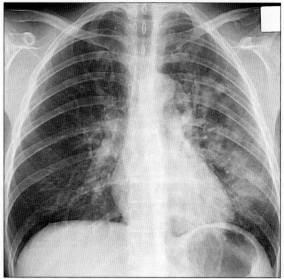

Figure 3. Multifocal consolidation was diagnosed in a 40-year-old man with bronchopneumonia. The posteroanterior chest radiograph shows patchy consolidation in the left upper and lower lobes. Notice the inhomogeneous increased opacity of the left heart compared with the region of the right atrium, which is consistent with consolidation in the retrocardiac region of the left lower lobe.

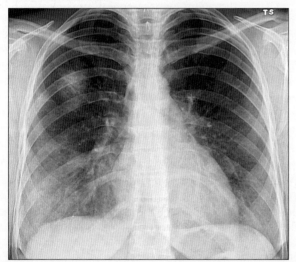

Figure 2. Multifocal consolidation was diagnosed in a 35-year-old man with Wegener granulomatosis who presented with hemoptysis. The posteroanterior chest radiograph shows consolidation in the right upper lobe and bilateral hazy areas of increased opacity (i.e., ground-glass opacities) that are consistent with pulmonary hemorrhage.

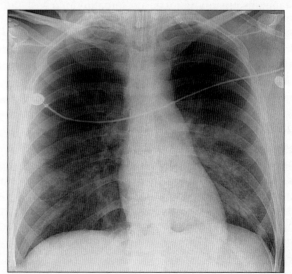

Figure 4. Aspiration pneumonia was diagnosed in a 32-year-old woman. The chest radiograph shows multifocal consolidation involving mainly the dependent lung regions.

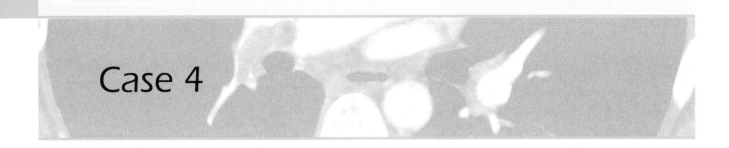

Case 4

DEMOGRAPHICS/CLINICAL HISTORY

A 41-year-old woman with a 7-week history of cough and recent laboratory tests showing peripheral eosinophilia, undergoing radiography and computed tomography (CT).

FINDINGS

Radiography shows bilateral, multifocal, peripheral, dense consolidation (Fig. 1) in a patient with chronic eosinophilic pneumonia. Coronal, reformatted CT shows bilateral, multifocal, peripheral consolidation and adjacent ground-glass opacities involving mainly the upper lung regions (Fig. 2). In a second patient, with cryptogenic organizing pneumonia, the posteroanterior chest radiograph shows patchy, bilateral areas of consolidation and hazy areas of increased opacity (Fig. 3). In a third patient with primary pulmonary lymphoma, CT shows bilateral, multiple, mass-like areas of consolidation containing air bronchograms (Fig. 4).

DISCUSSION

Definition/Background
Consolidation seen on the chest radiograph and CT scan is defined as a homogeneous increase in pulmonary parenchymal opacity that obscures the margins of vessels and airway walls. Air bronchograms may be present. Chronic, multifocal consolidation consists of unilateral patchy or confluent areas of consolidation present for several months.

Characteristic Clinical Features
Patients are often asymptomatic or have nonspecific symptoms of cough or fever. Most patients with eosinophilic lung disease have peripheral eosinophilia.

Characteristic Radiologic Findings
Patchy or confluent areas of increased opacity obscure the underlying vessels. Air bronchograms are commonly evident on the radiograph and CT scan.

Less Common Radiologic Manifestations
Ground-glass opacities are commonly seen adjacent to areas of consolidation on CT. Associated hilar or mediastinal lymphadenopathy may occur.

Differential Diagnosis
- Simple pulmonary eosinophilia (Loeffler syndrome)
- Chronic eosinophilic pneumonia
- Bronchiolitis obliterans organizing pneumonia
- Bronchioloalveolar cell carcinoma
- Lymphoma

Discussion
Simple pulmonary eosinophilia is characterized by blood eosinophilia and transient and migratory areas of consolidation that typically clear spontaneously within 1 month. Organizing pneumonia, also known as bronchiolitis obliterans organizing pneumonia (BOOP), most frequently manifests with patchy, nonsegmental, unilateral or bilateral areas of consolidation. The areas of consolidation may involve any lung zone. On CT, the areas of consolidation in BOOP often involve mainly the peribronchial and peripheral regions. BOOP may be idiopathic (e.g., cryptogenic organizing pneumonia) or result from a known cause such as infection, drug reaction, or collagen vascular disease.

The presence of consolidation that gradually increases over several months should raise the possibility of bronchioloalveolar cell carcinoma and lymphoma. The consolidation in bronchioloalveolar cell carcinoma may be focal or multifocal and confluent, and it is usually associated with air bronchograms. The consolidation results from tumor growth along the alveolar walls combined with secretion of mucin. Pulmonary lymphoma may result in single or multiple mass-like areas of consolidation or, less commonly, in extensive, confluent areas of consolidation. The areas of consolidation usually contain air bronchograms.

Diagnosis
Multifocal consolidation: chronic causes

Suggested Readings
Cordier JF: Cryptogenic organising pneumonia. Eur Respir J 28:422-446, 2006.

Jeong YJ, Kim KI, Seo IJ, et al: Eosinophilic lung diseases: A clinical, radiologic, and pathologic overview. Radiographics 27:617-637, 2007.

King LJ, Padley SP, Wotherspoon AC, et al: Pulmonary MALT lymphoma: Imaging findings in 24 cases. Eur Radiol 10:1932-1938, 2000.

Kjeldsberg KM, Oh K, Murray KA, Cannon G: Radiographic approach to multifocal consolidation. Semin Ultrasound CT MR 23:288-301, 2002.

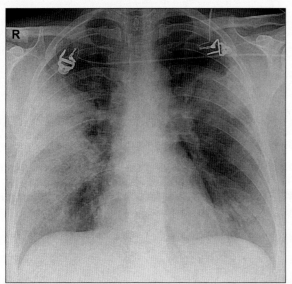

Figure 1. A 41-year-old woman had a 7-week history of cough and peripheral eosinophilia. The posteroanterior chest radiograph shows bilateral, multifocal, peripheral, dense consolidations. The patient had chronic eosinophilic pneumonia.

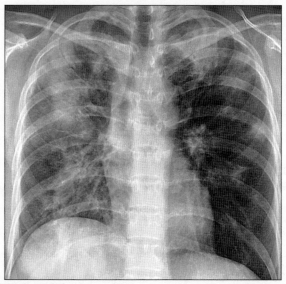

Figure 3. Multifocal consolidation is seen in a 50-year-old woman with idiopathic (cryptogenic) organizing pneumonia. The postero-anterior chest radiograph shows patchy, bilateral areas of consoli-dation and hazy areas of increased opacity.

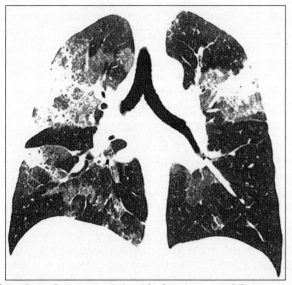

Figure 2. In the same patient with chronic eosinophilic pneumo-nia, coronal, reformatted CT shows bilateral, multifocal, periph-eral consolidations and adjacent ground-glass opacities involving mainly the upper lung regions.

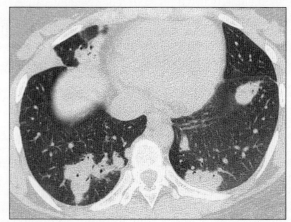

Figure 4. Multifocal consolidation is seen in an 18-year-old wom-an with primary pulmonary lymphoma. CT image shows bilat-eral, multiple, mass-like areas of consolidation containing air bronchograms.

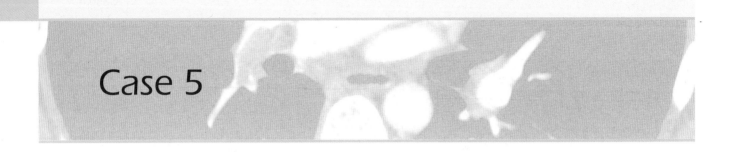

Case 5

DEMOGRAPHICS/CLINICAL HISTORY

A 31-year-old woman with acute onset of dyspnea after six cycles of bleomycin for Hodgkin lymphoma, undergoing radiography and computed tomography (CT).

FINDINGS

Chest radiograph shows extensive bilateral areas of consolidation (Fig. 1) that are consistent with diffuse alveolar damage resulting from a drug reaction and widening of the mediastinum. CT using soft tissue windows (Fig. 2) shows mediastinal lymph node enlargement caused by Hodgkin lymphoma. CT using lung window settings shows extensive consolidation that is most severe in the dependent lung regions, and extensive, bilateral areas of ground-glass opacities (Fig. 3).

DISCUSSION

Definition/Background

Consolidation on the chest radiograph and CT scan is defined as a homogeneous increase in pulmonary parenchymal opacity that obscures the margins of vessels and airway walls. A consolidation can be considered diffuse if the consolidation and accompanying ground-glass opacities occupy virtually all of the lung parenchyma.

Characteristic Clinical Features

Patients with acute diffuse consolidation typically present with acute shortness of breath. Pneumonia usually results in fever and productive cough, and diffuse pulmonary hemorrhage usually is associated with hemoptysis.

Characteristic Radiologic Findings

Diffuse parenchymal consolidation manifests as fairly homogenous, increased opacity of both lungs, with obscuration of the underlying vessels.

Less Common Radiologic Manifestations

Pleural effusions commonly are associated with hydrostatic pulmonary edema. They are relatively common in patients with severe pneumonia but occur in only a small percentage of patients with increased permeability edema or pulmonary hemorrhage. Enlarged hilar lymph nodes may be present in patients with pneumonia and enlarged mediastinal lymph nodes and in patients with chronic or recurrent hydrostatic pulmonary edema. On CT, ground-glass opacities are commonly seen adjacent to areas of consolidation.

Differential Diagnosis

- Pulmonary edema
- Acute respiratory distress syndrome (ARDS)
- Diffuse pulmonary hemorrhage
- Severe pneumonia

Discussion

Pulmonary edema may be hydrostatic (e.g., left heart failure, fluid overload) or caused by increased permeability. Increased permeability pulmonary edema is a characteristic manifestation of diffuse alveolar damage and results in the clinical entity of ARDS or, when less severe, acute lung injury (ALI). The characteristic radiologic manifestations of hydrostatic pulmonary edema consist of hazy perihilar increased opacity or consolidation associated with thickening of the interlobular septa (i.e., septal lines) and cardiomegaly. The consolidation in ARDS may be initially patchy but tends to become rapidly confluent and diffuse. Air bronchograms are commonly seen. Septal lines are seldom evident on the radiograph unless the patient has superimposed hydrostatic pulmonary edema. The main findings on CT consist of extensive, bilateral, ground-glass opacities and dependent areas of consolidation. Smooth thickening of the interlobular septa and intralobular lines may be seen superimposed on the ground-glass opacities, resulting in a pattern known as "crazy paving." Common causes of ARDS include shock, trauma, sepsis, pneumonia, and drug reactions. A similar pattern may be seen in acute interstitial pneumonia (AIP), which is essentially an idiopathic form of ARDS.

Diffuse pulmonary hemorrhage may result in patchy or confluent bilateral areas of consolidation that tend to involve mainly the middle and lower lung zones. The consolidation may have a predominantly perihilar distribution and typically spares the lung apices and the region of the costophrenic angles. Diffuse pulmonary hemorrhage is most commonly seen in patients with systemic vasculitis, including Goodpasture syndrome, Wegener granulomatosis, and microscopic polyangiitis. Diffuse hemorrhage can be seen in some collagen vascular diseases, particularly systemic lupus erythematosus.

Severe pneumonia may be caused by viruses, bacteria, or fungi (particularly *Pneumocystis jiroveci*). Although

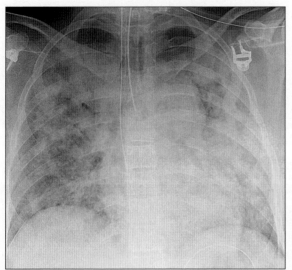

Figure 1. A 31-year-old woman has acute onset of dyspnea after six cycles of bleomycin for Hodgkin lymphoma. Chest radiograph shows extensive bilateral areas of consolidation that are consistent with diffuse alveolar damage resulting from a drug reaction and widening of the mediastinum.

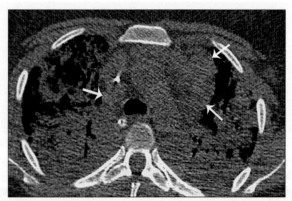

Figure 2. In the same patient, CT using soft tissue windows shows mediastinal lymph node enlargement *(arrows)* resulting from Hodgkin lymphoma and extensive consolidation involving mainly the dependent lung regions.

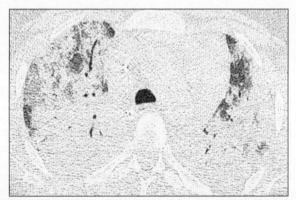

Figure 3. In the same patient, CT using lung windows shows extensive, bilateral areas of ground-glass opacities and consolidation, with the latter mainly in the dependent lung regions.

Pneumocystis may cause diffuse bilateral consolidation, it more commonly results in predominantly perihilar or diffuse ground-glass opacities.

Diagnosis
Diffuse consolidation: acute causes

Suggested Readings
Gluecker T, Capasso P, Schnyder P, et al: Clinical and radiologic features of pulmonary edema. Radiographics 19:1507-1531, 1999.

Ichikado K, Suga M, Muranaka H, et al: Prediction of prognosis for acute respiratory distress syndrome with thin-section CT: Validation in 44 cases. Radiology 238:321-329, 2006.

Johkoh T, Müller NL, Taniguchi H, et al: Acute interstitial pneumonia: Thin-section CT findings in 36 patients. Radiology 211:859-863, 1999.

Primack SL, Miller RR, Müller NL: Diffuse pulmonary hemorrhage: Clinical, pathologic, and imaging features. AJR Am J Roentgenol 164:295-300, 1995.

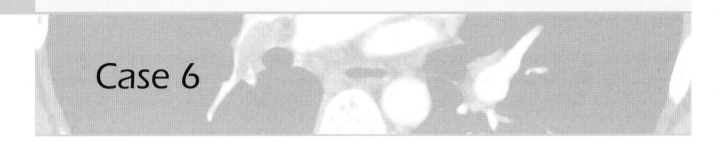

Case 6

DEMOGRAPHICS/CLINICAL HISTORY

A 46-year-old-man with chronic cough and progressive dyspnea, undergoing radiography.

FINDINGS

Chest radiograph shows extensive, bilateral consolidation and hazy areas of increased opacity (i.e. ground-glass opacities) in a patient with alveolar proteinosis (Fig. 1). In another patient with diffuse organizing pneumonia reaction due to amiodarone toxicity, the chest radiograph (Fig. 2) and CT (Fig. 3) show extensive consolidation and ground-glass opacities in a peribronchial distribution.

DISCUSSION

Definition/Background

Consolidation seen on the chest radiograph and CT scan is defined as a homogeneous increase in pulmonary parenchymal opacity that obscures the margins of vessels and airway walls. A consolidation can be considered diffuse if the consolidation and accompanying ground-glass opacities occupy virtually all of the lung parenchyma. A consolidation can be considered chronic if it is present for more than 1 month.

Characteristic Clinical Features

Patients have a chronic cough and progressive dyspnea.

Characteristic Radiologic Findings

Imaging shows extensive, bilateral consolidation and ground-glass opacities. Air bronchograms may be seen.

Less Common Radiologic Manifestations

Hilar and mediastinal lymphadenopathy may be present, particularly in patients with lymphoma and diffuse bronchoalveolar cell carcinoma.

Differential Diagnosis

- Pulmonary alveolar proteinosis
- Organizing pneumonia (bronchiolitis obliterans organizing pneumonia [BOOP])
- Eosinophilic pneumonia
- Lymphoma
- Bronchioloalveolar cell carcinoma

Discussion

Chronic, diffuse pulmonary consolidation is much less common than acute, diffuse consolidation. Chronic consolidation is usually focal or multifocal rather than diffuse.

Alveolar proteinosis is an uncommon condition of unknown origin that is often diffuse. Occasionally, alveolar proteinosis may be caused by inhalation of large quantities of silica dust (i.e., silicoproteinosis) or be associated with marked immunosuppression. Alveolar proteinosis is characterized on high-resolution CT by the presence of smooth septal lines and intralobular lines superimposed on the ground-glass opacities, resulting in a crazy-paving pattern.

Organizing pneumonia most commonly results in a patchy, bilateral consolidation that has a predominantly peribronchial and peripheral distribution on CT, but it occasionally may be diffuse. Similarly, chronic eosinophilic pneumonia typically results in consolidation mainly in the peripheral lung regions, but it may occasionally be diffuse.

Bilateral consolidation that progresses slowly over several months should raise the possibility of lymphoma or bronchioloalveolar cell carcinoma.

Diagnosis

Diffuse consolidation: chronic causes

Suggested Readings

Chung MJ, Lee KS, Franquet T, et al: Metabolic lung disease: Imaging and histopathologic findings. Eur J Radiol 54:233-245, 2005.

Jeong YJ, Kim KI, Seo IJ, et al: Eosinophilic lung diseases: A clinical, radiologic, and pathologic overview. Radiographics 27:617-637, 2007.

Lee KS, Kim EA: High-resolution CT of alveolar filling disorders. Radiol Clin North Am 39:1211-1230, 2001.

Lee KS, Kullnig P, Hartman TE, Muller NL: Cryptogenic organizing pneumonia: CT findings in 43 patients. AJR Am J Roentgenol 162:543-546, 1994.

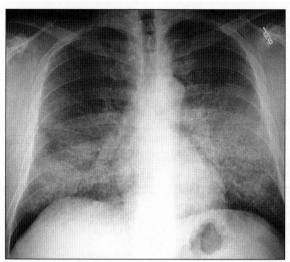

Figure 1. Chest radiograph shows extensive, bilateral consolidation and hazy areas of increased opacity (i.e., ground-glass opacities) in a 46-year-old patient with alveolar proteinosis.

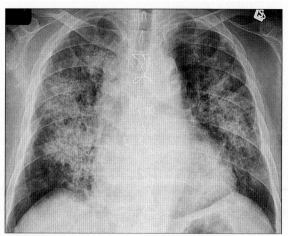

Figure 2. In a 59-year-old man with diffuse organizing pneumonia reaction due to amiodarone toxicity, the chest radiograph shows extensive consolidation. Other changes are related to a previous sternotomy.

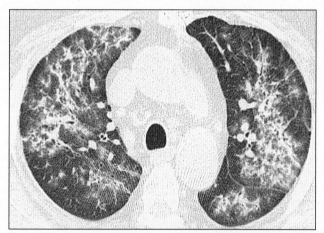

Figure 3. In a 59-year-old man with diffuse organizing pneumonia reaction due to amiodarone toxicity, CT shows extensive consolidation and ground-glass opacities in a peribronchial distribution.

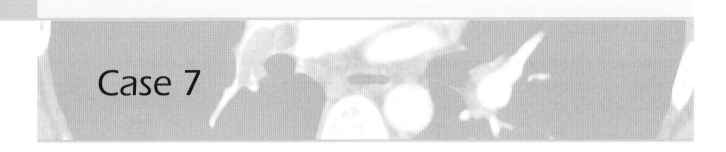

Case 7

DEMOGRAPHICS/CLINICAL HISTORY

A 58-year-old man with acute shortness of breath after coronary artery bypass graft surgery, undergoing radiography.

FINDINGS

Chest radiograph in a patient with acute pulmonary edema shows bilateral areas of consolidation involving mainly the perihilar regions of both lungs, creating a bat's wing or butterfly appearance; the cortex of both lungs is relatively unaffected (Fig. 1). Other findings are related to the sternotomy and the tube and lines in place. In another patient with diffuse pulmonary hemorrhage, CT shows extensive, bilateral areas of consolidation in a predominantly central and peribronchial distribution (Fig. 2).

DISCUSSION

Definition/Background

Consolidation seen on the chest radiograph and CT is defined as a homogeneous increase in pulmonary parenchymal opacity that obscures the margins of vessels and airway walls. Air bronchograms are often present. Central (i.e., butterfly or batwing distribution) refers to consolidation involving mainly the perihilar regions, with relative sparing of the outer third of the lungs.

Characteristic Clinical Features

Patients with central consolidation most commonly present with dyspnea. Other symptoms include fever (e.g., Pneumocystis pneumonia, organizing pneumonia) and hemoptysis (e.g., diffuse pulmonary hemorrhage). Patients with alveolar proteinosis may have relatively mild symptoms of chronic cough and shortness of breath despite extensive consolidation seen radiologically.

Characteristic Radiologic Findings

The characteristic findings of central consolidation consist of fairly homogeneous areas of increased opacity that obscure the underlying vessels and that spare the outer third of the lungs. In most patients, central consolidation is bilateral and symmetric.

Less Common Radiologic Manifestations

Patients may have associated findings of left heart failure or fluid overload (e.g., enlarged pulmonary vessels, septal lines, peribronchial cuffing, small pleural effusions) and reticulonodular opacities (e.g., resolving pulmonary hemorrhage, pulmonary alveolar proteinosis).

Differential Diagnosis

- Hydrostatic pulmonary edema
- Diffuse pulmonary hemorrhage
- Pneumocystis pneumonia
- Organizing pneumonia (bronchiolitis obliterans organizing pneumonia [BOOP])
- Pulmonary alveolar proteinosis

Discussion

The most common cause of central (i.e., butterfly or batwing) consolidation is hydrostatic pulmonary edema resulting from left heart failure or fluid overload associated with renal failure. These patients frequently have associated findings of left heart failure or fluid overload (e.g., enlarged pulmonary vessels, septal lines, peribronchial cuffing, small pleural effusions).

Diffuse pulmonary hemorrhage and Pneumocystis pneumonia frequently have no associated findings. Organizing pneumonia is a common reaction pattern that may result from infection or drugs or may be associated with collagen vascular diseases. In some cases, no cause is found (i.e., cryptogenic organizing pneumonia). It often has a predominantly peribronchial distribution on CT.

Alveolar proteinosis is characterized on high-resolution CT by the presence of smooth septal lines and intralobular lines superimposed on the ground-glass opacities, resulting in a crazy-paving pattern. A crazy-paving pattern also may be seen in a number of other conditions including the resolving phase of diffuse pulmonary hemorrhage and occasionally in pulmonary edema.

Diagnosis

Central consolidation (butterfly or batwing distribution)

Suggested Readings

Chung MJ, Lee KS, Franquet T, et al: Metabolic lung disease: Imaging and histopathologic findings. Eur J Radiol 54:233-245, 2005.

Gluecker T, Capasso P, Schnyder P, et al: Clinical and radiologic features of pulmonary edema. Radiographics 19:1507-1531, 1999.

Hiorns MP, Screaton NJ, Müller NL: Acute lung disease in the immunocompromised host. Radiol Clin North Am 39:1137-1151, 2001.

Kjeldsberg KM, Oh K, Murray KA, Cannon G: Radiographic approach to multifocal consolidation. Semin Ultrasound CT MR 23:288-301, 2002.

Primack SL, Miller RR, Müller NL: Diffuse pulmonary hemorrhage: Clinical, pathologic, and imaging features. AJR Am J Roentgenol 164:295-300, 1995.

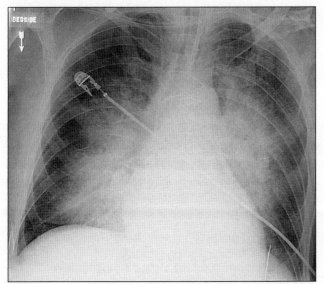

Figure 1. A 58-year-old man has acute hydrostatic pulmonary edema after coronary artery bypass graft surgery. The chest radiograph shows bilateral areas of consolidation involving mainly the perihilar regions and medullary portions of both lungs, creating a bat's wing or butterfly appearance; the cortex of both lungs is relatively unaffected. Other findings are related to the sternotomy and tubes lines in place.

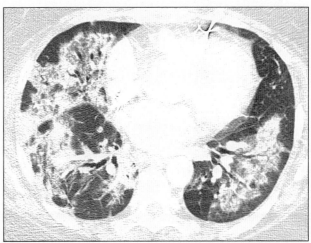

Figure 2. Diffuse pulmonary hemorrhage was diagnosed in a 36-year-old man with microscopic polyangiitis. CT shows extensive bilateral areas of consolidation in a predominantly central and peribronchial distribution.

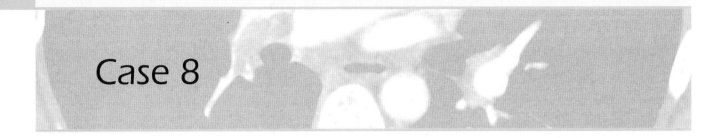

Case 8

DEMOGRAPHICS/CLINICAL HISTORY

A 39-year-old woman with chronic cough and progressive dyspnea, undergoing computed tomography.

FINDINGS

CT shows bilateral consolidation involving mainly the peripheral lung regions. Lung biopsy confirmed organizing pneumonia, and the final diagnosis was cryptogenic organizing pneumonia. In another patient who had chronic eosinophilic pneumonia, the chest radiograph shows bilateral consolidation involving mainly the peripheral lung regions of the upper lung zones (Fig. 2).

DISCUSSION

Definition/Background

Consolidation seen on the chest radiograph and CT scan is defined as a homogeneous increase in pulmonary parenchymal opacity that obscures the margins of vessels and airway walls. Air bronchograms are often present. Peripheral consolidation (i.e., reverse pulmonary edema pattern) is defined as consolidation involving predominantly the outer third of the lungs.

Characteristic Clinical Features

Common symptoms include cough and shortness of breath. Low-grade fever is common in chronic eosinophilic pneumonia and in cryptogenic organizing pneumonia. A history of atopy or asthma is elicited in approximately 50% of patients with chronic eosinophilic pneumonia. Most patients with chronic eosinophilic pneumonia have peripheral eosinophilia.

Characteristic Radiologic Findings

The characteristic findings of peripheral consolidation consist of fairly homogeneous areas of increased opacity that obscure the underlying vessels and that involve predominantly or exclusively the outer third of the lungs. The consolidation may be unilateral but is more commonly bilateral and fairly symmetric.

Less Common Radiologic Manifestations

Some patients may have associated pleural effusions or lymphadenopathy. Small, nodular opacities may be seen in patients with bronchioloalveolar cell carcinoma.

Differential Diagnosis

- Chronic eosinophilic pneumonia
- Organizing pneumonia (bronchiolitis obliterans organizing pneumonia [BOOP])
- Sarcoidosis
- Bronchioloalveolar cell carcinoma
- Radiation pneumonitis and fibrosis

Discussion

The most common causes of peripheral consolidation are chronic eosinophilic pneumonia and BOOP. Findings identical to chronic eosinophilic pneumonia may be seen in patients with Churg-Strauss syndrome. The consolidation in chronic eosinophilic pneumonia tends to involve mainly the upper lung zones and the outer third of the lungs. The peripheral distribution is apparent on the radiograph in 50% to 60% of cases and on CT in 90% to 95% of cases.

BOOP is a common reaction pattern associated with infection, drug toxicity, and collagen vascular diseases. In many patients, it is idiopathic (e.g., cryptogenic organizing pneumonia, idiopathic BOOP). The consolidation in organizing pneumonia frequently has a patchy distribution on the radiograph and a predominantly peribronchial and peripheral distribution on CT. In some patients, however, the consolidation may be predominantly or exclusively peripheral.

Sarcoidosis may result in a variety of parenchymal manifestations, including nodular opacities, ground-glass opacities, and consolidation. In most patients, the abnormalities have a perilymphatic distribution along the bronchi, vessels, septa, and pleura. Occasionally, sarcoidosis may manifest with predominantly or exclusively peripheral consolidation, usually in association with symmetric bilateral hilar and paratracheal lymphadenopathy.

Chronic eosinophilic pneumonia, organizing pneumonia, and sarcoidosis result in bilateral, fairly symmetric areas of consolidation. Causes of unilateral chronic peripheral consolidation include bronchioloalveolar cell carcinoma and radiation pneumonitis (typically after tangential beam irradiation for breast cancer).

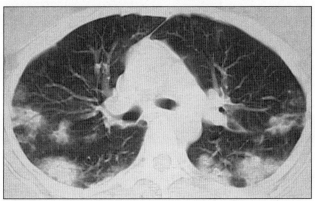

Figure 1. A 39-year-old woman has a chronic cough and progressive dyspnea. CT shows bilateral consolidations involving mainly the peripheral lung regions. Lung biopsy confirmed organizing pneumonia, and the final diagnosis was cryptogenic organizing pneumonia.

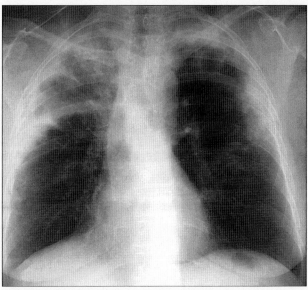

Figure 2. A 48-year-old woman has a chronic cough and peripheral eosinophilia. The chest radiograph shows bilateral consolidations involving mainly the peripheral lung regions of the upper lung zones. The final diagnosis was chronic eosinophilic pneumonia.

Diagnosis

Peripheral consolidation (reverse pulmonary edema pattern).

Suggested Readings

Allen JN, Davis WB: Eosinophilic lung diseases. Am J Respir Crit Care Med 150:1423-1438, 1994.

Cordier JF: Cryptogenic organising pneumonia. Eur Respir J 28: 422-446, 2006.

Kim Y, Lee KS, Choi DC, et al: The spectrum of eosinophilic lung disease: Radiologic findings. J Comput Assist Tomogr 21:920-930, 1997.

Lynch DA, Travis WD, Müller NL, et al: Idiopathic interstitial pneumonias: CT features. Radiology 236:10-21, 2005.

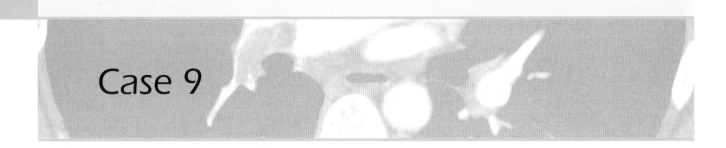

Case 9

DEMOGRAPHICS/CLINICAL HISTORY

A 40-year-old man with a mild, chronic cough, undergoing radiography.

FINDINGS

Chest radiograph shows hyperlucency and decreased vascularity of the left lung in a patient with Swyer-James-McLeod syndrome (Fig. 1). The mediastinum is shifted to the left, consistent with a decreased left lung volume. In other patients, CT shows a diffuse decrease in attenuation and vascularity of the right lung and an endoluminal tumor in right main bronchus (Fig. 2); decreased attenuation and vascularity of the left lung with associated bronchiectasis and mild volume loss, leading to an ipsilateral shift of the mediastinum and anterior junction line (Fig. 3); and air trapping in the left lung in a case of Swyer-James-McLeod syndrome (Fig. 4).

DISCUSSION

Definition/Background
Unilateral hyperlucency of a lung refers to increased lucency and usually decreased vascularity of one lung.

Characteristic Clinical Features
Patients may be asymptomatic or present with cough, dyspnea, and, occasionally, hemoptysis.

Characteristic Radiologic Findings
Radiologic findings include diffuse increased lucency of a lung, which usually is associated with decreased vascularity and decreased size of the hilum. The lung volume may be normal or decreased or may occasionally be increased. Expiratory chest radiography or CT frequently shows air trapping.

Less Common Radiologic Manifestations
Imaging may identify an absent hilum.

Differential Diagnosis
- Swyer-James-McLeod syndrome
- Partial bronchial obstruction
- Compensatory hyperinflation in lobar atelectasis or lobectomy
- Congenital lobar emphysema
- Proximal interruption of the pulmonary artery
- Fibrosing mediastinitis with narrowing of pulmonary artery
- Pneumothorax
- Congenital absence of pectoralis muscle (e.g., Poland syndrome)
- Mastectomy
- Scoliosis

Discussion
The main causes of unilateral hyperlucent lung in adults are Swyer-James-McLeod syndrome and partial obstruction of the main bronchus by a tumor or foreign body. Occasionally, it may result from hypoplasia or proximal interruption of the pulmonary artery.

In Swyer-James-McLeod syndrome, the ipsilateral hilum exists but is diminutive, a valuable feature in the differentiation from proximal interruption of a pulmonary artery (i.e., pulmonary artery agenesis). The diagnosis is confirmed by air trapping seen during expiration. This finding is a reflection of airway obstruction and is extremely valuable in differentiating the syndrome from other conditions that may give rise to unilateral or lobar hyperlucency.

Although several conditions can have a radiographic appearance similar to that of Swyer-James-McLeod syndrome, only one offers a serious potential difficulty. A partly obstructing lesion situated within a main bronchus can create a triad of radiographic signs that are indistinguishable from Swyer-James-McLeod syndrome: a smaller than normal lung volume, air trapping on expiration, and diffuse oligemia as a result of hypoxic vasoconstriction. In any patient with these signs, the presence of a lesion within the ipsilateral main bronchus must be excluded before a diagnosis of the syndrome is accepted; the easiest way to accomplish exclusion is by performing CT.

On the chest radiograph, it is important to exclude extrapulmonary abnormalities that may result in unilateral lucency of a hemithorax, such as pneumothorax, congenital absence of the pectoralis muscle, mastectomy, scoliosis, or hyperlucency due to technical artifacts such as patient rotation.

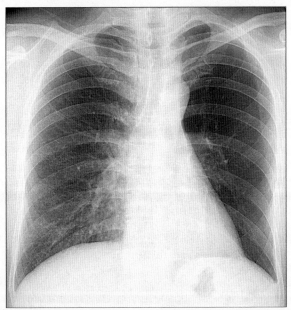

Figure 1. Chest radiograph shows hyperlucency and decreased vascularity of the left lung. The mediastinum is shifted to the left, consistent with a decreased left lung volume. The patient was a 40-year-old man with Swyer-James-McLeod syndrome.

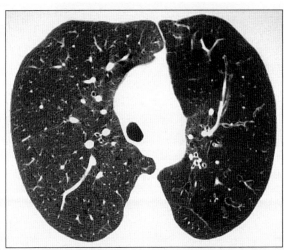

Figure 3. High-resolution CT shows decreased attenuation and vascularity of the left lung with associated bronchiectasis and mild volume loss, leading to an ipsilateral shift of the mediastinum and anterior junction line. The patient was a 61-year-old woman with Swyer-James-McLeod syndrome.

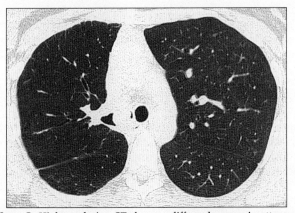

Figure 2. High-resolution CT shows a diffuse decrease in attenuation and vascularity of the right lung and an endoluminal tumor in the right main bronchus. The patient was a 31-year-old woman with a typical carcinoid tumor.

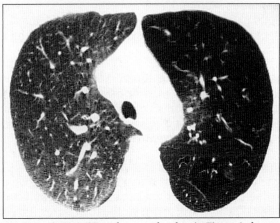

Figure 4. Expiratory CT at the same level as in Figure 3 shows air trapping in the left lung. The mediastinum and anterior junction line are in the midline in a 61-year-old woman with Swyer-James-McLeod syndrome.

Diagnosis
Hyperlucent lung, unilateral hyperlucent lung

Suggested Readings
Bouros D, Pare P, Panagou P, et al: The varied manifestation of pulmonary artery agenesis in adulthood. Chest 108:670-676, 1995.
Lucaya J, Gartner S, Garcia-Pena P, et al: Spectrum of manifestations of Swyer-James-MacLeod syndrome. J Comput Assist Tomogr 22:592-597, 1998.

Moore ADA, Godwin JD, Dietrich PA, et al: Swyer-James syndrome: CT findings in eight patients. AJR Am J Roentgenol 158:1211-1215, 1992.

Case 10

DEMOGRAPHICS/CLINICAL HISTORY

A 55-year-old man with acute shortness of breath, undergoing computed tomography (CT).

FINDINGS

CT shows extensive, bilateral, smooth, interlobular septal thickening (i.e., septal pattern) in a patient with interstitial pulmonary edema. Small, bilateral pleural effusions also can be seen (Fig. 1).

DISCUSSION

Definition/Background

A septal pattern results from thickening of the interlobular septa (i.e., connective tissue that separates the secondary pulmonary lobules).

Characteristic Clinical Features

Patients with a septal pattern most commonly present with progressive shortness of breath. Symptoms may be acute (e.g., hydrostatic pulmonary edema) or chronic (e.g., lymphangitic carcinomatosis).

Characteristic Radiologic Findings

On the chest radiograph, septal lines typically appear as thin, linear opacities at right angles to and in contact with the lateral pleural surfaces near the lung bases (i.e., Kerley B lines) (Fig. 2). On high-resolution CT, septal thickening can also be seen in the central lung parenchyma, where it results in characteristic polygonal arcades (Fig. 1).

Less Common Radiologic Manifestations

In hydrostatic pulmonary edema and lymphangitic carcinomatosis, septal thickening is frequently associated with small pleural effusions. Less common associated findings include hilar and mediastinal lymphadenopathy (Fig. 3). In most patients with septal thickening, the architecture of the lung is preserved. Distortion of architecture, such as traction bronchiectasis and bronchiolectasis, is seen in septal thickening associated with pulmonary fibrosis.

Differential Diagnosis
- Pulmonary edema
- Lymphatic spread of tumor (e.g. lymphangitic carcinomatosis, lymphoma, leukemia)
- Sarcoidosis
- Metabolic lung disease (e.g., alveolar proteinosis, amyloidosis, alveolar microlithiasis, Niemann-Pick syndrome)
- Interstitial pulmonary fibrosis (e.g., idiopathic pulmonary fibrosis, nonspecific interstitial pneumonia, asbestosis, chronic hypersensitivity pneumonitis)
- Pulmonary veno-occlusive disease
- Churg-Strauss syndrome
- Pleural inflammation

Discussion

Thickening of the interlobular septa may be caused by edema, cellular infiltration, or fibrosis. The differential diagnosis on high-resolution CT is based on the characteristics of the septal thickening (e.g., smooth, nodular, irregular) and the presence of associated findings.

Smooth septal thickening is commonly caused by hydrostatic pulmonary edema (Fig. 1). Less common causes of smooth septal thickening include lymphatic spread of carcinoma, lymphoma, leukemia, Churg-Strauss syndrome, acute lung rejection, pulmonary veno-occlusive disease, congenital lymphangiectasia, and Niemann-Pick syndrome (Fig. 4). These conditions tend to result in extensive septal thickening that is usually bilateral and often symmetric. Localized, smooth septal thickening often occurs adjacent to pleural inflammation, particularly in patients with empyema or after pleurodesis.

Nodular septal thickening occurs most commonly in patients with lymphangitic carcinomatosis and sarcoidosis. Less common causes include lymphoma, Kaposi sarcoma, leukemia, and amyloidosis. It is important to distinguish veins normally present in the interlobular septa, particularly when they are seen in cross section, from nodular septal thickening.

Irregular septal thickening is seen most commonly in patients with interstitial fibrosis, particularly idiopathic pulmonary fibrosis, asbestosis, and sarcoidosis. It is usually associated with other findings of fibrosis, such as reticulation, traction bronchiectasis, and bronchiolectasis and is seldom the predominant pattern.

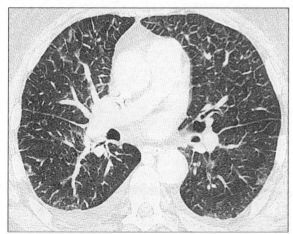

Figure 1. CT shows extensive, bilateral, smooth, interlobular septal thickening (i.e., septal pattern) in a 55-year-old man with interstitial pulmonary edema. Small, bilateral pleural effusions can be seen.

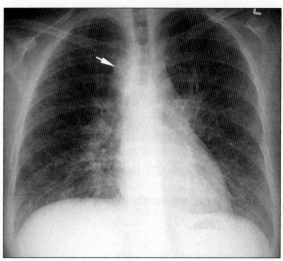

Figure 3. Posteroanterior chest radiograph shows a septal pattern in the lymphangitic carcinomatosis of a 36-year-old woman with breast cancer. The radiograph shows extensive, bilateral, linear opacities and right paratracheal lymph node enlargement *(arrow)*.

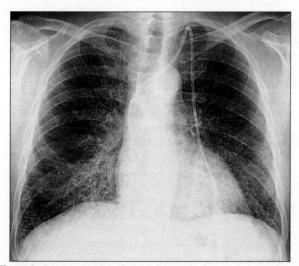

Figure 2. Posteroanterior chest radiograph shows the septal pattern in a 54-year-old man with interstitial pulmonary edema. Extensive, bilateral linear opacities are 1 to 2 cm long and perpendicular to the pleura (i.e., Kerley B lines). A central venous line is in place.

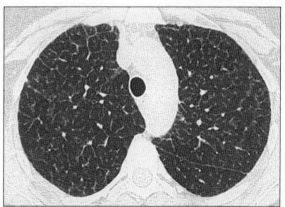

Figure 4. CT shows the septal pattern in Niemann-Pick syndrome. High-resolution CT shows diffuse, bilateral, and symmetric interlobular septal thickening in a 54-year-old woman.

Diagnosis
Septal pattern: definition and differential diagnosis

Suggested Readings

Kang EY, Grenier P, Laurent F, Müller NL: Interlobular septal thickening: Patterns at high-resolution computed tomography. J Thorac Imaging 11:260-264, 1996.

Müller NL, Miller RR: Computed tomography of chronic diffuse infiltrative lung disease. Part 1. Am Rev Respir Dis 142:1206-1215, 1990.

Webb WR: Thin-section CT of the secondary pulmonary lobule: Anatomy and the image—the 2004 Fleischner lecture. Radiology 239:322-338, 2006.

Case 11

DEMOGRAPHICS/CLINICAL HISTORY

A 47-year-old woman with progressive shortness of breath, undergoing radiography and computed tomography (CT).

FINDINGS

Posteroanterior chest radiograph (Fig. 1) shows hyperlucency of both lungs, which is most noticeable in the peripheral lung regions and lower lung zones, and hyperinflation with flattening of the diaphragm due to panacinar emphysema. Coronal, reformatted, high-resolution CT (Fig. 2) shows extensive areas of decreased attenuation mainly in the lower lobes, which is consistent with panacinar emphysema. In another patient with severe bronchiolitis obliterans, a posteroanterior chest radiograph (Fig. 3) shows hyperlucency of both lungs, marked decrease in the peripheral vascular markings, and increased lung volumes. Coronal, reformatted, high-resolution CT (Fig. 4) in a different patient shows extensive areas of decreased attenuation and vascularity and areas of slightly increased attenuation and vascularity, resulting in a mosaic pattern of attenuation and perfusion.

DISCUSSION

Definition/Background
Bilateral hyperlucency refers to increased lucency and usually decreased vascularity of both lungs. The lung volumes may be normal, or more commonly, they are increased.

Characteristic Clinical Features
Patients usually have chronic symptoms of cough and progressive shortness of breath.

Characteristic Radiologic Findings
Findings include diffuse, increased lucency of both lungs, which usually is associated with decreased vascularity and increased lung volumes.

Less Common Radiologic Manifestations
Imaging may show central pulmonary arteries that are enlarged by chronic pulmonary arterial hypertension.

Differential Diagnosis
- Emphysema
- Asthma
- Bronchiolitis in infants
- Bronchiolitis obliterans
- Pulmonary arterial hypertension
- Kyphosis
- Bilateral mastectomy
- Overexposed chest radiograph

Discussion
The most common cause of generalized bilateral hyperlucency and overinflation of both lungs is emphysema. Radiographic manifestations of emphysema include irregular areas of radiolucency, local avascular areas, distortion of vessels, bullae, and hyperinflation. On CT, emphysema is characterized by areas of abnormally low attenuation. The areas of low attenuation usually have no visible walls, although occasionally, walls 1 mm or less are seen, particularly in patients with paraseptal emphysema and bulla formation.

The most common radiographic abnormalities of asthma are bronchial wall thickening and hyperinflation. Hyperinflation in asthma is more common in children than in adults. High-resolution CT may show areas of decreased attenuation and vascularity; expiratory CT commonly shows focal areas of air trapping.

The radiographic manifestations of severe bronchiolitis obliterans (i.e., obliterative bronchiolitis) consist of hyperinflation and a decrease in peripheral vascular markings. Areas of decreased attenuation and vascularity can be seen on inspiratory CT scans, and air trapping can be seen on expiratory CT scans. Redistribution of blood flow to uninvolved lung results in a heterogeneous pattern of attenuation and vascularity (i.e., mosaic perfusion). Common associated findings include bronchial dilatation and bronchial wall thickening.

Increased lucency on the chest radiograph can result from chest wall abnormalities (e.g., kyphosis, bilateral mastectomy) or technical artifacts (e.g., overexposed radiograph).

Diagnosis
Hyperlucent lung, bilateral

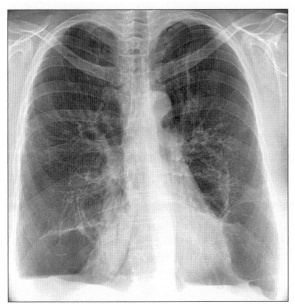

Figure 1. Posteroanterior chest radiograph shows hyperlucency of both lungs, which is most noticeable in the peripheral lung regions and lower lung zones, and hyperinflation with flattening of the diaphragm. The patient was a 47-year-old woman with panacinar emphysema due to α1-antitrypsin deficiency.

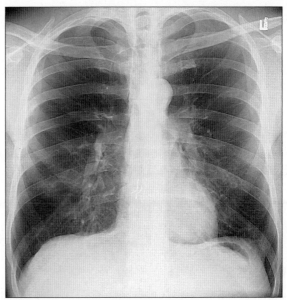

Figure 3. Posteroanterior chest radiograph shows hyperlucency of both lungs, a marked decrease in the peripheral vascular markings, and increased lung volumes. The patient was a 44-year-old man with severe bronchiolitis obliterans after bilateral lung transplantation.

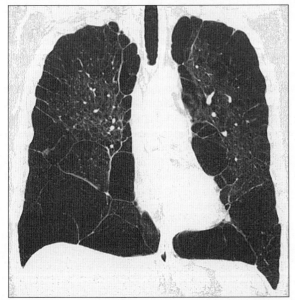

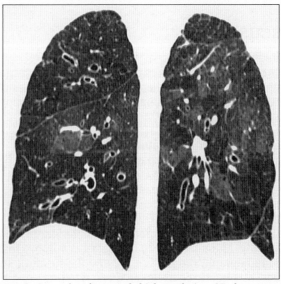

Figure 2. In the same patient, coronal, reformatted, high-resolution CT shows extensive areas of decreased attenuation mainly in the lower lobes, which is consistent with panacinar emphysema. Several bullae and upper lobe centrilobular emphysema can be seen.

Figure 4. Coronal, reformatted, high-resolution CT shows extensive areas of decreased attenuation and vascularity and areas of slightly increased attenuation and vascularity, resulting in a mosaic pattern of attenuation and perfusion. Extensive bronchiectasis can be seen. The patient was a 20-year-old woman with severe bronchiolitis obliterans after bilateral lung transplantation.

Suggested Readings

Bankier AA, Madani A, Gevenois PA: CT quantification of pulmonary emphysema: Assessment of lung structure and function. Crit Rev Comput Tomogr 43:399-417, 2002.

Pratt PC: Role of conventional chest radiography in diagnosis and exclusion of emphysema. Am J Med 82:998-1006, 1987.

Silva CI, Colby TV, Müller NL: Asthma and associated conditions: High-resolution CT and pathologic findings. AJR Am J Roentgenol 183:817-824, 2004.

Thurlbeck WM, Müller NL: Emphysema: Definition, imaging, and quantification. AJR Am J Roentgenol 163:1017-1025, 1994.

Case 12

DEMOGRAPHICS/CLINICAL HISTORY

A 76-year-old man with progressive shortness of breath, undergoing chest radiography and computed tomography (CT).

FINDINGS

Posteroanterior chest radiograph shows an extensive bilateral reticular pattern, which is worse in the lower lung zones, and reduced lung volumes (Fig. 1). The reticular pattern in this patient with idiopathic pulmonary fibrosis was caused by summation of irregular linear opacities and honeycombing, as demonstrated on a coronal high-resolution CT image (Fig. 2).

DISCUSSION

Definition/Background

A reticular pattern (i.e., reticulation) on the chest radiograph is defined as a collection of innumerable, small, linear opacities that by summation produce an appearance resembling a net.

Characteristic Clinical Features

Patients with a reticular pattern most commonly present with slowly progressive shortness of breath and dry cough. Occasionally, the patients may be asymptomatic.

Characteristic Radiologic Findings

The characteristic appearance is that of innumerable, interlacing line shadows that suggest a mesh. On the chest radiograph, the pattern may be the result of summation of smooth or irregular linear opacities or cystic spaces, or both. In most patients, the reticular pattern involves mainly the lower lung zones.

Less Common Radiologic Manifestations

The reticular pattern is often the only finding on the radiograph. Associated findings may be related to the underlying disease, such as pleural thickening or effusion in collagen vascular disease, esophageal dilatation in scleroderma, or pleural plaques in asbestosis. Idiopathic pulmonary fibrosis is more common in smokers, and these patients often have associated findings of emphysema. Enlarged central pulmonary arteries suggest associated pulmonary arterial hypertension.

Differential Diagnosis

- Pulmonary edema
- Interstitial pulmonary fibrosis: Idiopathic pulmonary fibrosis (IPF), nonspecific interstitial pneumonia (NSIP), asbestosis-related, hypersensitivity pneumonitis (chronic), sarcoidosis
- Pulmonary Langerhans histiocytosis
- Lymphangioleiomyomatosis

Discussion

A reticular pattern usually reflects the presence of interstitial lung disease. The most common cause of a reticular pattern on the chest radiograph is pulmonary interstitial edema due to left heart failure or fluid overload. The reticular pattern in this case results from superimposition of numerous, thickened, interlobular septa. The diagnosis can usually be made by the presence of smooth, short lines perpendicular to the pleura and extending to the pleura (i.e., septal or Kerley B lines), enlarged upper lobe vessels due to blood flow redistribution, bronchial wall thickening (i.e., peribronchial cuffing due to edema), cardiomegaly, and small pleural effusions. The second most common cause of a reticular pattern is chronic interstitial pulmonary fibrosis. Common underlying diseases include idiopathic pulmonary fibrosis, fibrosis associated with collagen vascular disease, asbestosis, sarcoidosis, drug reaction, and chronic hypersensitivity pneumonitis. A reticular pattern on the radiograph may result from diseases characterized by predominantly cystic changes on CT, particularly pulmonary Langerhans histiocytosis, and lymphangioleiomyomatosis. Idiopathic pulmonary fibrosis, fibrosis associated with collagen vascular disease (mainly scleroderma and rheumatoid arthritis), and asbestosis typically involve mainly the lower lung zones and are frequently associated with decreased lung volumes. The reticulation in sarcoidosis and pulmonary Langerhans histiocytosis tends to involve mainly the upper and middle lung zones with relative sparing of the lung bases. Lymphangioleiomyomatosis, seen almost exclusively in women of childbearing age, typically results in a subtle, fine reticular pattern with occasional cystic spaces evident on the radiograph and normal or increased lung volumes (Figs. 3 and 4). With the exception of pulmonary edema, chest radiograph plays.

A limited role in the differential diagnosis of the various interstitial lung diseases. In most cases, high-resolution CT is required for assessment of these patients.

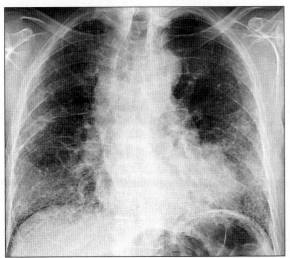

Figure 1. Posteroanterior chest radiograph shows extensive bilateral reticular pattern, which is worse in the lower lung zones, and reduced lung volumes in a 76-year-old man with idiopathic pulmonary fibrosis.

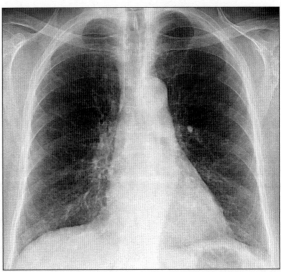

Figure 3. Posteroanterior chest radiograph shows a diffuse, fine reticular pattern and normal lung volumes in a 45-year-old woman with long-standing lymphangioleiomyomatosis.

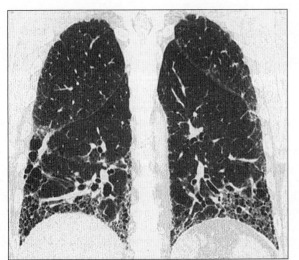

Figure 2. In the same patient, coronal reformation, high-resolution CT image shows bilateral, irregular, linear opacities and honeycombing involving mainly the subpleural lung regions of the lower lobes, resulting in a reticular pattern on the chest radiograph.

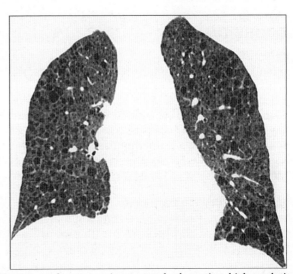

Figure 4. In the same patient, coronal reformation, high-resolution CT image shows bilateral, numerous, thin-walled cysts consistent with long-standing lymphangioleiomyomatosis.

Diagnosis
Reticular pattern on a chest radiograph

Suggested Readings

Aziz ZA, Wells AU, Bateman ED, et al: Interstitial lung disease: Effects of thin-section CT on clinical decision making. Radiology 238:725-733, 2006.

Miller WT Jr: Chest radiographic evaluation of diffuse infiltrative lung disease: Review of a dying art. Eur J Radiol 44:182-197, 2002.

McLoud TC, Carrington CB, Gaensler EA: Diffuse infiltrative lung disease: A new scheme for description. Radiology 149:353-363, 1983.

Case 13

DEMOGRAPHICS/CLINICAL HISTORY

A 73-year-old woman with shortness of breath, undergoing computed tomography (CT).

FINDINGS

The reticular pattern seen on CT is caused by intralobular linear opacities (Figs. 1 and 2) involving mainly the peripheral lung regions and associated architectural lung distortion. The patient had idiopathic pulmonary fibrosis.

DISCUSSION

Definition/Background

A reticular pattern on high-resolution CT refers mainly to reticulation caused by intralobular linear opacities. A reticular pattern caused by thickening of interlobular septa is considered separately under septal pattern, and a reticular pattern caused by smooth interlobular and intralobular lines superimposed on ground-glass opacities is considered separately under crazy-paving pattern.

Characteristic Clinical Features

Patients with a reticular pattern commonly present with slowly progressive shortness of breath and dry cough. Occasionally, patients may be asymptomatic.

Characteristic Radiologic Findings

The characteristic appearance is that of innumerable, interlacing line shadows a few millimeters apart due to intralobular lines. A reticular pattern caused by pulmonary fibrosis typically is associated with distortion of lung architecture (Figs. 1 and 2), volume loss, and traction bronchiectasis and bronchiolectasis (i.e., bronchial or bronchiolar dilatation caused by surrounding retractile pulmonary fibrosis).

Less Common Radiologic Manifestations

The reticular pattern may be the predominant or only abnormality on high-resolution CT or be associated with other parenchymal findings, including ground-glass opacities, consolidation, and small nodules. Associated extrapulmonary findings (IPF) may be related to the underlying disease, such as pleural thickening or effusion in collagen vascular disease, esophageal dilatation in scleroderma, and pleural plaques in asbestosis.

Idiopathic pulmonary fibrosis (IPF) is more common in smokers; these patients often have associated findings of emphysema. Enlarged central pulmonary arteries suggest associated pulmonary arterial hypertension.

Differential Diagnosis

- Idiopathic pulmonary fibrosis
- Nonspecific interstitial pneumonia (NSIP)
- Interstitial fibrosis associated with connective tissue disease
- Asbestosis
- Chronic hypersensitivity pneumonitis
- Sarcoidosis
- Drug reaction

Discussion

IPF is an idiopathic, chronic interstitial fibrosis limited to the lung and associated with the histologic appearance of usual interstitial pneumonia (UIP). The characteristic high-resolution CT findings of IPF consist of a reticular pattern in a patchy distribution and that involves all lobes but is most severe in the subpleural lung regions and in the lung bases (Fig. 3). Honeycombing occurs in 80% to 90% of patients. NSIP is a chronic interstitial lung disease characterized histologically by a combination of interstitial fibrosis and inflammation that resembles IPF clinically but has a considerably better prognosis. NSIP may be idiopathic but occurs most commonly in patients with connective tissue disease, particularly scleroderma, and in those with drug reactions. The high-resolution CT findings most commonly consist of ground-glass opacities and a fine reticular pattern. Evidence of architectural distortion with traction bronchiectasis and bronchiolectasis is commonly seen on high-resolution CT, but honeycombing is uncommon at presentation. The abnormalities may be diffuse, but they involve mainly the lower lung zones in 60% to 90% of cases. Although the fibrosis in NSIP is often predominantly peripheral and basal in approximately 50% of patients, there is relative sparing of the immediate subpleural lung in the dorsal regions of the lower lobes.

The most common collagen vascular diseases associated with a reticular pattern on the chest radiograph and high-resolution CT are scleroderma and rheumatoid arthritis. The histologic, radiographic, and high-resolution CT manifestations of scleroderma are usually those of NSIP; rheumatoid arthritis tends to result in findings of UIP and, less commonly, NSIP.

In chronic hypersensitivity pneumonitis (HP), fibrosis occurs predominantly in the middle lung zones or shows

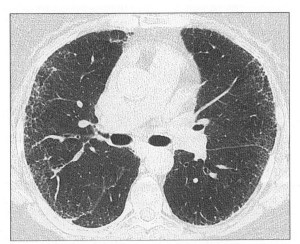

Figure 1. In a 73-year-old woman with idiopathic pulmonary fibrosis, high-resolution CT at the level of bronchus intermedius shows a reticular pattern caused by intralobular linear opacities involving mainly the peripheral lung regions. Notice the associated architectural distortion.

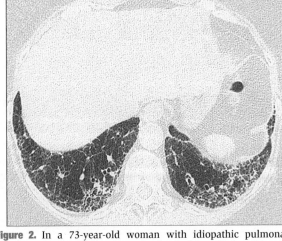

Figure 2. In a 73-year-old woman with idiopathic pulmonary fibrosis, high-resolution CT at the level of lung bases shows reticular pattern caused by intralobular linear opacities involving mainly the peripheral lung regions. Notice the associated architectural distortion.

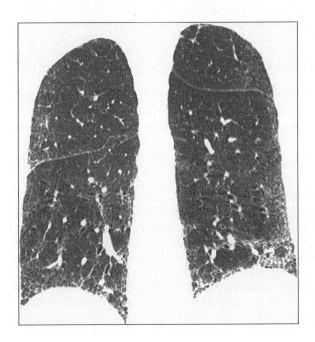

Figure 3. Coronal reformation image shows that the reticular pattern involves mainly the peripheral lung regions and lower lung zones in a 73-year-old woman with idiopathic pulmonary fibrosis.

no zonal predominance. Lung apices and bases are relatively spared. In most cases, there are superimposed findings of subacute disease, typically poorly defined centrilobular nodular opacities, extensive bilateral ground-glass opacities, and lobular areas of decreased attenuation and vascularity with air trapping on expiratory images.

The fibrosis in sarcoidosis typically involves mainly the upper and middle lung zones and is associated with superior retraction of the hila, traction bronchiectasis of the central bronchi, and compensatory overinflation of the lower lobes.

The reticular pattern in asbestosis usually is mild and involves predominantly or exclusively the lower lung zones. Almost all patients have associated pleural plaques or diffuse pleural thickening.

Diagnosis

Reticular pattern on high-resolution computed tomography

Suggested Readings

Devaraj A, Wells AU, Hansell DM: Computed tomographic imaging in connective tissue diseases. Semin Respir Crit Care Med 28:389-397, 2007.

Lynch DA, Travis WD, Müller NL, et al: Idiopathic interstitial pneumonias: CT features. Radiology 236:10-21, 2005.

Silva CI, Churg A, Müller NL: Hypersensitivity pneumonitis: Spectrum of high-resolution CT and pathologic findings. AJR Am J Roentgenol 188:334-344, 2007.

Silva CI, Müller NL, Lynch DA, et al: Chronic hypersensitivity pneumonitis: Differentiation from idiopathic pulmonary fibrosis and nonspecific interstitial pneumonia by using thin-section CT. Radiology 246:288-297, 2008.

Case 14

DEMOGRAPHICS/CLINICAL HISTORY

A 39-year-old woman with shortness of breath, undergoing computed tomography (CT).

FINDINGS

Bilateral, thin-walled cysts are surrounded by normal lung parenchyma in a patient with lymphangioleiomyomatosis (Figs. 1 and 2).

DISCUSSION

Definition/Background

A cystic pattern on high-resolution CT is characterized by numerous cysts that are air-containing parenchymal spaces with well-defined walls.

Characteristic Clinical Features

Patients with a cystic pattern most commonly present with slowly progressive shortness of breath and dry cough. Occasionally, the patients may be asymptomatic.

Characteristic Radiologic Findings

By definition, a cystic pattern on high-resolution CT is characterized by the presence of numerous cysts. The cysts may be diffuse (Figs. 1 and 2) or involve mainly the upper or lower lung zones. Common associated findings in patients with pulmonary Langerhans cell histiocytosis include small nodules, ground-glass opacities, and emphysema. Cysts in patients with *Pneumocystis* pneumonia, lymphoid interstitial pneumonia (LIP), or hypersensitivity pneumonitis are usually seen in areas of ground-glass opacification.

Less Common Radiologic Manifestations

Pneumothorax is a common complication in pulmonary Langerhans cell histiocytosis, lymphangioleiomyomatosis, and lung cysts from *Pneumocystis* pneumonia. Pleural effusion is relatively common in lymphangioleiomyomatosis but uncommon in other cystic lung diseases. Slightly enlarged mediastinal lymph nodes are common in patients with extensive pulmonary fibrosis and in those with lymphangioleiomyomatosis.

Differential Diagnosis

- Lymphangioleiomyomatosis
- Pulmonary Langerhans cell histiocytosis
- Birt-Hogg-Dubé syndrome
- Honeycombing in end-stage fibrosis
- Lymphoid interstitial pneumonia (LIP)
- Hypersensitivity pneumonitis
- *Pneumocystis jiroveci* pneumonia

Discussion

Lymphangioleiomyomatosis is a rare disease limited to women and characterized by cyst formation and an interstitial proliferation of smooth muscle–like cells. The characteristic high-resolution CT finding consists of numerous, thin-walled, air-filled cysts surrounded by normal lung parenchyma (Fig. 1). The cysts usually are between 0.2 and 2 cm in diameter and are distributed diffusely throughout the lungs without any zonal predominance (Fig. 2).

Pulmonary Langerhans cell histiocytosis is a disease characterized histologically by infiltration of the lung by Langerhans cells that typically manifests in young adults and is seen almost exclusively in smokers. The characteristic findings on high-resolution CT consist of cysts (approximately 80% of patients) and nodules (60% to 80% of patients). The nodules range from 1 to 10 mm in diameter, and the cysts range from a few millimeters to several centimeters in diameter and may be round, oval, or have bizarre shapes with bilobed, cloverleaf, and branching configurations. Regardless of the stage of the disease, the abnormalities are diffuse throughout the middle and upper lung zones, with relative sparing of the lung bases.

Birt-Hogg-Dubé syndrome is a rare autosomal dominant disorder characterized by facial papules, which represent fibrofolliculomas; multiple, thin-walled, cystic spaces that occur mainly in the lower lobes; and an increased risk for renal tumors (Fig. 3).

Honeycombing refers to the presence of cystic spaces between 0.3 and 1 cm in diameter whose walls consist of various amounts of fibrous tissue. Honeycombing is seen in end-stage pulmonary fibrosis and tends to be most severe in the subpleural regions and along the interlobar fissures (Fig. 4). The most common diseases in which the abnormality is identified are idiopathic pulmonary fibrosis (Fig. 4), connective tissue disease, and sarcoidosis.

Single or multiple cysts that are typically superimposed on ground-glass opacities are seen in approximately 60% of patients with LIP and 13% to 40% of patients with hypersensitivity pneumonitis. The cysts in LIP are usually few and tend to involve mainly the lower lung zones; occasionally, LIP may result in extensive cyst formation. Cystic spaces are seen in approximately

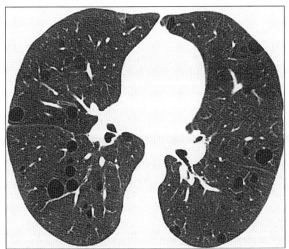

Figure 1. High-resolution CT image shows bilateral, thin-walled cysts surrounded by normal lung parenchyma in a 39-year-old woman with lymphangioleiomyomatosis

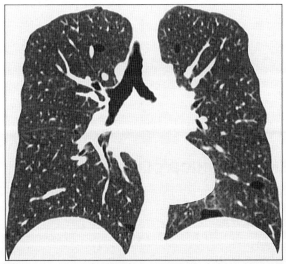

Figure 3. Coronal reformation image shows a few, thin-walled cysts in a 56-year-old woman with Birt-Hogg-Dubé syndrome.

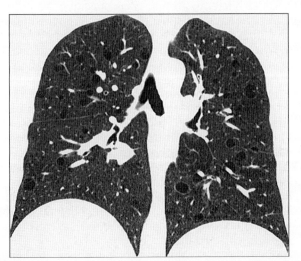

Figure 2. Coronal reformation image shows bilateral, thin-walled cysts throughout the lungs that are surrounded by normal lung parenchyma in a 39-year-old woman with lymphangioleiomyomatosis.

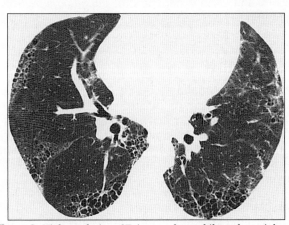

Figure 4. High-resolution CT image shows bilateral, peripheral honeycombing and associated reticulation in a 67-year-old man with idiopathic pulmonary fibrosis.

30% of patients with *Pneumocystis* pneumonia, and they may be single or multiple, occur mainly in the upper lobes, and are typically superimposed on ground-glass opacities.

Diagnosis
Cystic pattern on high-resolution computed tomography

Suggested Readings

Abbott GF, Rosado-de-Christenson ML, Franks TJ, et al: From the archives of the AFIP: Pulmonary Langerhans cell histiocytosis. Radiographics 24:821-841, 2004.

Bonelli FS, Hartman TE, Swensen SJ, Sherrick A: Accuracy of high-resolution CT in diagnosing lung diseases. AJR Am J Roentgenol 170:1507-1512, 1998.

Koyama M, Johkoh T, Honda O, et al: Chronic cystic lung disease: Diagnostic accuracy of high-resolution CT in 92 patients. AJR Am J Roentgenol 180:827-835, 2003.

Niku S, Stark P, Levin DL, Friedman PJ: Lymphangioleiomyomatosis: clinical, pathologic, and radiologic manifestations. J Thorac Imaging 20:98-102, 2005.

Case 15

DEMOGRAPHICS/CLINICAL HISTORY

A 46-year-old woman who is human immunodeficiency virus (HIV) positive and has fever and shortness of breath, undergoing computed tomography (CT).

FINDINGS

CT shows extensive, bilateral ground-glass opacities (Figs. 1 and 2) in a patient with *Pneumocystis jiroveci* pneumonia.

DISCUSSION

Definition/Background

Ground-glass opacity is defined on high-resolution CT as a hazy, increased opacity of lung, with preservation of bronchial and vascular margins. Ground-glass opacity on a chest radiograph is defined as hazy, increased lung opacity, within which margins of pulmonary vessels may be indistinct.

Characteristic Clinical Features

Acute ground-glass opacities due to infection are seen most commonly in immunocompromised patients, who usually present with fever and progressive shortness of breath. Patients with diffuse pulmonary hemorrhage usually present with hemoptysis.

Characteristic Radiologic Findings

Patients have a focal, multifocal, or diffuse, hazy, increased opacity without obscuration of underlying vascular markings. If the vessels are obscured, the term *consolidation* is used.

Less Common Radiologic Manifestations

Associated findings can include cysts (e.g., *Pneumocystis* pneumonia), small nodules (e.g., cytomegalovirus infection, *Pneumocystis* pneumonia), and reticular opacities (e.g., resolving or recurrent hemorrhage).

Differential Diagnosis

- *Pneumocystis jiroveci* pneumonia
- Cytomegalovirus pneumonia
- Acute respiratory distress syndrome (ARDS)
- Acute interstitial pneumonia (AIP)
- Focal or diffuse pulmonary hemorrhage
- Aspiration

Discussion

Pneumocystis jiroveci pneumonia occurs almost exclusively in immunocompromised patients, particularly patients with acquired immunodeficiency syndrome (AIDS) and patients on chronic immunosuppressive therapy. The characteristic high-resolution CT finding consists of bilateral, ground-glass opacities, which may be diffuse or have a distinct mosaic pattern with areas of normal lung intervening between the ground-glass opacities. With time, the areas of ground-glass attenuation progress to consolidation. Common ancillary findings include cyst formation (approximately 30% of patients) and reticulation. Less commonly, acute, diffuse ground-glass opacities may result from cytomegalovirus pneumonia.

The high-resolution CT manifestations of ARDS consist of bilateral ground-glass opacities commonly associated with dependent areas of consolidation. Similar findings are seen in AIP, which is idiopathic ARDS.

Pulmonary hemorrhage may result in focal, patchy, unilateral or bilateral or in symmetric, bilateral ground-glass opacities (Figs. 3 and 4). When severe, it may progress to consolidation.

Ground-glass opacities occurring mainly in the dependent regions should raise the possibility of aspiration. Aspiration frequently results in dependent centrilobular nodules (e.g., aspiration bronchiolitis) or areas of consolidation (e.g., aspiration pneumonia).

Diagnosis

Ground-glass pattern in acute lung disease

Suggested Readings

Boiselle PM, Crans CA Jr, Kaplan MA: The changing face of Pneumocystis carinii pneumonia in AIDS patients. AJR Am J Roentgenol 172:1301-1309, 1999.

Collins J, Stern EJ: Ground-glass opacity at CT: The ABCs. AJR Am J Roentgenol 169:355-367, 1997.

Nowers K, Rasband JD, Berges G, Gosselin M: Approach to ground-glass opacification of the lung. Semin Ultrasound CT MR 23:302-323, 2002.

Primack SL, Miller RR, Müller NL: Diffuse pulmonary hemorrhage: clinical, pathologic, and imaging features. AJR Am J Roentgenol 164:295-300, 1995.

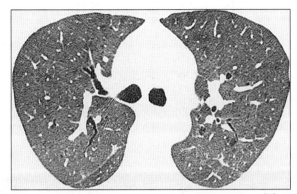

Figure 1. High-resolution CT image shows extensive, bilateral ground-glass opacities in a 46-year-old, HIV-positive woman with *Pneumocystis jiroveci* pneumonia.

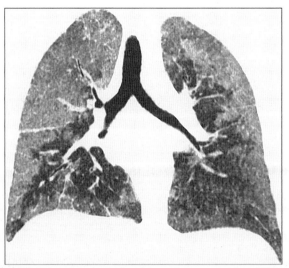

Figure 3. Coronal re-formation image shows extensive, bilateral ground-glass opacities involving mainly the upper and middle lung regions in a 38-year-old man with diffuse pulmonary hemorrhage resulting from angiosarcoma.

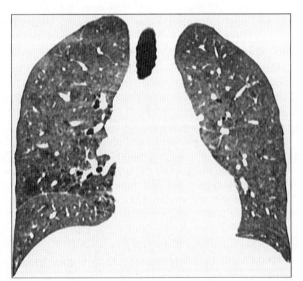

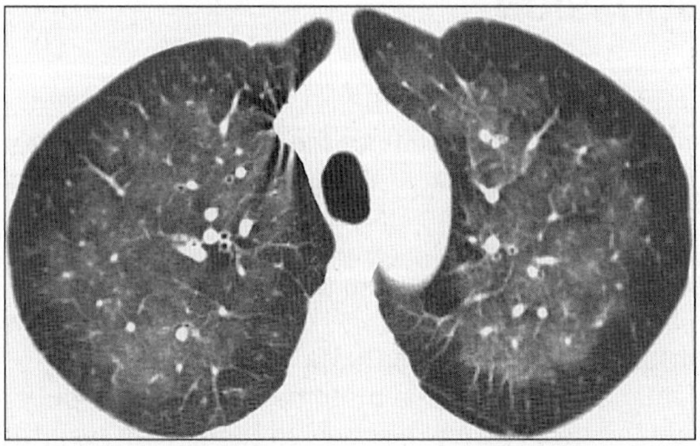

Figure 2. Coronal reformation image shows extensive, bilateral ground-glass opacities in a 46-year-old, HIV-positive woman with *Pneumocystis jiroveci* pneumonia.

Figure 4. High-resolution CT image shows bilateral, central ground-glass opacities in a 34-year-old man with pulmonary hemorrhage resulting from Goodpasture syndrome.

Case 16

DEMOGRAPHICS/CLINICAL HISTORY

A 65-year-old, immunocompetent woman with progressive dyspnea and dry cough, undergoing computed tomography (CT).

FINDINGS

CT shows extensive bilateral ground-glass opacities (Figs. 1 and 2) and lobular areas of decreased attenuation and vascularity (Fig. 1). The patient was a bird breeder with hypersensitivity pneumonitis.

DISCUSSION

Definition/Background

Ground-glass opacity is defined on high-resolution CT as hazy, increased opacity of the lung, with preservation of bronchial and vascular margins. Ground-glass opacity on a chest radiograph is defined as hazy, increased lung opacity that is usually extensive and within which margins of pulmonary vessels may be indistinct.

Characteristic Clinical Features

Patients have chronic symptoms, most commonly dry cough and progressive dyspnea. Patients with respiratory bronchiolitis–interstitial lung disease (RBILD) typically have a history of more than 30 pack-years of smoking.

Characteristic Radiologic Findings

Findings include focal, multifocal, or diffuse, hazy increased opacity without obscuration of underlying vascular markings. If the vessels are obscured, the term *consolidation* is used.

Less Common Radiologic Manifestations

Associated findings can include cysts (e.g., lymphoid interstitial pneumonia, hypersensitivity pneumonitis), centrilobular nodules (hypersensitivity pneumonitis, RBILD), reticular opacities (e.g., nonspecific interstitial pneumonia, chronic hypersensitivity pneumonitis), and lobular areas of air trapping (e.g., RBILD, hypersensitivity pneumonitis).

Differential Diagnosis

- Hypersensitivity pneumonitis (HP)
- Nonspecific interstitial pneumonia (NSIP)
- Connective tissue disease
- Drug reaction
- Respiratory bronchiolitis–interstitial lung disease (RBILD)
- Desquamative interstitial pneumonia (DIP)
- Lymphoid interstitial pneumonia (LIP)
- Alveolar proteinosis
- Bronchioloalveolar cell carcinoma

Discussion

The differential diagnoses for patients with chronic respiratory symptoms and predominantly or exclusively ground-glass opacities include subacute and chronic HP (Figs. 1 and 2), NSIP (Figs. 3 and Fig. 4), DIP, RBILD, and LIP. HP is probably the most common cause of diffuse ground-glass opacities in normal hosts. The areas of ground-glass attenuation in HP may be diffuse but frequently involve mainly the middle and lower lung zones. Localized areas of decreased attenuation and perfusion often exist in conjunction with areas of ground-glass attenuation (Fig. 1). These show air trapping on CT scans performed at end expiration. Ground-glass opacities may be seen in conjunction with centrilobular nodules. Approximately 13% of patients with subacute HP have 1 to 15, thin-walled lung cysts ranging from 3 to 25 mm in maximal diameter and occurring in a random distribution.

NSIP may be idiopathic or association with connective tissue disease or a drug reaction. It usually manifests with bilateral, symmetric ground-glass opacities mainly in the lower lung zones (Figs. 3 and 4). Most patients have a fine reticular pattern superimposed on the ground-glass opacities, traction bronchiectasis, and architectural distortion consistent with pulmonary fibrosis (Figs. 3 and 4).

Patients who have RBILD typically are current smokers with more than 30 pack-years of cigarette smoking. High-resolution CT manifestations of RBILD typically consist of ground-glass opacities and poorly defined centrilobular nodules. The abnormalities can be diffuse or involve mainly the upper or lower lung zones. Most patients have associated centrilobular emphysema.

DIP is an uncommon condition seen mainly in current cigarette smokers. The most common radiographic and high-resolution CT finding consists of symmetric, bilateral ground-glass opacities. The ground-glass opacities may be patchy or diffuse, but in approximately 60% of patients, they involve mainly the lower lung zones. A mild reticular pattern in a predominantly subpleural and basal distribution is seen in 60% to 80% of patients.

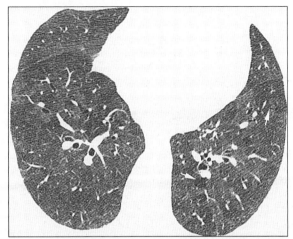

Figure 1. High-resolution CT image shows extensive, bilateral ground-glass opacities and lobular areas of decreased attenuation and vascularity *(arrows)* in a 65-year-old woman who was a bird breeder with subacute hypersensitivity pneumonitis.

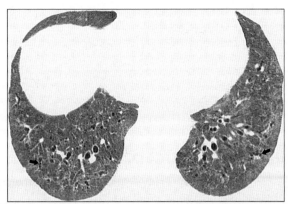

Figure 3. High-resolution CT image shows diffuse, bilateral ground-glass opacities and mild superimposed reticulation in a 60-year-old woman with nonspecific interstitial pneumonia. The bronchi within the areas of ground-glass opacities are dilated and distorted bronchi (i.e., traction bronchiectasis; *arrows*).

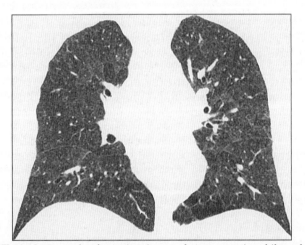

Figure 2. Coronal reformation image shows extensive, bilateral ground-glass opacities and lobular areas of decreased attenuation and vascularity in a 65-year-old woman who was a bird breeder with subacute hypersensitivity pneumonitis.

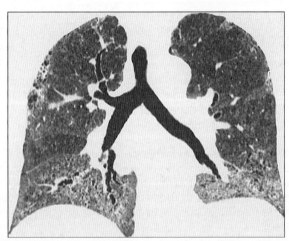

Figure 4. Coronal reformation image shows diffuse, bilateral ground-glass opacities involving mainly the lower lung zones in a 60-year-old woman with nonspecific interstitial pneumonia. Findings of fibrosis include reticulation, traction bronchiectasis, and subpleural honeycombing.

Occasionally, bronchioloalveolar cell carcinoma may result in focal, patchy, or confluent unilateral or bilateral ground-glass opacities.

Diagnosis
Ground-glass pattern in chronic lung disease

Suggested Readings

Collins J, Stern EJ: Ground-glass opacity at CT: The ABCs. AJR Am J Roentgenol 169:355-367, 1997.

Lynch DA, Travis WD, Müller NL, et al: Idiopathic interstitial pneumonias: CT features. Radiology 236:10-21, 2005.

Nowers K, Rasband JD, Berges G, Gosselin M: Approach to ground-glass opacification of the lung. Semin Ultrasound CT MR 23:302-323, 2002.

Park CM, Goo JM, Lee HJ, et al: Nodular ground-glass opacity at thin-section CT: Histologic correlation and evaluation of change at follow-up. Radiographics 27:391-408, 2007.

Silva CIS, Müller NL, Churg A: Hypersensitivity pneumonitis: Spectrum of high-resolution CT and pathologic findings. AJR Am J Roentgenol 188:334-344, 2007.

Case 17

DEMOGRAPHICS/CLINICAL HISTORY

A 55-year-old man with slowly progressive shortness of breath, undergoing computed tomography (CT).

FINDINGS

CT shows bilateral, ground-glass opacities with superimposed smooth septal lines and intralobular lines, resulting in a pattern known as crazy paving (Figs. 1 and 2) in a patient with alveolar proteinosis.

DISCUSSION

Definition/Background

The crazy paving pattern represents thickened interlobular septa and intralobular lines superimposed on a background of ground-glass opacity, resembling irregularly shaped paving stones.

Characteristic Clinical Features

Symptoms may be acute or chronic, depending on the cause of the crazy paving pattern. Common symptoms include cough and dyspnea. Hemoptysis due to pulmonary hemorrhage occurs in patients with crazy paving pattern.

Characteristic Radiologic Findings

Smoothly thickened interlobular septa and intralobular lines superimposed on a background of ground-glass opacity. The crazy paving pattern is often sharply demarcated from more normal lung and may have a geographical outline (Fig. 2).

Less Common Radiologic Manifestations

Associated findings can include reticulation, traction bronchiectasis, and bronchiolectasis due to fibrosis (i.e., chronic disease); small nodules and septal lines (i.e., recurrent or resolving pulmonary hemorrhage); consolidation (i.e., acute respiratory distress syndrome, pneumonia, and hemorrhage).

Differential Diagnosis

- Alveolar proteinosis
- *Pneumocystis* pneumonia
- Bacterial pneumonia
- Acute respiratory distress syndrome (ARDS)
- Acute interstitial pneumonia (AIP)
- Acute eosinophilic pneumonia
- Pulmonary hemorrhage
- Pulmonary edema
- Nonspecific interstitial pneumonia (NSIP)
- Lipoid pneumonia
- Bronchioloalveolar cell carcinoma
- Radiation pneumonitis

Discussion

The crazy paving pattern was first described in patients with pulmonary alveolar proteinosis, for which it is typical (Figs. 1 and 2), but it also may be seen in patients with a variety of other diseases. Causes of the pattern include acute conditions, such as ARDS, AIP, pulmonary edema, pulmonary hemorrhage (Fig. 3), bacterial pneumonia, *Pneumocystis* pneumonia, *Mycoplasma* pneumonia, and acute eosinophilic pneumonia, and subacute or chronic conditions, such as radiation pneumonitis, lipoid pneumonia, alveolar proteinosis, Churg-Strauss syndrome, and bronchioloalveolar cell carcinoma. The differential diagnosis is broad, and like the differential diagnosis for ground-glass opacities, it is based largely on the presence and distribution of associated findings, such as consolidation, and the clinical findings.

Diagnosis

Crazy paving pattern on high-resolution computed tomography

Suggested Readings

Chung MJ, Lee KS, Franquet T, et al: Metabolic lung disease: Imaging and histopathologic findings. Eur J Radiol 54:233-245, 2005.

Franquet T, Giménez A, Bordes R, et al: The crazy-paving pattern in exogenous lipoid pneumonia: CT-pathologic correlation. AJR Am J Roentgenol 170:315-317, 1998.

Hansell DM, Bankier AA, MacMahon H, et al: Fleischner Society: Glossary of terms for thoracic imaging. Radiology 246:697-722, 2008.

Johkoh T, Itoh H, Müller NL, et al: Crazy-paving appearance at thin-section CT: Spectrum of disease and pathologic findings. Radiology 211:155-160, 1999.

Murayama S, Murakami J, Yabuuchi H, et al: "Crazy paving appearance" on high resolution CT in various diseases. J Comput Assist Tomogr 23:749-752, 1999.

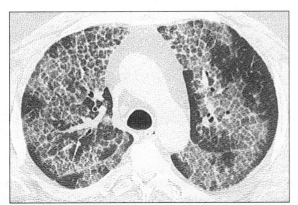

Figure 1. High-resolution CT image shows bilateral ground-glass opacities with superimposed smooth septal lines and intralobular lines, resulting in a crazy paving pattern. The patient was a 55-year-old man with alveolar proteinosis.

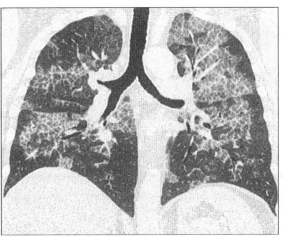

Figure 2. Coronal reformation image shows bilateral ground-glass opacities with superimposed smooth septal lines and intralobular lines, resulting in a crazy paving pattern. Notice the sharp demarcation between normal and abnormal parenchyma, a feature that usually reflects lobular boundaries. The patient was a 55-year-old man with alveolar proteinosis.

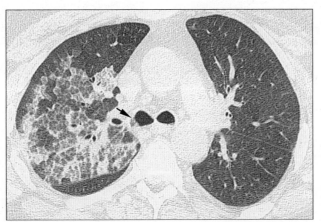

Figure 3. High-resolution CT image shows the crazy paving pattern in the right upper lobe, characterized by thickened interlobular septa and intralobular lines superimposed on a background of ground-glass opacity. Notice presence of blood in the right main bronchus (arrow). The patient was a 51-year-old man with pulmonary hemorrhage who presented with hemoptysis.

Case 18

DEMOGRAPHICS/CLINICAL HISTORY

A 75-year-old woman with progressive shortness of breath, undergoing computed tomography (CT).

FINDINGS

Combination of areas of decreased attenuation and vascularity and areas of increased attenuation and vascularity (i.e., mosaic attenuation/perfusion pattern) occurred in a patient with chronic thromboembolic pulmonary hypertension (Fig. 1). Notice the eccentric thrombus in the lateral wall of the right interlobar artery (Fig. 2).

DISCUSSION

Definition/Background

A mosaic attenuation pattern refers to a heterogeneous appearance on high-resolution CT with a patchwork of regions of two or more different attenuations: increased attenuation, normal attenuation, and decreased attenuation. A mosaic perfusion pattern refers to areas of decreased attenuation and vascularity (i.e., decreased size and number of vessels) and areas of normal or increased attenuation and vascularity.

Characteristic Clinical Features

Patients with a mosaic attenuation pattern due to ground-glass opacities (Fig. 3) typically present with symptoms related to the underlying interstitial or air space disease. Patients with a mosaic perfusion pattern due to vascular abnormality usually present with signs of pulmonary arterial hypertension, and those with a mosaic perfusion pattern due to airway disease usually present with findings of airway obstruction.

Characteristic Radiologic Findings

The characteristic feature of the mosaic attenuation pattern is the heterogeneous appearance of the lung parenchyma. A mosaic attenuation pattern resulting from patchy ground-glass opacities due to interstitial or air space disease typically is associated with similar vessel size in the areas with normal and increased attenuation (Fig. 3), and in these patients, the abnormal lung regions are the ones with the ground-glass opacities. Mosaic attenuation due to vascular (Fig. 1) or airway obstruction (Fig. 4) typically is associated with increased size and number of blood vessels in the areas with increased attenuation and decreased size and number of vessels in the remaining parenchyma, and in these patients, the abnormal lung regions are those with decreased attenuation and vascularity. Because decreased attenuation and vascularity are related to decreased blood flow and the areas of increased attenuation and vascularity are related to blood flow redistribution, this pattern is commonly referred to as mosaic perfusion pattern.

Less Common Radiologic Manifestations

Bronchiectasis is commonly present in patients with mosaic perfusion pattern due to small airway obstruction (Fig. 4), and enlarged central pulmonary arteries are commonly present in patients with mosaic perfusion pattern due to chronic thromboembolic pulmonary arterial hypertension.

Differential Diagnosis

- Bronchiolitis obliterans
- Asthma
- Chronic thromboembolic pulmonary hypertension
- Primary hypertension
- Hypersensitivity pneumonitis
- Respiratory bronchiolitis–interstitial lung disease (RBILD)
- *Pneumocystis* pneumonia (AIDS)

Discussion

The differential diagnosis of a mosaic attenuation pattern due to patchy ground-glass opacities is that of ground-glass opacities (Fig. 3). The differential diagnosis of a mosaic perfusion pattern includes various airway and vascular abnormalities. A mosaic perfusion pattern is seen most commonly in patients with bronchiolitis obliterans and with chronic thromboembolic pulmonary arterial hypertension. Bronchiolitis obliterans (i.e., obliterative bronchiolitis) is characterized by areas of decreased attenuation and vascularity seen on inspiratory CT scans and air trapping on expiratory scans. Bronchiectasis is commonly present. High-resolution CT findings of asthma include thickening and narrowing of the bronchi, bronchial dilatation, patchy areas of decreased attenuation and vascularity on inspiratory images, and air trapping on expiratory CT. Chronic pulmonary thromboembolic pulmonary arterial hypertension usually results in a mosaic perfusion pattern of increased diameter of the main, lobar, and segmental pulmonary arteries. Contrast-enhanced CT shows eccentric, flattened mural thrombi, which may be occlusive or have areas of recanalization. A mosaic perfusion pattern

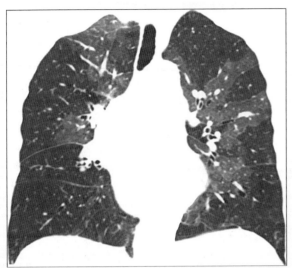

Figure 1. Coronal reformation CT image shows areas of decreased attenuation and vascularity and areas of increased attenuation and vascularity (i.e., mosaic attenuation/perfusion pattern) in 75-year-old woman with chronic thromboembolic pulmonary hypertension

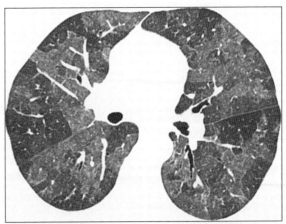

Figure 3. High-resolution CT image shows bilateral ground-glass opacities in a geographic distribution and areas of normal intervening lung resulting in a mosaic attenuation pattern. The patient was a 50-year-old woman with *Pneumocystis* pneumonia.

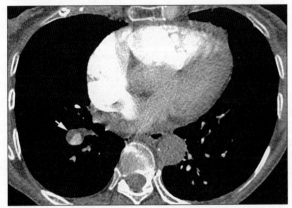

Figure 2. Soft tissue image shows eccentric thrombus in the lateral wall of the right interlobar artery *(arrow)* in 75-year-old woman with chronic thromboembolic pulmonary hypertension

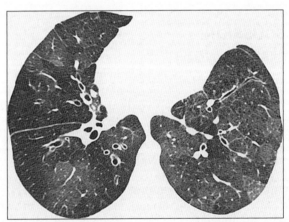

Figure 4. Mosaic attenuation (perfusion) pattern occurred after bilateral lung transplantation in a 20-year-old woman with obliterative bronchiolitis. High-resolution CT image shows areas of decreased attenuation and vascularity and areas of normal or increased attenuation and vascularity. Notice bronchiectasis within the areas of decreased attenuation.

also may be seen in patients with severe primary pulmonary hypertension. Hypersensitivity pneumonitis, respiratory bronchiolitis–associated interstitial lung disease (RBILD), and *Pneumocystis* pneumonia may result in a mosaic attenuation pattern with a combination of ground-glass opacities, areas of normal lung, and areas of decreased attenuation and vascularity, a combination of findings referred to as the head cheese sign.

Diagnosis
Mosaic attenuation and mosaic perfusion pattern

Suggested Readings

Silva CI, Colby TV, Müller NL: Asthma and associated conditions: High-resolution CT and pathologic findings. AJR Am J Roentgenol 183:817-824, 2004.

Pipavath SJ, Lynch DA, Cool C, et al: Radiologic and pathologic features of bronchiolitis. AJR Am J Roentgenol 185:354-363, 2005.

Worthy SA, Müller NL, Hartman TE, et al: Mosaic attenuation pattern on thin-section CT scans of the lung: Differentiation among infiltrative lung, airway, and vascular diseases as a cause. Radiology 205:465-470, 1997.

Case 19

DEMOGRAPHICS/CLINICAL HISTORY

A 55-year-old woman with progressive shortness of breath 1 year after stem cell transplantation, undergoing computed tomography (CT).

FINDINGS

Inspiratory CT image (Fig. 1) shows no definite abnormality. Expiratory CT image (Fig. 2) shows extensive air trapping in a patient with bronchiolitis obliterans after stem cell transplantation for multiple myeloma.

DISCUSSION

Definition/Background

Air trapping is the retention of air in lung distal to obstruction (usually partial). The diagnosis of air trapping is made on end-expiration CT based on the presence of areas with a less than normal increase in attenuation and lack of volume reduction, and it is easiest to make when the abnormality is patchy in distribution and abnormal lung regions can be contrasted with normal lung regions.

Characteristic Clinical Features

The patients may be asymptomatic or present with cough and progressive shortness of breath caused by airway obstruction.

Characteristic Radiologic Findings

The characteristic feature of air trapping is the presence of decreased attenuation and lack of volume reduction of the affected lung compared with the normal lung on imaging performed at the end of maximal expiration (i.e., expiratory CT or radiograph).

Less Common Radiologic Manifestations

The affected lung may appear normal (Figs. 1 and 2) or have decreased attenuation and vascularity on inspiratory CT (Figs. 3 and 4). Bronchiectasis is common in patients with bronchiolitis obliterans.

Differential Diagnosis

- Bronchiolitis obliterans (obliterative bronchiolitis)
- Asthma
- Chronic obstructive pulmonary disease (COPD)
- Partial bronchial obstruction of any cause
- Bronchomalacia
- Bronchial atresia
- Congenital lobar emphysema
- Sarcoidosis
- Hypersensitivity pneumonitis
- Normal pattern in dependent lung regions

Discussion

Air trapping is typically seen in patients with obstructive lung disease, including bronchiolitis obliterans (i.e., obliterative bronchiolitis) (Figs. 1 and 2), asthma (Figs. 3 and Fig. 4), and COPD and in association with some interstitial lung diseases, particularly sarcoidosis and hypersensitivity pneumonitis. It may result from partial bronchial obstruction by a tumor or foreign body, in which case it is typically limited to a lung, lobe, or segment. Congenital causes of air trapping include bronchial atresia, congenital lobar emphysema, and bronchomalacia. Some air trapping is common in normal individuals (Fig. 5), in whom it usually involves a small portion of lung (less than 25% of the cross-sectional area of one lung at one scan level) and is most typically seen in the superior segments of the lower lobes, the anterior middle lobe, or lingula, or involving individual pulmonary lobules, particularly in the dependent regions of the lower lobes. Air trapping can be considered abnormal when it affects a volume of lung equal to or greater than a pulmonary segment and is not limited to the superior segment of the lower lobe or the lingula tip.

Diagnosis

Air trapping

Suggested Readings

Arakawa H, Webb WR: Air trapping on expiratory high-resolution CT scans in the absence of inspiratory scan abnormalities: Correlation with pulmonary function tests and differential diagnosis. AJR Am J Roentgenol 170:1349-1353, 1998.

de Jong PA, Dodd JD, Coxson HO, et al: Bronchiolitis obliterans following lung transplantation: Early detection using computed tomographic scanning. Thorax 61:799-804, 2006.

Silva CI, Colby TV, Müller NL: Asthma and associated conditions: High-resolution CT and pathologic findings. AJR Am J Roentgenol 183:817-824, 2004.

Pipavath SJ, Lynch DA, Cool C, et al: Radiologic and pathologic features of bronchiolitis. AJR Am J Roentgenol 185:354-363, 2005.

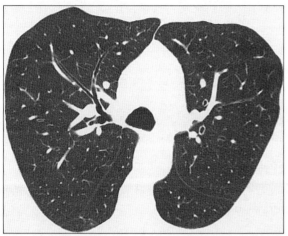

Figure 1. Inspiratory CT image in a 55-year-old woman with bronchiolitis obliterans after stem cell transplantation for multiple myeloma shows no definite abnormality.

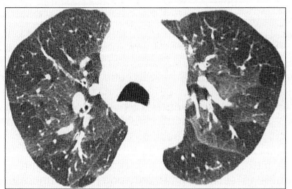

Figure 2. Expiratory CT image shows extensive air trapping in a 55-year-old woman with bronchiolitis obliterans after stem cell transplantation for multiple myeloma.

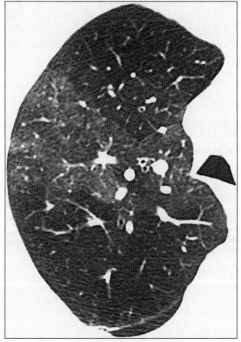

Figure 3. Inspiratory CT image of air trapping in a 54-year-old woman with severe asthma shows a mosaic attenuation pattern.

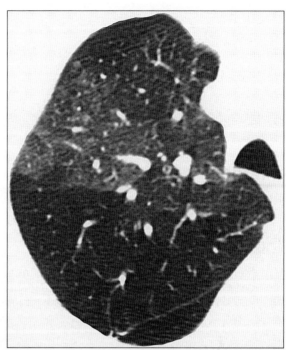

Figure 4. Expiratory CT image of a 54-year-old woman with severe asthma shows extensive air trapping accentuating the areas of decreased attenuation and vascularity seen on the inspiratory image.

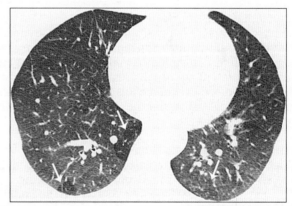

Figure 5. Expiratory, high-resolution CT of a 41-year-old man shows air trapping (*arrows*) in a few pulmonary lobules in the lower lobes. The patient was an asymptomatic, lifelong nonsmoker.

Case 20

DEMOGRAPHICS/CLINICAL HISTORY

A 24-year-old woman, progressive exertional dyspnea.

FINDINGS

Posteroanterior chest radiograph (Fig. 1) shows numerous nodules measuring between 1 and 5 mm in diameter throughout both lungs, most profuse in the lower lobes.

DISCUSSION

Definition/Background

The nodular pattern is characterized by the presence of numerous round opacities measuring less than 1 cm in diameter. It results from expansion of the parenchymal interstitium by a roughly spherical cellular infiltrate, fibrous tissue, or both.

Characteristic Clinical Features

Small nodular opacities per se are seldom diffuse enough to result in substantial functional impairment. The patients therefore are often asymptomatic. The symptoms when present are usually related to the underlying condition, namely fever and chills in acute infection and cough and progressive shortness of breath in chronic interstitial lung disease.

Characteristic Radiologic Findings

By definition, the characteristic radiologic finding is the presence of numerous round opacities measuring less than 1 cm in diameter (Figs. 1, 2, 3, and 4). The nodules may be well defined or poorly defined and may have smooth or spiculated margins.

Less Common Radiologic Manifestations

Patients may have associated findings, including hilar and mediastinal lymphadenopathy and pleural thickening or effusion.

Differential Diagnosis

- Infection: tuberculosis, fungi, viral pneumonia
- Neoplasms: metastases, bronchioloalveolar carcinoma
- Inhalational diseases: silicosis, coalworker's pneumoconiosis
- Miscellaneous conditions: sarcoidosis, talcosis in intravenous drug users

Discussion

The differential diagnosis is based on clinical history (acute, chronic, exposure history), pattern and distribution of the nodules, and presence of associated findings such as cavity formation, calcification, lymphadenopathy (Fig. 2), and pleural effusion or thickening. For example, a diffuse small nodular pattern in a febrile patient with acute disease is most suggestive of hematogenous infection, particularly miliary tuberculosis (Fig. 3). A similar pattern in a patient with chronic symptoms may result from silicosis, coalworker's pneumoconiosis, intravenous talcosis, metastatic carcinoma (particularly from the thyroid), and bronchioloalveolar carcinoma. The overall distribution of nodules on the radiograph often helps narrow the differential diagnosis. For example, the nodules in silicosis and coalworker's pneumoconiosis may be diffuse but most commonly involve mainly the middle and upper lung zones (Fig. 4), whereas those resulting from hematogenous processes, such as miliary tuberculosis and metastatic carcinoma, are diffuse or involve mainly the lower lung zones (where blood flow is greater) (Fig. 1). The nodules in miliary tuberculosis and miliary fungal infection typically measure 1–3 mm in diameter. Nodules in endobronchial spread of tuberculosis or nontuberculous mycobacterial infection usually measure 3 to 10 mm in diameter and tend to be unilateral or to have an asymmetric bilateral distribution.

Diagnosis

Small nodular pattern, chest radiograph

Suggested Readings

Miller WT Jr: Chest radiographic evaluation of diffuse infiltrative lung disease: Review of a dying art. Eur J Radiol 44:182-197, 2002.

McLoud TC, Carrington CB, Gaensler EA: Diffuse infiltrative lung disease: A new scheme for description. Radiology 149:353-363, 1983.

Raoof S, Raoof S, Naidich DP: Imaging of unusual diffuse lung diseases. Curr Opin Pulm Med 10:383-389, 2004.

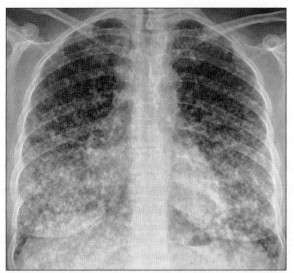

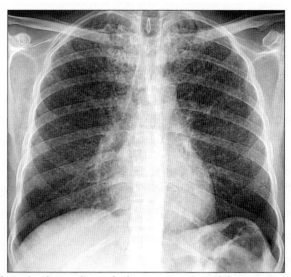

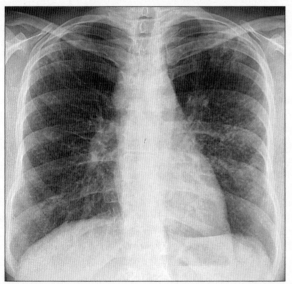

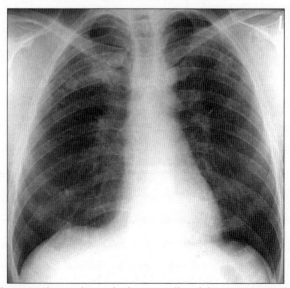

Figure 1. Posteroanterior chest radiograph shows numerous nodules measuring between 1 and 5 mm in diameter throughout both lungs, most profuse in the lower lobes. The patient was a 24-year-old woman with metastatic thyroid carcinoma.

Figure 3. Chest radiograph shows numerous nodules, 1 to 2 mm in diameter, throughout both lungs (miliary pattern). The patient was a 50-year-old man with miliary tuberculosis.

Figure 2. Posteroanterior chest radiograph shows numerous nodules involving mainly the middle and upper lung zones. Also noted is increased opacity in the right paratracheal region consistent with lymphadenopathy. The patient was a 45-year-old woman with sarcoidosis.

Figure 4. Chest radiograph shows small nodular opacities in the upper lobes. The patient was a 48-year-old man with silicosis.

Case 21

DEMOGRAPHICS/CLINICAL HISTORY

A 42-year-old man with shortness of breath, undergoing computed tomography (CT).

FINDINGS

Small perilymphatic nodules (Figs. 1 and 2) are located mainly along the bronchi, vessels, interlobar fissures, and subpleural lung regions

DISCUSSION

Definition/Background

A perilymphatic distribution refers to distribution along the lymphatic vessels in the lung, along bronchovascular bundles, interlobular septa, and pulmonary veins and in the pleura. A perilymphatic distribution of nodules may result in nodular thickening of these structures on high-resolution CT.

Characteristic Clinical Features

Patients may be asymptomatic or have nonspecific symptoms of dry cough and shortness of breath.

Characteristic Radiologic Findings

A perilymphatic distribution is characterized by the presence of nodules along the bronchovascular interstitium, interlobular septa, and subpleural lung regions (Figs. 1 to 3). The nodules tend to be well defined and usually are 2 to 5 mm in diameter. Nodules in a perilymphatic distribution are frequently associated with nodular thickening of the bronchovascular bundles. Another sign that is helpful in assessing the perilymphatic distribution is the presence of subpleural nodules in relation to the interlobar fissures (Fig. 2), a characteristic finding in sarcoidosis, silicosis, and coalworker's pneumoconiosis.

Less Common Radiologic Manifestations

Patients with sarcoidosis and silicosis frequently have associated bilateral hilar lymphadenopathy. Eggshell calcification of hilar and mediastinal lymph nodes is seen in a small percentage of patients with silicosis and sarcoidosis.

Differential Diagnosis

- Sarcoidosis
- Lymphatic spread of tumor (e.g., lymphangitic carcinomatosis, lymphoma)
- Silicosis
- Coalworker's pneumoconiosis
- Lymphoid interstitial pneumonia (LIP)
- Lymphoid hyperplasia
- Amyloidosis

Discussion

The most common radiologic manifestation of sarcoidosis is symmetric bilateral hilar and mediastinal lymph node enlargement with or without associated parenchymal abnormalities. Parenchymal involvement typically results in a nodular or reticulonodular pattern involving mainly the upper and middle lung zones. On high-resolution CT, nodules are seen at initial evaluation in 90% to 100% of patients who have parenchymal abnormalities. The nodules are typically most numerous along the bronchoarterial and pleural interstitium and adjacent to the interlobar fissures, a distribution that suggests sarcoidosis. Although nodular septal thickening (Fig. 3) is often evident on high-resolution CT, it seldom is the predominant finding. In most patients with lymphangitic spread of tumor, the main finding is interlobular septal thickening. The septal thickening may be smooth or, less commonly, nodular. Peribronchovascular and subpleural nodules may be seen but they are typically not as profuse as in patients with sarcoidosis. Other common findings seen in patients with lymphatic spread of tumor are unilateral or asymmetric hilar lymph node enlargement and pleural effusion. Silicosis and coalworker's pneumoconiosis are associated with the presence of small, well-defined nodules that usually are 2 to 5 mm in diameter. Similar to sarcoidosis, silicosis and coalworker's pneumoconiosis can be diffuse, but they usually involve mainly the middle and upper lung zones and are frequently associated with hilar and mediastinal lymph node enlargement. Similar to sarcoidosis, nodules are frequently seen in the subpleural regions and along the interlobar fissures. However, the nodules in silicosis and coalworker's pneumoconiosis have a predominantly centrilobular distribution and typically are most numerous in the dorsal half of the upper lobes. The diagnosis is readily made based on the radiographic or CT findings and exposure history.

Diagnosis

Perilymphatic nodular pattern on high-resolution

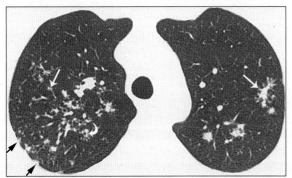

Figure 1. In a 42-year-old man with sarcoidosis, high-resolution CT at the level of the aortic arch shows small perilymphatic nodules located mainly along the bronchi *(curved arrow)*, vessels *(straight white arrows)*, and subpleural regions *(short black arrows)*.

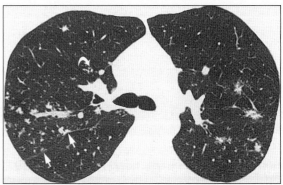

Figure 2. In a 42-year-old man with sarcoidosis, high-resolution CT at the level of the main bronchi shows small perilymphatic nodules located mainly along the bronchi *(curved arrow)*, vessels, and interlobar fissures *(straight arrows)*.

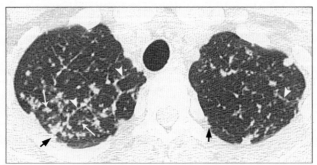

Figure 3. In a 41-year-old man with sarcoidosis, high-resolution CT at the level of the upper lobes shows numerous small, perilymphatic nodules located mainly along the interlobular septa *(arrowheads)*, centrilobular regions *(long white arrows)*, and subpleural regions *(short black arrows)*.

Suggested Readings

Chong S, Lee KS, Chung MJ, et al: Pneumoconiosis: Comparison of imaging and pathologic findings. Radiographics 26:59-77, 2006.

Honda O, Johkoh T, Ichikado K, et al: Comparison of high resolution CT findings of sarcoidosis, lymphoma, and lymphangitic carcinoma: Is there any difference of involved interstitium? J Comput Assist Tomogr 23:374-379, 1999.

Lee KS, Kim TS, Han J, et al: Diffuse micronodular lung disease: HRCT and pathologic findings. J Comput Assist Tomogr 23:99-106, 1999.

Nunes H, Brillet PY, Valeyre D, et al: Imaging in sarcoidosis. Semin Respir Crit Care Med 28:102-120, 2007.

Case 22

DEMOGRAPHICS/CLINICAL HISTORY

A 50-year-old man with progressive shortness of breath, undergoing computed tomography (CT).

FINDINGS

Bilateral, symmetric, poorly defined centrilobular nodular opacities (Figs. 1 and 2). The centrilobular opacities typically are a few millimeters away from the pleura, interlobular septa, and large vessels and bronchi. The patient was a bird breeder with subacute hypersensitivity pneumonitis.

DISCUSSION

Definition/Background

The centrilobular region is located in the center of the secondary lobule, adjacent to the bronchiolovascular core. A centrilobular nodular pattern is characterized by numerous, small nodules in a centrilobular distribution.

Characteristic Clinical Features

The patients may be asymptomatic (e.g., respiratory bronchiolitis), present with acute fever and cough (e.g., infectious bronchiolitis), have a more indolent course with fever and cough (e.g., tuberculosis), or have progressive shortness of breath (e.g., hypersensitivity pneumonitis).

Characteristic Radiologic Findings

Centrilobular nodules are characterized on high-resolution CT by their location several millimeters away from the pleural surfaces, interlobar fissures, and interlobular septa (Figs. 1 and 2). The nodules usually are 3 to 7 mm in diameter and may have well-defined or poorly defined margins. Patients frequently have associated bronchial wall thickening. Differentiating centrilobular, perilymphatic, and random distribution of small nodules is most easily accomplished by looking for pleural nodules and nodules arising in relation to the interlobar fissures. If subpleural nodules are absent, the pattern is centrilobular. If numerous subpleural or fissural nodules are present, the pattern is perilymphatic or random.

Less Common Radiologic Manifestations

Associated findings can include areas of decreased attenuation and vascularity and air trapping (particularly in hypersensitivity pneumonitis), branching linear and nodular opacities (mainly in infectious bronchiolitis), extensive ground-glass opacities (e.g., hypersensitivity pneumonitis, respiratory bronchiolitis-interstitial lung disease), lobular areas of consolidation (e.g., bronchopneumonia), and bronchi filled with secretions (e.g., aspiration) (Fig. 3).

Differential Diagnosis

- Infectious bronchiolitis due to viral, mycoplasmal, bacterial, or fungal infection
- Panbronchiolitis
- Aspiration bronchiolitis
- Hypersensitivity pneumonitis
- Pneumoconiosis: silicosis or coal worker's pneumoconiosis
- Respiratory bronchiolitis
- Respiratory bronchiolitis–interstitial lung disease (RBILD)
- Severe pulmonary arterial hypertension
- Pulmonary capillary hemangiomatosis
- Intravascular metastases

Discussion

Centrilobular nodules indicate bronchiolitis or bronchiolocentric interstitial lung disease. The centrilobular nodules in infectious bronchiolitis usually are well defined and have a patchy, unilateral or bilateral distribution. Infectious bronchiolitis may be caused by viral, mycoplasmal, bacterial, or fungal infection. The centrilobular nodules in infectious bronchiolitis are commonly associated with branching linear and nodular opacities, resulting in a tree-in-bud pattern. Similar findings are seen in endobronchial spread of tuberculosis and in nontuberculous mycobacterial infections. In aspiration bronchiolitis, the centrilobular nodules are located mainly in the dependent lung regions (Fig. 3).

Centrilobular nodules in hypersensitivity pneumonitis, respiratory bronchiolitis, and RBILD typically have poorly defined margins, whereas those associated with infectious bronchiolitis and endobronchial spread of tuberculosis usually have well-defined margins and are commonly associated with branching opacities, resulting in a tree-in-bud appearance. In hypersensitivity pneumonitis, the nodules are usually diffuse throughout the lungs (Fig. 2) or involve mainly the middle and lower lung zones and are frequently associated with ground-glass opacities and lobular areas of decreased attenuation and vascularity with air trapping on expiratory CT. The centrilobular nodules in respiratory bronchiolitis and RBILD tend to involve predominantly or exclusively

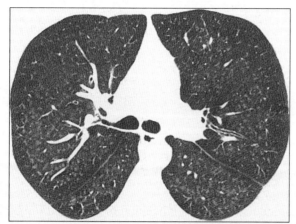

Figure 1. High-resolution CT image shows numerous, bilateral, poorly defined, centrilobular nodular opacities in a symmetric distribution. The centrilobular opacities typically are a few millimeters away from the pleura, interlobular septa, and large vessels and bronchi. The 50-year-old man was a bird breeder and developed subacute hypersensitivity pneumonitis.

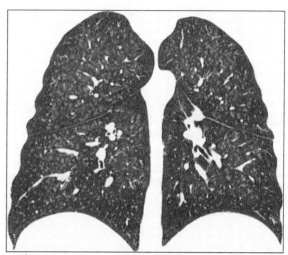

Figure 2. Coronal reformation image shows diffuse, poorly defined, centrilobular nodular opacities in a 50-year-old man who was a bird breeder and developed subacute hypersensitivity pneumonitis. The centrilobular opacities typically are a few millimeters away from the pleura, interlobular septa, and large vessels and bronchi.

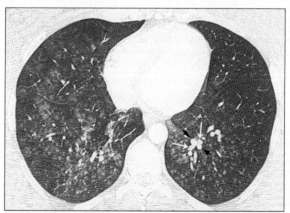

Figure 3. In a 26-year-old man with aspiration bronchiolitis resulting from a closed head injury, high-resolution CT shows bilateral, poorly defined, centrilobular nodular opacities and lobular areas of ground-glass opacity. Notice the bronchi filled with secretions (*white arrows*) adjacent to the accompanying pulmonary arteries (*black arrows*) in the left lower lobe.

the upper lobes, and because these conditions are seen exclusively in cigarette smokers, they frequently are associated with centrilobular emphysema.

Diagnosis

Centrilobular nodules on high-resolution computed tomography

Suggested Readings

Heyneman LE, Ward S, Lynch DA, et al: Respiratory bronchiolitis, respiratory bronchiolitis-associated interstitial lung disease, and desquamative interstitial pneumonia: Different entities or part of the spectrum of the same disease process? AJR Am J Roentgenol 173:1617-1622, 1999.

Okada F, Ando Y, Yoshitake S, et al: Clinical/pathologic correlations in 553 patients with primary centrilobular findings on high-resolution CT scan of the thorax. Chest 132:1939-1948, 2007.

Pipavath SJ, Lynch DA, Cool C, et al: Radiologic and pathologic features of bronchiolitis. AJR Am J Roentgenol 185:354-363, 2005.

Silva CIS, Müller NL, Churg A: Hypersensitivity pneumonitis: Spectrum of high-resolution CT and pathologic findings. AJR Am J Roentgenol 188:334-344, 2007.

Case 23

DEMOGRAPHICS/CLINICAL HISTORY

A 57-year-old man with fever and cough, undergoing computed tomography (CT).

FINDINGS

High-resolution CT images (Figs. 1 and 2) show centrilobular branching nodular and linear opacities, resulting in a tree-in-bud appearance.

DISCUSSION

Definition/Background
The tree-in-bud pattern refers to centrilobular branching structures that resemble a budding tree. It is usually associated with small centrilobular nodules.

Characteristic Clinical Features
Clinical features include fever and cough in infectious bronchiolitis and endobronchial spread of tuberculosis; chronic cough in patients with mucoid impaction associated with bronchiectasis; worsening of symptoms of asthma in patients with allergic bronchopulmonary aspergillosis; history of impaired consciousness or esophageal motility disorder in aspiration bronchiolitis; and dyspnea and weight loss in patients with intravascular metastases.

Characteristic Radiologic Findings
The tree-in-bud pattern is characterized on high-resolution CT by branching opacities several millimeters away from the pleural surfaces, interlobar fissures, and interlobular septa. Patients frequently have associated centrilobular nodules and bronchial wall thickening.

Less Common Radiologic Manifestations
Associated findings may include lobular or confluent areas of consolidation (i.e., bronchopneumonia), bronchiectasis, and areas of decreased attenuation and vascularity and air trapping. Patients with infectious bronchiolitis and bronchopneumonia may have hilar and mediastinal lymphadenopathy or pleural effusions.

Differential Diagnosis
- Infectious bronchiolitis (i.e., bacterial, fungal, or viral)
- Endobronchial spread of Mycobacterium tuberculosis or Mycobacterium avium-intracellulare complex (MAI)
- Mucoid impaction distal to bronchiectasis
- Allergic bronchopulmonary aspergillosis
- Aspiration bronchiolitis
- Bronchiolitis due to inhalation of gases and fumes
- Intravascular metastases

Discussion
The tree-in-bud pattern usually reflects the presence of dilated centrilobular bronchioles with their lumina impacted with mucus, fluid, or pus and often associated with peribronchiolar inflammation. The pattern usually is associated with infection of the small airways, and the most common causes are infectious bronchiolitis (Fig. 3), bronchopneumonia, and endobronchial spread of tuberculosis (Fig. 4) or MAI. It also reflects the presence of mucoid impaction distal to bronchiectasis, bronchial obstruction, or associated allergic bronchopulmonary aspergillosis. The various forms of infectious bronchiolitis and endobronchial spread of mycobacterial infection tend to result in a focal or multifocal, unilateral or bilateral tree-in-bud pattern. Centrilobular nodules and a tree-in-bud pattern involving mainly the dependent regions suggest aspiration bronchiolitis. Panbronchiolitis typically results in a bilateral, symmetric tree-in-bud pattern that may be diffuse but tends to have lower lobe predominance and is commonly associated with air trapping and bronchiectasis. Panbronchiolitis is a common condition in East Asia, particularly Japan, but it is uncommon in Europe and North America. Occasionally, a tree-in-bud pattern may result from abnormalities of the centrilobular pulmonary arteries. Causes include intravascular metastases and microangiopathy. Intravascular metastases are seen most commonly in carcinoma of the breast or kidney.

Diagnosis
Tree-in-bud pattern on high-resolution computed tomography

Suggested Readings
Collins J, Blankenbaker D, Stern EJ: CT patterns of bronchiolar disease: What is "tree-in-bud"? AJR Am J Roentgenol 171:365-370, 1998.

Gruden JF, Webb WR, Naidich DP, McGuinness G: Multinodular disease: anatomic localization at thin-section CT—multireader evaluation of a simple algorithm. Radiology 210:711-720, 1999.

Rossi SE, Franquet T, Volpacchio M, et al: Tree-in-bud pattern at thin-section CT of the lungs: Radiologic-pathologic overview. Radiographics 25:789-801, 2005.

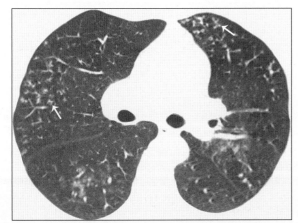

Figure 1. High-resolution CT image at the level of the bronchus intermedius shows bilateral centrilobular branching nodular and linear opacities, resulting in a tree-in-bud appearance *(arrows)*. The patient was a 57-year-old man with infectious bronchiolitis.

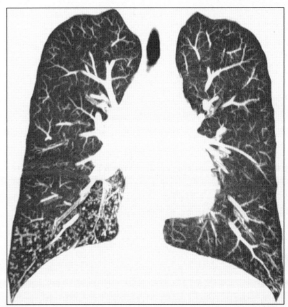

Figure 3. In a 20-year-old woman with recurrent respiratory infection, a coronal maximum-intensity projection (MIP) image shows centrilobular nodules in the lower lobes with a tree-in-bud appearance.

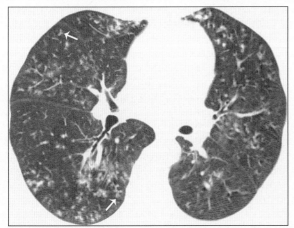

Figure 2. High-resolution CT image at the level of the right middle lobe bronchus shows bilateral centrilobular branching nodular and linear opacities, resulting in a tree-in-bud appearance *(arrows)*. The patient was a 57-year-old man with infectious bronchiolitis.

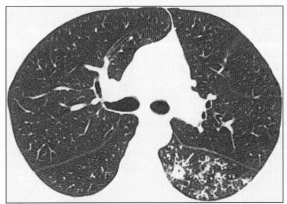

Figure 4. In a 30-year-old woman with endobronchial spread of tuberculosis, high-resolution CT shows centrilobular branching nodular and linear opacities, resulting in a tree-in-bud appearance in the left lower lobe, and a cavitated nodule *(arrow)*.

Case 24

DEMOGRAPHICS/CLINICAL HISTORY

A 74-year-old man with progressive shortness of breath, undergoing computed tomography (CT).

FINDINGS

Numerous, well-defined, small nodules are randomly distributed in relation to structures of the lung and a secondary lobule (Figs. 1 and 2). A left pleural effusion (Fig. 1) and a left upper lobe mass (Fig. 2) are consistent with pulmonary carcinoma.

DISCUSSION

Definition/Background

Small nodules occur in a random distribution in relation to structures of the lung and secondary lobule. They are usually of hematogenous origin and therefore tend to involve mainly the lower lobes.

Characteristic Clinical Features

Acute presentation includes fever and shortness of breath in patients with miliary infection (e.g., tuberculosis, histoplasmosis, coccidioidomycosis). Asymptomatic or, less commonly, progressive shortness of breath occur in patients with hematogenous spread of metastases.

Characteristic Radiologic Findings

Small nodules occur with a random distribution in relation to the secondary pulmonary lobules. Differentiation of perilymphatic, centrilobular, and random distribution of small nodules is most easily accomplished by looking for pleural nodules and nodules arising in relation to the fissures. If subpleural nodules are absent, the pattern is centrilobular. If numerous subpleural or fissural nodules are present, the pattern is perilymphatic or random. These two patterns are distinguished by looking at the distribution of other nodules. If they are patchy in distribution and particularly if a distinct predominance is observed relative to the peribronchovascular interstitium, interlobular septa, or subpleural regions, the nodules are perilymphatic. If the nodules are distributed in a diffuse and uniform manner, the pattern is random (Figs. 1 and 2).

Less Common Radiologic Manifestations

Associated findings that may be seen in some patients include septal thickening (e.g., miliary infection, lymphangitic carcinomatosis) and lymphadenopathy or mass (e.g., infection, metastases) (Fig. 2).

Differential Diagnosis

- Miliary tuberculosis
- Miliary fungal infection (e.g., coccidioidomycosis, cryptococcosis, histoplasmosis)
- Pulmonary metastases
- Septic embolism

Discussion

Small nodules in a random distribution in relation to structures of the lung and secondary lobule are seen most commonly in miliary tuberculosis (Fig. 3), miliary fungal infections, and pulmonary metastases (Figs. 1 and 2). Hematogenous miliary infections and metastases tend to be most numerous in the lung periphery and lung bases. Randomly distributed nodules can be seen in relation to interlobular septa, small vessels, and pleural surfaces (Fig. 3) but do not have consistent or predominant distribution in relation to any of these structures. Lung involvement tends to be bilateral and symmetric. The random distribution of nodules usually can be recognized on high-resolution CT images but may be easier to appreciate on maximum intensity projection (MIP) reconstructions (Fig. 4).

Diagnosis

Randomly distributed nodules on high-resolution computed tomography

Suggested Readings

Hansell DM, Bankier AA, MacMahon H, et al: Fleischner Society: Glossary of terms for thoracic imaging. Radiology 246:697-722, 2008.
Lee KS, Kim TS, Han J, et al: Diffuse micronodular lung disease: HRCT and pathologic findings. J Comput Assist Tomogr 23:99-106, 1999.
McGuinness G, Naidich DP, Jagirdar J, et al: High resolution CT findings in miliary lung disease. J Comput Assist Tomogr 16:384-390, 1992.
Murata K, Takahashi M, Mori M, et al: Pulmonary metastatic nodules: CT-pathologic correlation. Radiology 182:331-335, 1992.

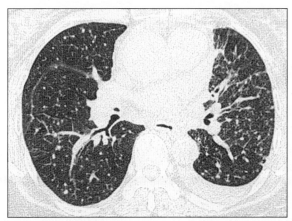

Figure 1. High-resolution CT image shows numerous, bilateral, well-defined, small nodules in a random distribution. A left pleural effusion also can be seen in this 74-year-old man with metastatic pulmonary carcinoma.

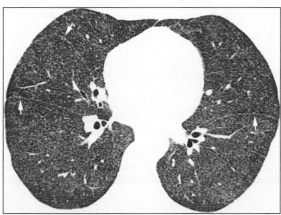

Figure 3. High-resolution CT image shows numerous, small, well-defined nodules that can be seen in relation to interlobular septa, small vessels, and pleural surfaces *(arrows)* but do not have consistent or predominant distribution in relation to any of these. The patient was a 47-year-old woman with biopsy-proven miliary tuberculosis.

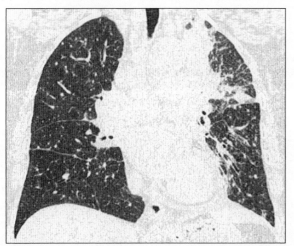

Figure 2. Coronal reformation image shows a random distribution of numerous, well-defined, small nodules and a left upper lobe mass in a 74-year-old man with metastatic pulmonary carcinoma.

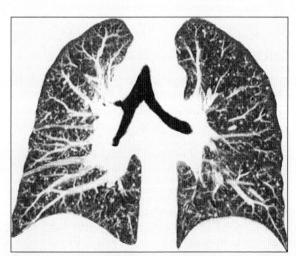

Figure 4. Coronal MIP image shows numerous, bilateral, small nodules in a random distribution. The patient was a 46-year-old man with biopsy-proven miliary tuberculosis.

Case 25

DEMOGRAPHICS/CLINICAL HISTORY

A 57-year-old man with fever and neutropenia after hematopoietic stem cell transplantation, undergoing computed tomography (CT).

FINDINGS

Bilateral nodules (Figs. 1 and 2) are surrounded by a halo of ground-glass attenuation (i.e., CT halo sign) in a patient with angioinvasive aspergillosis.

DISCUSSION

Definition/Background

A CT halo sign is a ground-glass opacity surrounding a nodule or mass. The halo of ground-glass attenuation may result from hemorrhage (e.g., invasive aspergillosis), less dense infiltration by the inflammatory process (e.g., organizing pneumonia) or tumor (e.g., pulmonary lymphoma), or the characteristic lepidic growth of bronchioalveolar carcinoma.

Characteristic Clinical Features

Patients may be asymptomatic or present with nonspecific symptoms of cough and fever. Patients with CT halo sign due to pulmonary adenocarcinoma are usually asymptomatic smokers. Patients with CT halo sign caused by angioinvasive aspergillosis typically have severe neutropenia, most commonly in the setting of leukemia, chemotherapy, or stem cell transplantation.

Characteristic Radiologic Findings

Single or multiple nodules or masses are surrounded by a rim of ground-glass opacity on CT.

Less Common Radiologic Manifestations

Most nodules with a CT halo sign have soft tissue density. Occasionally, they may be cavitated.

Differential Diagnosis

- Infection: aspergillosis, candidiasis, mucormycosis, cytomegalovirus, herpes simplex
- Neoplasm: pulmonary adenocarcinoma, metastatic angiosarcoma, metastatic mucinous adenocarcinoma, Kaposi sarcoma, lymphoma
- Vasculitis: Wegener granulomatosis
- Organizing pneumonia (i.e., bronchiolitis obliterans organizing pneumonia [BOOP])

Discussion

Although the differential diagnosis is broad, the CT halo sign can strongly suggest a specific diagnosis in the proper clinical context. In immunocompromised patients with severe neutropenia, the presence of one or more nodules with a halo sign suggests angioinvasive aspergillosis (Figs. 1 and 2). In a patient with AIDS, multiple lung nodules with a halo sign most often suggest Kaposi sarcoma. In an asymptomatic smoker, the presence of a nodule with ground-glass opacity surrounding a solid component suggests bronchogenic carcinoma, most commonly adenocarcinoma (Fig. 3).

Diagnosis

Lung nodules with computed tomography halo sign

Suggested Readings

Kim Y, Lee KS, Jung KJ, et al: Halo sign on high resolution CT: Findings in spectrum of pulmonary diseases with pathologic correlation. J Comput Assist Tomogr 23:622-626, 1999.

Lee YR, Choi YW, Lee KJ, et al: CT halo sign: The spectrum of pulmonary diseases. Br J Radiol 78:862-865, 2005.

Primack SL, Hartman TE, Lee KS, Müller NL: Pulmonary nodules and the CT halo sign. Radiology 190:513-515, 1994.

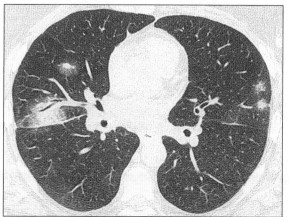

Figure 1. High-resolution CT image shows bilateral nodules surrounded by a rim of ground-glass attenuation (i.e., CT halo sign) in a 57-year-old man with angioinvasive aspergillosis and severe neutropenia after hematopoietic stem cell transplantation.

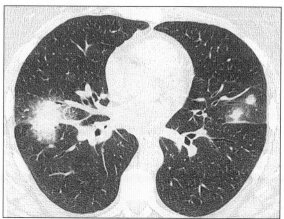

Figure 2. High-resolution CT image shows bilateral nodules surrounded by a rim of ground-glass attenuation (i.e., CT halo sign) in a 57-year-old man with angioinvasive aspergillosis and severe neutropenia after hematopoietic stem cell transplantation.

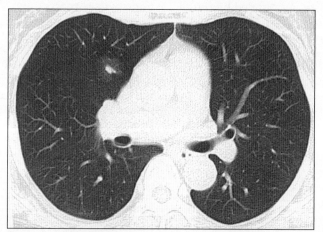

Figure 3. High-resolution CT image shows a small nodule surrounded by a rim of ground-glass attenuation (i.e., CT halo sign) in a 58-year-old smoker with pulmonary adenocarcinoma.

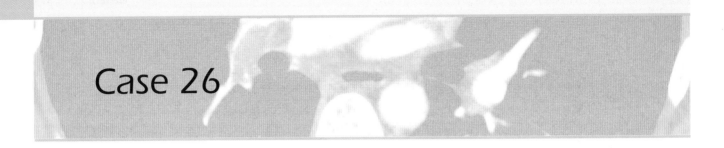

Case 26

DEMOGRAPHICS/CLINICAL HISTORY

A 47-year-old man, hemoptysis.

FINDINGS

Magnified view of the left lung apex from a posteroanterior chest radiograph (Fig. 1) shows large cavity containing homogeneous soft tissue mass surrounded by rim of air (air crescent sign). Also noted is left apical pleural thickening, left upper lobe scarring, and superior retraction of the left hilum.

DISCUSSION

Definition/Background

A cavity is a gas-filled space that may be seen within an area of consolidation, within a mass, or within a nodule. An intracavitary mass can usually be readily recognized on the radiograph and CT because of the presence of a meniscus or air crescent sign, which refers to a collection of gas with a crescentic shape that separates the wall of the cavity from the intracavitary mass.

Characteristic Clinical Features

The patients may be asymptomatic or present with nonspecific symptoms of cough and fever. Recurrent hemoptysis may also occur.

Characteristic Radiologic Findings

Usually thin-walled cystic lesion representing a cavity or focal area of bronchiectasis and containing an intracavitary soft tissue opacity, which is typically separated from the inner wall by a crescentic lucency (air crescent sign) (Figs. 1, 2, 3, and 4).

Less Common Radiologic Manifestations

Patients with intracavitary fungus ball usually have findings of fibrosis including reticular opacities, architectural distortion, and traction bronchiectasis. Intracavitary masses may also be seen in angioinvasive fungal infection, in which case the patient may present with multiple cavitating nodules containing intracavitary masses and no other radiologic findings.

Differential Diagnosis

- Fungus ball, usually aspergilloma, rarely *Candida*
- Active infection: angioinvasive aspergillosis, *Candida,* hydatid cyst, paragonimiasis abscess with inspissated pus, lung gangrene
- Blood clot in cavity, bullae, or bronchiectasis
- Neoplasm: pulmonary carcinoma, metastasis

Discussion

Intracavitary masses and the air crescent sign are seen in two main situations: fungal colonization of a pre-existing cavity and angioinvasive fungal infection. In the vast majority of cases, colonization of previous cavities is caused by *Aspergillus* (aspergilloma) and occurs in the setting of residual cavitation or bronchiectasis as the result of previous tuberculosis or sarcoidosis. These patients typically have a history of previous tuberculosis or long-standing sarcoidosis with unilateral or bilateral upper lobe fibrosis and bronchiectasis. Occasionally the intracavitary mass may represent intracavitary hemorrhage rather than a fungus ball.

Angioinvasive fungal infection typically occurs in severely immunocompromised patients, most commonly in leukemia and following hematopoietic stem cell transplantation (Fig. 4). In this setting the intracavitary mass represents retraction of infarcted lung. The vast majority of cases are the result of angioinvasive aspergillosis; occasionally similar findings may be seen in candidiasis and mucormycosis.

Unusual causes of an air crescent sign include necrotizing pneumonia, hydatid disease, Wegener granulomatosis, and pulmonary carcinoma.

Diagnosis

Intracavitary mass (meniscus or air crescent sign)

Suggested Readings

Abramson S: The air crescent sign. Radiology 218:230-232, 2001.
Franquet T, Müller NL, Giménez A, Guembe P, de La Torre J, Bagué S: Spectrum of pulmonary aspergillosis: Histologic, clinical, and radiologic findings. Radiographics 21:825-837, 2001.
Koul PA, Koul AN, Wahid A, Mir FA: CT in pulmonary hydatid disease: Unusual appearances. Chest 118:1645-1647, 2000.

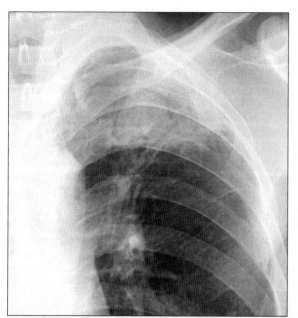

Figure 1. Magnified view of the left lung apex from a posteroanterior chest radiograph shows large cavity containing homogeneous soft tissue mass surrounded by rim of air (air crescent sign). Also noted is left apical pleural thickening, left upper lobe scarring, and superior retraction of the left hilum. The patient was a 47-year-old man with previous tuberculosis and left upper lobe intracavitary aspergilloma.

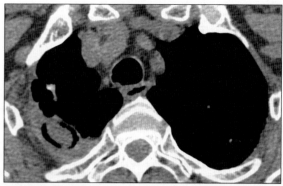

Figure 3. High-resolution CT image photographed at soft tissue windows shows right upper lobe cavity containing oval soft tissue mass surrounded by rim of air. Also noted is right pleural thickening and small focus of calcification in the right upper lobe. The patient was a 68-year-old man with previous tuberculosis and right upper lobe intracavitary aspergilloma.

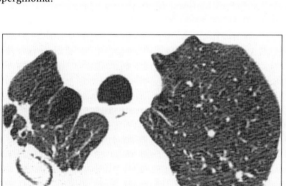

Figure 2. High-resolution CT image demonstrates right upper lobe cavity containing oval soft tissue mass surrounded by rim of air. Also noted are areas of scarring in the right upper lobe and bilateral centrilobular emphysema. The patient was a 68-year-old man with previous tuberculosis and right upper lobe intracavitary aspergilloma.

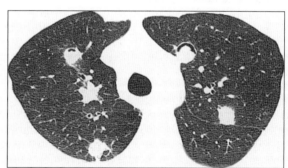

Figure 4. High-resolution CT image demonstrates several bilateral nodules. One of the nodules on the right and one on the left are cavitated and contain soft tissue opacity with crescent of air density. The patient was a 24-year-old man with leukemia and angio-invasive aspergillosis.

Case 27

DEMOGRAPHICS/CLINICAL HISTORY

A 79-year-old man, cough, low-grade fever.

FINDINGS

Posteroanterior chest radiograph (Fig. 1) shows cavity with well-defined smooth margins and a fluid level in the right middle lung zone. Poorly defined areas of consolidation are present in the right upper lobe and nodular opacities in the right upper and left middle lung zones.

DISCUSSION

Definition/Background

A cavity is defined radiologically as a gas-containing space within the lung surrounded by a wall whose thickness is greater than 1 mm. In most cases, it is formed by necrosis of the central portion of a lesion and drainage of the resultant, partially liquefied material via communicating airways.

Characteristic Clinical Features

Patients with a solitary cavitated lung nodule or mass may be asymptomatic or may have systemic symptoms suggestive of infection (fever, chills) or symptoms related to the cavitary lesion (productive cough, hemoptysis).

Characteristic Radiologic Findings

A cavitary nodule or mass may have smooth, lobulated, or spiculated, well-defined or ill-defined margins (Figs. 1, 2, 3, and 4). The inner wall may be smooth, irregular, or nodular. These features can be helpful in the differential diagnosis (see below). A cavity caused by tuberculosis may occur in any lobe but is most commonly located in the upper lobes or superior segments of lower lobes and is frequently associated with other findings such as patchy consolidation and small nodules (Figs. 1 and 2).

Less Common Radiologic Manifestations

Cavitating nodules may be associated with hilar or mediastinal lymphadenopathy and with pleural complications including pneumothorax, effusion, empyema, and bronchopleural fistula.

Differential Diagnosis

- Infection (tuberculosis, fungal infection, lung abscess)
- Neoplasm (pulmonary carcinoma, solitary metastasis)
- Congenital abnormalities (bronchogenic cyst, congenital cystic adenomatoid malformation)
- Inflammatory processes (Wegener granulomatosis, rheumatoid nodule)
- Trauma: pulmonary laceration (post-traumatic pneumatocele)

Discussion

The cavity wall is usually thick in an acute lung abscess, primary and metastatic carcinoma, and Wegener granulomatosis and is often thin in chronic infection such as coccidioidomycosis (Figs. 3, 4). Assessment of cavity wall thickness is useful in distinguishing between a benign and a malignant lesion. In one study of 65 solitary cavities in the lung, all lesions in which the thickest part of the cavity wall was 1 mm or less were benign; of the lesions whose thickest measurement was 4 mm or less, 92% were benign; of those that were 5 to 15 mm in their thickest part, benign and malignant lesions were equally divided; and 92% of lesions whose cavity wall was greater than 15 mm in thickness were malignant.

The inner lining of the cavity is usually nodular in carcinoma, shaggy in acute lung abscess, and smooth in most other cavitary lesions. When material is identified within a cavity, it usually represents pus or partially liquefied necrotic neoplasm and appears as a flat, smooth air-fluid level without specific radiologic features. Occasionally, intracavitary material has characteristics that are strongly suggestive of a specific disease. Examples include an intracavitary fungus ball, which may form a mobile mass, and the collapsed membranes of a ruptured *Echinococcus* cyst, which float on top of the fluid within the cyst and create the characteristic water lily sign).

Occasionally a thin-walled cavitary lesion may represent a bronchogenic cyst or a congenital cystic adenomatoid malformation that has communicated with an airway, or a traumatic or post-infectious pneumatocele. Pneumatoceles are thin-walled gas-filled spaces within the lung, most frequently caused by acute pneumonia, trauma, or aspiration of hydrocarbon fluid, and usually transient. Pneumatoceles are believed to result from check-valve airway obstruction. They may be single or multiple and typically have smooth, thin walls.

Diagnosis

Solitary cavitary lung nodule or mass

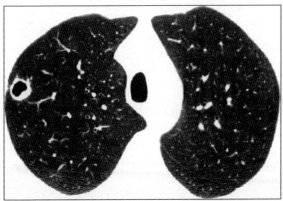

Figure 3. CT image shows thin-walled cavity in the right upper lobe. The patient was a 44-year-old man with coccidioidomycosis.

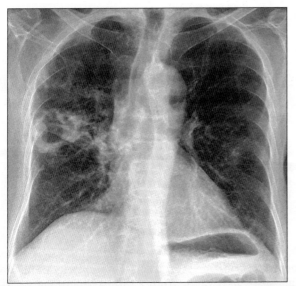

Figure 1. Posteroanterior chest radiograph shows cavity with well-defined smooth margins and a fluid level in the right middle lung zone. Poorly defined areas of consolidation are present in the right upper lobe and nodular opacities in the right upper and left middle lung zones. The patient was a 79-year-old man with pulmonary tuberculosis.

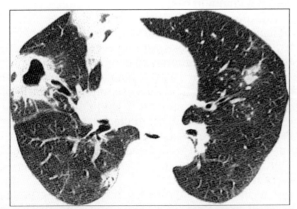

Figure 2. High-resolution CT image demonstrates cavity in the right middle lobe, focal areas of consolidation in the right middle and lower lobes and lingula, and centrilobular nodular opacities in the right middle lobe and lingula. The patient was a 79-year-old man with pulmonary tuberculosis.

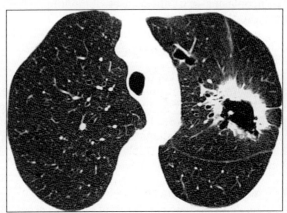

Figure 4. CT image demonstrates large cavitating mass with spiculated margins and nodular inner walls in the left upper lobe. The patient was a 64-year-old woman with pulmonary adenocarcinoma.

Suggested Readings

Erasmus JJ, Connolly JE, McAdams HP, Roggli VL: Solitary pulmonary nodules: Part I: Morphologic evaluation for differentiation of benign and malignant lesions. Radiographics 20:43-58, 2000.

Erasmus JJ, McAdams HP, Connolly JE: Solitary pulmonary nodules: Part II: Evaluation of the indeterminate nodule. Radiographics 20:59-66, 2000.

Ryu JH, Swensen SJ: Cystic and cavitary lung diseases: Focal and diffuse. Mayo Clin Proc 78(6):744-752, 2003.

Case 28

DEMOGRAPHICS/CLINICAL HISTORY

A 79-year-old man, weight loss, malaise, cough.

FINDINGS

Posteroanterior chest radiograph (Fig. 1) shows numerous smoothly marginated nodules and masses measuring 0.5 cm to approximately 4 cm in diameter. The nodules are most numerous in the lower lung zones.

DISCUSSION

Definition/Background

Multiple pulmonary nodules and masses may result from infection (e.g., tuberculosis, fungal infection, septic embolism), neoplasms (e.g., metastases, lymphoma), inflammatory processes (Wegener granulomatosis, rheumatoid nodules), or trauma (multiple pulmonary hematomas) or may be congenital (arteriovenous malformations).

Characteristic Clinical Features

Patients with multiple lung nodules are often asymptomatic or present with nonspecific symptoms of cough, malaise, and weight loss. In some cases, the symptoms may be suggestive of a diagnosis. For example, multiple nodules in a patient with sinusitis and renal abnormalities are most suggestive of Wegener granulomatosis.

Characteristic Radiologic Findings

Approximately circular opacities of various sizes may have smooth, lobulated or spiculated, well-defined or ill-defined margins. In the majority of cases, multiple nodules are of soft tissue density (Figs. 1 and 2). Surrounding halo of ground-glass opacity may be seen in patients with hemorrhagic nodules or nodules associated with inflammatory reaction or mucus production (Fig. 3).

Less Common Radiologic Manifestations

Occasionally multiple nodules may be cavitated (Fig. 4) or contain areas of calcification. Pleural effusions may occur in association with pulmonary metastases, Wegener granulomatosis, and pulmonary infection (e.g., septic embolism).

Differential Diagnosis

- Pulmonary metastases
- Lymphoma
- Infection (tuberculosis, fungal infection, septic embolism)
- Congenital abnormalities (arteriovenous malformations)
- Inflammatory processes (Wegener granulomatosis, rheumatoid nodules)
- Trauma: post-traumatic hematomas

Discussion

The radiologic manifestations of multiple pulmonary metastases may range from a diffuse micronodular pattern resembling miliary disease to large, well-defined cannonball masses. The nodules may be of uniform size, indicating a simultaneous origin in one shower of emboli, or may differ, suggesting embolic events of different ages. On CT, pulmonary metastases are most commonly seen in the outer third of the lungs, particularly the subpleural regions of the lower zones.

Another common cause of multiple nodules is pulmonary infection. Multiple nodules may be seen in septic embolism, tuberculosis, histoplasmosis, coccidioidomycosis, and cryptococcosis. Multiple nodules in tuberculosis result from endobronchial or miliary spread and are usually less than 1 cm in diameter. Similarly histoplasmosis and coccidioidomycosis often present with a single nodule measuring up to 3 cm in diameter or multiple nodules less than 1 cm in diameter.

Septic embolism is characterized by the presence of multiple nodules and wedge-shaped peripheral opacities that measure approximately 1 to 3 cm in diameter and that are frequently cavitated.

In the immunocompromised host, multiple nodules may result from invasive aspergillosis, candidiasis, and cytomegalovirus pneumonia. Angioinvasive aspergillosis usually presents with multiple nodules ranging from a few millimeters to approximately 3 cm in diameter. These tend to have ill-defined margins on the chest radiograph and to be surrounded by a rim of ground-glass attenuation on CT, known as the CT halo sign (Fig. 3). This rim is the result of pulmonary hemorrhage. The findings of candidiasis may be identical to those of invasive aspergillosis. The nodules in cytomegalovirus and herpes virus pneumonia usually measure less than 1 cm in diameter.

The most common vascular abnormalities resulting in multiple nodules are congenital arteriovenous malformations often seen in patients with Osler-Weber-Rendu syndrome. CT demonstrates characteristic large feeding arteries and draining veins.

Multiple nodules and masses may also be a manifestation of inflammatory processes, including Wegener granulomatosis and necrobiotic pulmonary nodules,

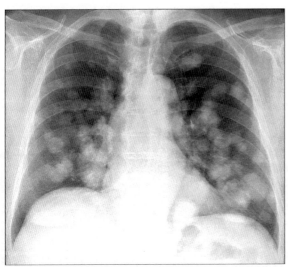

Figure 1. Posteroanterior chest radiograph shows numerous smoothly marginated nodules measuring 0.5 cm to approximately 4 cm in diameter. The nodules are most numerous in the lower lung zones. The patient was a 79-year-old man with pulmonary metastases from adenocarcinoma of the colon.

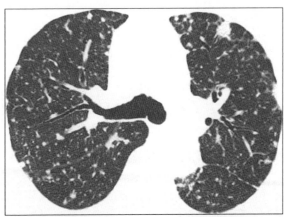

Figure 2. CT image shows numerous bilateral nodules ranging from approximately 2 to 15 mm in diameter. The nodules have a random distribution in the lungs. Some of the nodules have smooth margins, but many of them have spiculated margins. The patient was an 80-year-old woman with metastatic adenocarcinoma.

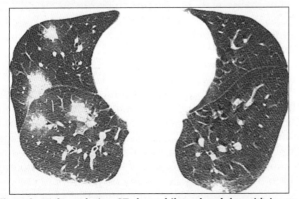

Figure 3. High-resolution CT shows bilateral nodules with irregular margins and a rim of ground-glass attenuation (CT halo sign). Also noted are septal lines resulting from fluid overload. The patient was a 24-year-old man with leukemia, severe neutropenia, and angioinvasive aspergillosis.

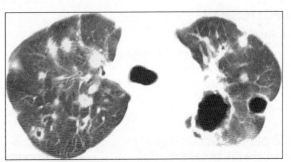

Figure 4. CT image shows numerous bilateral nodules and masses of various sizes, most of them solid and with irregular or ill-defined margins. Two of the lesions in the left upper lobe and a smaller one in the right upper lobe are cavitated. The patient was a 21-year-old man with pulmonary metastases from carcinoma of the tongue.

in patients with rheumatoid arthritis. Wegener granulomatosis typically presents with multiple nodules and masses ranging from a few millimeters up to 10 cm in diameter. Approximately 50% cavitate. Rheumatoid nodules are an uncommon manifestation of rheumatoid arthritis. They may be single or multiple and range from a few millimeters to 5 cm in diameter.

Diagnosis
Multiple lung nodules and masses

Suggested Readings

Dodd JD, Souza CA, Müller NL: High-resolution MDCT of pulmonary septic embolism: Evaluation of the feeding vessel sign. AJR Am J Roentgenol 187:623-629, 2006.

Primack SL, Hartman TE, Lee KS, Müller NL: Pulmonary nodules and the CT halo sign. Radiology 190:513-515, 1994.

Seo JB, Im JG, Goo JM, Chung MJ, Kim MY: Atypical pulmonary metastases: Spectrum of radiologic findings. Radiographics 21:403-417, 2001.

Sheehan RE, Flint JD, Müller NL: Computed tomography features of the thoracic manifestations of Wegener granulomatosis. J Thorac Imaging 18:34-41, 2003.

Case 29

DEMOGRAPHICS/CLINICAL HISTORY

A 36-year-old man who is an intravenous drug user with fever, undergoing computed tomography (CT).

FINDINGS

Axial (Fig. 1) and coronal (Fig. 2) CT images show multiple, bilateral, peripheral nodules, most of which are cavitated. The patient had septic emboli caused by *Staphylococcus aureus.*

DISCUSSION

Definition/Background

A cavity is defined radiologically as a gas-containing space within the lung surrounded by a wall whose thickness is greater than 1 mm. In most cases, it is formed by necrosis of the central portion of a lesion and drainage of the resultant, partially liquefied material through communicating airways.

Characteristic Clinical Features

Patients with multiple cavitary lung nodules usually are symptomatic. Patients with multiple cavities due to infection often present with fever and cough, and patients with cavitary metastases often present with weight loss and malaise. The presentation of patients with infection may be acute (e.g., septic embolism, angioinvasive aspergillosis) or indolent (e.g., tuberculosis and nontuberculous mycobacterial infections).

Characteristic Radiologic Findings

Multiple cavitated nodules caused by hematogenous dissemination of infection (i.e., septic embolism) or tumor (i.e., metastases) tend to involve mainly the peripheral regions of the lower lobes. Cavities in tuberculosis and nontuberculous mycobacterial infections tend to involve mainly the upper lobes and superior segments of the lower lobes.

Less Common Radiologic Manifestations

Cavitating nodules may be associated with hilar or mediastinal lymphadenopathy and with pleural complications, including pneumothorax, effusion, empyema, and bronchopleural fistula.

Differential Diagnosis

- Infection (e.g., tuberculosis, fungal infection, septic embolism)
- Neoplasm (e.g., metastatic squamous cell carcinoma)
- Congenital abnormalities (e.g., congenital cystic adenomatoid malformation)
- Inflammatory processes (e.g., Wegener granulomatosis, rheumatoid nodules)
- Trauma: pulmonary lacerations (e.g., post-traumatic pneumatoceles)

Discussion

Cavitation occurs in approximately 4% of pulmonary metastases (Fig. 3). It is seen most often in squamous cell carcinoma, and the primary sites usually are in the head and neck in men and the cervix in women. Although uncommon, cavitation can occur in patients with metastatic adenocarcinoma or metastatic sarcoma.

The cavity wall is usually thick in an acute lung abscess, primary and metastatic carcinoma, and Wegener granulomatosis, and it often is thin in septic embolism. However, thin-walled cavities may develop in metastatic squamous cell carcinomas, particularly from primary tumors in the head and neck.

Septic embolism occurs most commonly in intravenous drug abusers and in immunocompromised patients with central venous lines. Septic embolism is characterized by the presence of multiple nodules and wedge-shaped peripheral opacities measuring approximately 1 to 3 cm in diameter and that often are cavitated. The nodules tend to be most numerous in the peripheral lung regions and the lower lobes. Other infections that may result in multiple cavitary nodules include angioinvasive aspergillosis, tuberculosis, nontuberculous mycobacterial infections, coccidioidomycosis, and Wegener granulomatosis. Angioinvasive aspergillosis is seen almost exclusively in neutropenic immunocompromised patients. Tuberculosis and other mycobacteria tend to involve mainly the upper lobes and superior segments of the lower lobes. Wegener granulomatosis can manifest with several nodules and masses, approximately 50% of which cavitate, and with areas of consolidation that may also cavitate.

Pneumatoceles are thin-walled, gas-filled spaces within the lung that commonly are caused by acute pneumonia, trauma, or aspiration of hydrocarbon fluid; they are usually transient. Pneumatoceles likely result from check-valve airway obstruction. They may be single or multiple; typically have smooth, thin walls; and may contain fluid levels.

Diagnosis

Multiple cavitary lung nodules

Suggested Readings

Ryu JH, Swensen SJ: Cystic and cavitary lung diseases: Focal and diffuse. Mayo Clin Proc 78:744-752, 2003.

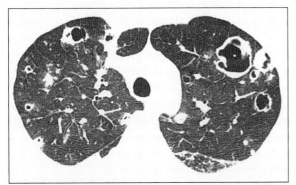

Figure 1. In a 36-year-old man, an intravenous drug user, with fever, axial CT shows multiple, bilateral, peripheral nodules, most of which are cavitated. The patient had septic emboli caused by *Staphylococcus aureus.*

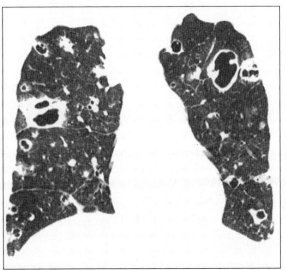

Figure 2. In a 36-year-old man, an intravenous drug user with fever, coronal CT shows multiple, bilateral, peripheral nodules, most of which are cavitated. The patient had septic emboli caused by *Staphylococcus aureus.*

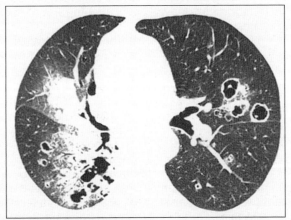

Figure 3. In a 67-year-old man with metastatic squamous cell carcinoma, CT shows multiple, bilateral, cavitated nodules. Notice the focal consolidation in the right middle lobe and ground-glass opacities in the right lung.

Case 30

DEMOGRAPHICS/CLINICAL HISTORY

An 82-year-old woman with recurrent hemoptysis, undergoing radiography and computed tomography (CT).

FINDINGS

Posteroanterior chest radiograph shows right upper lobe atelectasis (Fig. 1). The focal convexity with a downward bulge in the medial portion of the displaced minor fissure and a concave appearance of the lateral aspect of the minor fissure result in a reverse S configuration, known as the S sign of Golden. The right hemidiaphragm is mildly elevated. CT shows an atelectatic right upper lobe as a soft tissue density lying against the mediastinum and outlined laterally by the minor fissure that is displaced superiorly and medially (Fig. 2). Contrast-enhanced CT image right upper lobe atelectasis and a central tumor proven to be a bronchogenic carcinoma (Fig. 3).

DISCUSSION

Definition/Background
Lobar atelectasis is reduced inflation of a lobe. The term collapse is often used interchangeably with atelectasis, but it should be reserved for severe atelectasis.

Characteristic Clinical Features
Patients with lobar atelectasis may be asymptomatic or present with nonspecific symptoms of cough and shortness of breath. The symptoms may be acute (e.g., aspiration of foreign body) or chronic (e.g., endobronchial tumor). Endobronchial tumors may result in hemoptysis.

Characteristic Radiologic Findings
The chest radiograph is usually sufficient for diagnosis. Direct signs of right upper lobe atelectasis include superior displacement of the minor fissure and crowding of bronchi and vessels within the area of atelectasis; indirect signs include pulmonary opacification, cephalad displacement of the hilum, and elevation or tenting of the hemidiaphragm (i.e., juxtaphrenic peak). The latter consists of a small, sharply defined triangular opacity that projects upward from the medial half of the hemidiaphragm at or near the highest point of the dome. In most cases, the juxtaphrenic peak is related to an inferior accessory fissure. CT may be used when the chest radiograph findings are difficult to interpret and to establish the cause. Contrast-enhanced CT may show obstructing central lesion.

Less Common Radiologic Manifestations
Hilar and mediastinal lymphadenopathy may be seen and should raise the possibility of malignancy.

Differential Diagnosis
- Consolidation of the right upper lobe

Discussion
The main distinguishing feature between lobar atelectasis and consolidation is volume loss. Lobar atelectasis typically is caused by obstruction of a lobar bronchus by tumor, mucus, blood, or foreign body. Obstructive pneumonitis (e.g., distal to pulmonary carcinoma) frequently leads to consolidation severe enough to limit the loss of volume. The characteristic radiographic picture of obstructive atelectasis and pneumonitis (i.e., homogeneous opacification of a segment, lobe, or lung without air bronchograms) strongly suggests an obstructing endobronchial lesion. Lobar consolidation is most commonly caused by pneumonia and typically is associated with air bronchograms.

Diagnosis
Atelectasis of the right upper lobe

Suggested Readings
Molina PL, Hiken JN, Glazer HS: Imaging evaluation of obstructive atelectasis. J Thorac Imaging 11:176-186, 1996.
Woodring JH, Reed JC: Radiographic manifestations of lobar atelectasis. J Thorac Imaging 11:109-144, 1996.

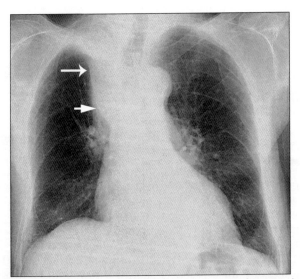

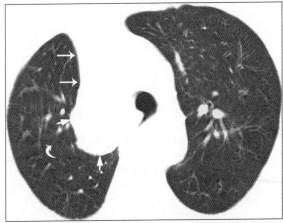

Figure 1. In an 82-year-old woman with recurrent hemoptysis, the posteroanterior chest radiograph shows right upper lobe atelectasis. Notice the focal convexity with downward bulge *(short arrow)* in the medial portion of the displaced minor fissure and concave appearance of the lateral aspect of the minor fissure *(long arrow)*, resulting in a reverse S configuration known as the S sign of Golden. The right hemidiaphragm is mildly elevated.

Figure 2. CT shows an atelectatic right upper lobe as a soft tissue density lying against the mediastinum and outlined laterally by the minor fissure *(long arrows)* that is displaced superiorly and medially. Notice the anterior and superior displacement of the major fissure *(curved arrow)* and a right hilar mass *(short arrows)* associated with the focal convexity.

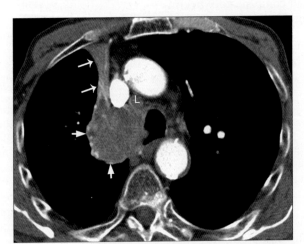

Figure 3. Contrast-enhanced CT shows right upper lobe atelectasis *(long arrows)* and a central tumor *(short arrows)* confirmed to be a bronchogenic carcinoma. Notice the right paratracheal lymph node enlargement.

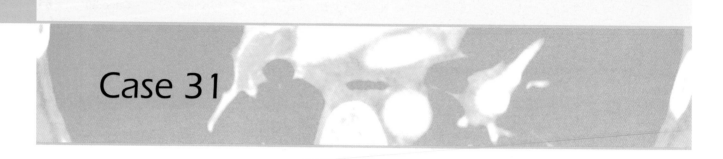

Case 31

DEMOGRAPHICS/CLINICAL HISTORY

A 65-year-old man with a cough, undergoing radiography.

FINDINGS

Posteroanterior chest radiograph shows a poorly defined increased opacity of the left hemithorax associated with obliteration of the left heart border (i.e., silhouette sign), volume loss of the left hemithorax, elevation of the left hemidiaphragm, and superior displacement of the left hilum characteristic of left upper lobe atelectasis (Fig. 1). Notice the crescentic lucency between the aortic arch and the apex of the atelectatic left upper lobe (i.e., Luftsichel sign). Lateral chest radiograph shows anterior displacement of the left major fissure and compensatory overinflation of the left lower lobe (Fig. 2). In another patient, CT shows complete atelectasis of the left upper lobe with anterior displacement of the left major fissure resulting from the tumor in the left main bronchus (Fig. 3).

DISCUSSION

Definition/Background

Lobar atelectasis is reduced inflation of a lobe. The term collapse often is used interchangeably with atelectasis, but it should be reserved for severe atelectasis.

Characteristic Clinical Features

Patients with lobar atelectasis may be asymptomatic or present with nonspecific symptoms of cough and shortness of breath. The symptoms may be acute (e.g., aspiration of foreign body) or chronic (e.g., endobronchial tumor). Endobronchial tumors may result in hemoptysis.

Characteristic Radiologic Findings

The chest radiograph is usually sufficient for diagnosis. Direct signs of lobar atelectasis include displacement of the interlobar fissures and crowding of bronchi and vessels within the area of atelectasis; indirect signs include pulmonary opacification, cephalad displacement of the hilum, ipsilateral diaphragmatic elevation, mediastinal shift, and compensatory overinflation of the lower lobe. Left upper lobe atelectasis typically includes the lingula and results in obscuration of the left heart border. Compensatory overinflation of the superior segment of the lower lobe often results in a crescent of hyperlucency adjacent to the aortic arch known as the Luftsichel ("air crescent") sign. CT may be used when the chest radiographic findings are difficult to interpret and to evaluate the cause. Contrast-enhanced CT may show an enhancing endobronchial lesion.

Less Common Radiologic Manifestations

Hilar and mediastinal lymphadenopathy may be seen and should raise the possibility of malignancy.

Differential Diagnosis

- Left upper lobe consolidation

Discussion

The main distinguishing feature between lobar atelectasis and consolidation is the presence of volume loss. The main cause of lobar atelectasis is obstruction of a lobar bronchus by tumor, mucus, blood, or foreign body. Obstructive pneumonitis (e.g., distal to pulmonary carcinoma) frequently leads to consolidation severe enough to limit the loss of volume. The characteristic radiographic picture of obstructive atelectasis and pneumonitis (i.e., homogeneous opacification of a segment, lobe, or lung without air bronchograms) strongly suggests an obstructing endobronchial lesion.

Diagnosis

Atelectasis of the left upper lobe

Suggested Readings

Molina PL, Hiken JN, Glazer HS: Imaging evaluation of obstructive atelectasis. J Thorac Imaging 11:176-186, 1996.

Woodring JH, Reed JC: Radiographic manifestations of lobar atelectasis. J Thorac Imaging 11:109-144, 1996.

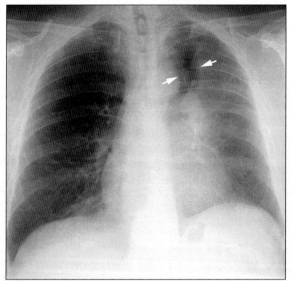

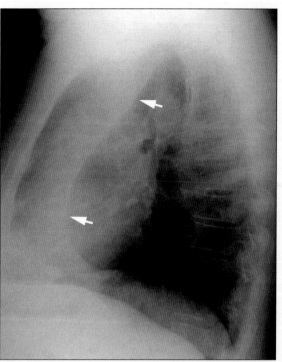

Figure 1. In a 65-year-old man with a cough, the posteroanterior chest radiograph shows poorly defined, increased opacity of the left hemithorax that is associated with obliteration of the left heart border (i.e., silhouette sign), volume loss of the left hemithorax, elevation of the left hemidiaphragm, and superior displacement of the left hilum, which is characteristic of left upper lobe atelectasis. Notice the crescentic lucency between the aortic arch and the atelectatic left upper lobe (i.e., Luftsichel sign) *(arrows)*.

Figure 2. In the same patient, the lateral chest radiograph shows anterior displacement of the left major fissure *(arrows)* and overinflation of the left lower lobe.

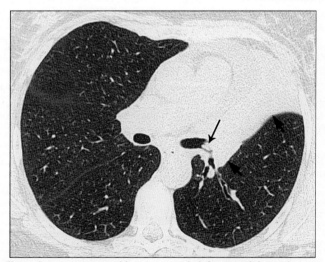

Figure 3. In a 61-year-old woman with left upper lobe atelectasis caused by an endobronchial tumor, CT shows complete atelectasis of the left upper lobe with anterior displacement of the left major fissure *(short arrows)* caused by tumor in left main bronchus *(long arrow)*.

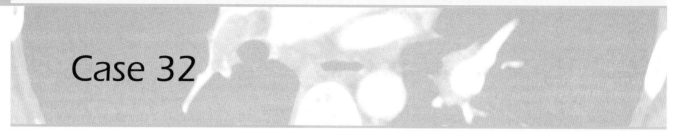

Case 32

DEMOGRAPHICS/CLINICAL HISTORY

An 86-year-old woman, chronic cough.

FINDINGS

Posteroanterior chest radiograph (Fig. 1) shows poorly defined area of increased opacity, associated with obscuration of the right heart border ("silhouette" sign). Lateral view (Fig. 2) shows downward shift of the minor fissure and forward shift of the right major fissure, resulting in a thin wedge-shaped area of increased opacity characteristic of right middle lobe atelectasis.

DISCUSSION

Definition/Background

Lobar atelectasis is reduced inflation of a lobe. The term *collapse* is often used interchangeably with *atelectasis,* but should be reserved for severe atelectasis.

Characteristic Clinical Features

Patients with lobar atelectasis may be asymptomatic or present with nonspecific symptoms of cough and shortness of breath. The symptoms may be acute (e.g., aspiration of foreign body) or chronic (endobronchial tumor). Endobronchial tumors may result in hemoptysis.

Characteristic Radiologic Findings

The diagnosis of right middle lobe atelectasis is one of the most difficult to make on the frontal radiograph and one of the easiest on the lateral radiograph. With progressive loss of volume, the minor fissure and the lower half of the major fissure approximate forming a triangular "pancake." In PA projection there may be no discernible increase in opacity, the only evidence of disease being obliteration of part of the right cardiac border as a result of contiguity of the right atrium with the medial segment of the atelectatic lobe (the silhouette sign) (Fig. 1). On the lateral radiograph, the minor fissure can be seen to move downward and the major fissure to move anteriorly, resulting in a triangular or wedge-shaped opacity, the thinnest portion of which is in the hilar region (Fig. 2). The diagnosis can be readily made on CT (Figs. 3 and 4).

Less Common Radiologic Manifestations

Hilar and mediastinal lymphadenopathy may be seen and should raise the possibility of malignancy.

Differential Diagnosis

- Right middle lobe consolidation

Discussion

The main distinguishing feature between lobar atelectasis and consolidation is the presence of volume loss. Right middle lobe atelectasis is commonly seen in patients with bronchiectasis and in obstruction of a lobar bronchus by tumor, mucus, blood, or foreign body. Obstructive pneumonitis (e.g., distal to pulmonary carcinoma) frequently leads to consolidation severe enough to limit loss of volume. The characteristic radiographic picture of obstructive atelectasis and pneumonitis (i.e., homogeneous opacification of a segment, lobe, or lung without air bronchograms) is highly suggestive of an obstructing endobronchial lesion. Lobar consolidation is most commonly caused by pneumonia and is typically associated with air bronchograms.

Diagnosis

Atelectasis of the right middle lobe

Suggested Readings

Molina PL, Hiken JN, Glazer HS: Imaging evaluation of obstructive atelectasis. J Thorac Imaging 11:176-186, 1996.
Woodring JH, Reed JC: Radiographic manifestations of lobar atelectasis. J Thorac Imaging 11:109-144, 1996.

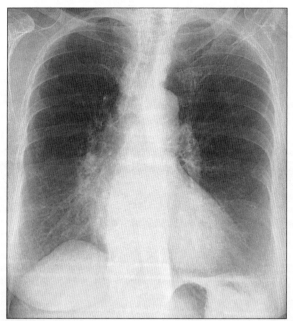

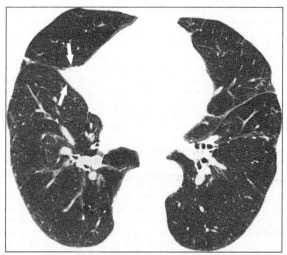

Figure 3. High-resolution CT image shows characteristic triangular opacity *(arrows)* abutting the right heart border, caused by posterior displacement of the minor fissure and anterior displacement of the major fissure. The patient was an 86-year-old woman with right middle lobe atelectasis.

Figure 1. Posteroanterior chest radiograph shows poorly defined area of increased opacity, associated with obscuration of the right heart border ("silhouette" sign). The patient was an 86-year-old woman with right middle lobe atelectasis.

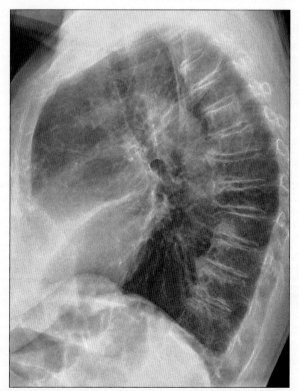

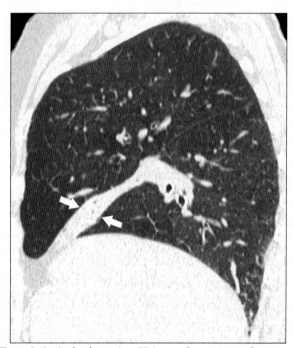

Figure 4. Sagittal reformation CT image demonstrates downward displacement of the minor fissure and forward shift of the right major fissure, resulting in a thin wedge-shaped area of increased attenuation *(arrows)*. The patient was an 86-year-old woman with right middle lobe atelectasis.

Figure 2. Lateral view demonstrates downward shift of the minor fissure and forward shift of the right major fissure, resulting in a thin wedge-shaped area of increased opacity. The patient was an 86-year-old woman with right middle lobe atelectasis.

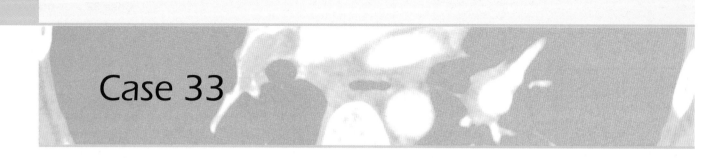

Case 33

DEMOGRAPHICS/CLINICAL HISTORY

A 73-year-old man, incidental finding on CT.

FINDINGS

CT images at the level of the left upper lobe bronchus (Fig. 1) and lingular bronchus (Fig. 2) show oval right upper lobe mass abutting the pleura and pulmonary vessels curving toward the opacity and pleura (comet tail sign). Also noted are marked volume loss of the upper lobe with forward displacement of the right major fissure and left upper lobe scarring. CT image photographed at soft tissue windows (Fig. 3) demonstrates that the oval opacity abuts a focal area of pleural thickening. Also noted are left pleural and right paravertebral pleural plaques. Coronal reformation CT image (Fig. 4) better demonstrates the curving of the vessels and other structures toward the focal area of pleural thickening and the associated volume loss.

DISCUSSION

Definition/Background

Rounded atelectasis is reduced inflation of a lung resulting in a rounded opacity abutting a pleural surface, associated with pleural thickening, and with distorted vessels that have a curvilinear disposition as they converge on the mass.

Characteristic Clinical Features

Rounded atelectasis is usually asymptomatic.

Characteristic Radiologic Findings

Round atelectasis manifests as a fairly homogeneous, round, oval, wedge-shaped, or irregularly shaped mass in the peripheral lung adjacent to thickened pleura and associated with volume loss of the affected lung. Pulmonary vessels and bronchi can be seen to curve and converge toward the mass and the area of pleural thickening ("comet tail" sign) (Figs. 1, 2, 3, and 4).

Less Common Radiologic Manifestations

Pleural effusion

Differential Diagnosis

- Pulmonary carcinoma
- Granuloma
- Pneumonia

Discussion

The main differential diagnosis is pulmonary carcinoma. The distinction can usually be made using CT, which shows the characteristic features of round atelectasis: bronchi and vessels curving into the periphery and converging toward a mass and area of pleural thickening ("comet tail" sign) that abuts an area of pleural thickening and that is associated with evidence of volume loss in the affected lobe. The hilar (central) aspect of the mass usually has indistinct margins as a result of blurring by the entering vessels. FDG-PET imaging typically shows no uptake. Occasionally, needle biopsy may be required to rule out carcinoma.

Diagnosis

Rounded atelectasis

Suggested Readings

Batra P, Brown K, Hayashi K, Mori M: Rounded atelectasis. J Thorac Imaging 11:187-197, 1996.

Ludeman N, Elicker BM, Reddy GP, et al: Atypical rounded atelectasis: Diagnosis and management based on results of F-18 FDG positron emission tomography. Clin Nucl Med 30:734-735, 2005.

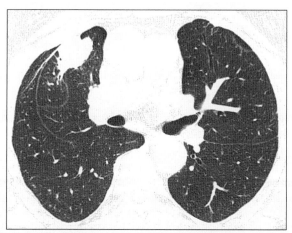

Figure 1. CT image at the level of the left upper lobe bronchus shows right upper lobe oval opacity abutting the pleura and pulmonary vessels curving toward the opacity and pleura (comet tail sign). Also noted is marked volume loss of the upper lobe with forward displacement of the right major fissure and left upper lobe scarring. The patient was a 73-year-old man with previous asbestos exposure, bilateral pleural plaques, and rounded atelectasis in the right upper lobe.

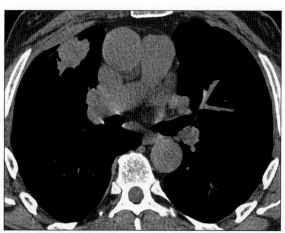

Figure 3. CT image photographed at soft tissue windows demonstrates oval soft tissue mass abutting focal area of pleural thickening. Also noted are left pleural and right paravertebral pleural plaques. The patient was a 73-year-old man with previous asbestos exposure, bilateral pleural plaques, and rounded atelectasis in the right upper lobe.

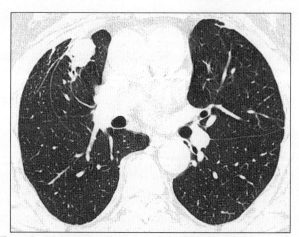

Figure 2. CT image at the level of the lingular bronchus shows right upper lobe oval opacity abutting the pleura and pulmonary vessels curving toward the opacity and pleura (comet tail sign). Also noted is marked volume loss of the upper lobe with forward displacement of the right major fissure and left upper lobe scarring. The patient was a 73-year-old man with previous asbestos exposure, bilateral pleural plaques, and rounded atelectasis in the right upper lobe.

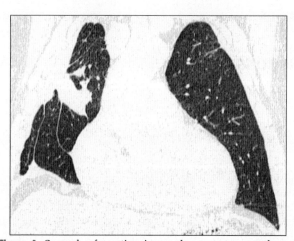

Figure 4. Coronal reformation image demonstrates vessels and other structures curving toward the focal area of pleural thickening and associated volume loss. The patient was a 73-year-old man with previous asbestos exposure, bilateral pleural plaques, and rounded atelectasis in the right upper lobe.

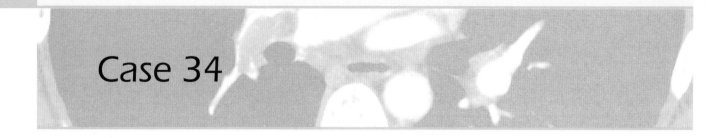

Case 34

DEMOGRAPHICS/CLINICAL HISTORY

A 37-year-old woman with chronic cough, undergoing radiography.

FINDINGS

Posteroanterior chest radiograph shows downward displacement of the major fissure and medial displacement of the right hilum consistent with right lower lobe atelectasis (Fig. 1). Calcified granulomas incidentally identified in the right apex are consistent with previous tuberculosis.

DISCUSSION

Definition/Background

Lobar atelectasis is defined as reduced inflation of a lobe. The term collapse is often used interchangeably with atelectasis but should be reserved for severe atelectasis.

Characteristic Clinical Features

Patients with lobar atelectasis may be asymptomatic or present with nonspecific symptoms of cough and shortness of breath. The symptoms may be acute (e.g., aspiration of foreign body) or chronic (e.g., endobronchial tumor), and endobronchial tumors may result in hemoptysis.

Characteristic Radiologic Findings

Right lower lobe atelectasis results in downward displacement of the major fissure, which usually becomes evident on a posteroanterior (PA) projection as a well-defined interface extending obliquely downward and laterally from the region of the hilum. As atelectasis progresses, the lobe moves posteromedially to occupy a position in the posterior costophrenic gutter and medial costovertebral angle. On the PA view, the hilum and main bronchus are displaced inferiorly and medially; the interlobar artery is displaced medially and often is not visible because it is obscured by the surrounding airless lung. The atelectatic lobe also obscures the hemidiaphragm.

Less Common Radiologic Manifestations

Hilar and mediastinal lymphadenopathy may be seen and should raise the possibility of malignancy.

Differential Diagnosis

- Right lower lobe consolidation

Discussion

Lobar atelectasis can be differentiated from consolidation by the presence of volume loss. Right lower lobe atelectasis is commonly seen in patients with bronchiectasis and in those with obstruction of a lobar bronchus by tumor, mucus, blood, or foreign body. Obstructive pneumonitis (e.g., distal to pulmonary carcinoma) frequently leads to consolidation severe enough to limit loss of volume. The characteristic radiographic picture of obstructive atelectasis and pneumonitis (i.e., homogeneous opacification of a segment, lobe, or lung without air bronchograms) suggests an obstructing endobronchial lesion. Lobar consolidation most commonly results from pneumonia and is typically associated with air bronchograms.

Diagnosis

Atelectasis of the right lower lobe

Suggested Readings

Molina PL, Hiken JN, Glazer HS: Imaging evaluation of obstructive atelectasis. J Thorac Imaging 11:176-186, 1996.
Woodring JH, Reed JC: Radiographic manifestations of lobar atelectasis. J Thorac Imaging 11:109-144, 1996.

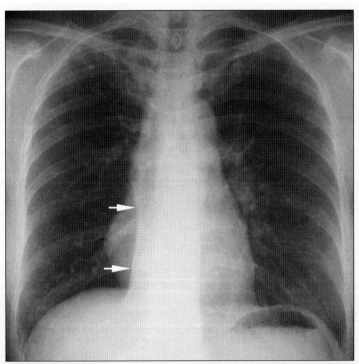

Figure 1. Posteroanterior chest radiograph shows downward displacement of the major fissure *(arrows)* and medial displacement of the right hilum, which are findings consistent with right lower lobe atelectasis. Calcified granulomas incidentally identified in the right apex are consistent with previous tuberculosis.

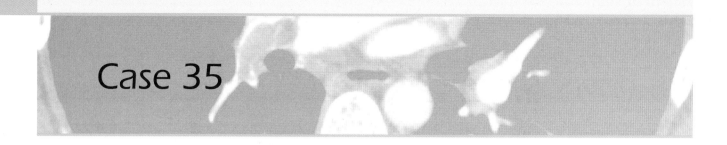

Case 35

DEMOGRAPHICS/CLINICAL HISTORY

A 79-year-old man with acute shortness of breath, undergoing radiography.

FINDINGS

Chest radiograph shows opacification and decreased volume of the right hemithorax. The trachea and mediastinum are shifted to the right. The lack of air bronchograms within the opacified atelectatic right lung is consistent with obstructive atelectasis (Fig. 1). Bronchoscopy showed complete obstruction by mucus. Chest radiograph 2 days later after bronchoscopy and physiotherapy shows complete re-expansion of the right lung (Fig. 2). In another patient, the chest radiograph shows complete opacification of the right hemithorax with only mild volume loss and abrupt termination of the right main bronchus due to bronchogenic carcinoma (Fig. 3).

DISCUSSION

Definition/Background

Opacification of a hemithorax refers to a homogenous increase in the opacity of an entire hemithorax, usually in association with a relatively normal contralateral hemithorax.

Characteristic Clinical Features

Patients usually present with progressive dyspnea and cough. Patients with endobronchial tumors may present with hemoptysis, and those with bronchial, pulmonary, or pleural malignancy present with anorexia, malaise, and weight loss. Patients with acute bronchial obstruction by mucus or foreign body present with acute shortness of breath and cough.

Characteristic Radiologic Findings

On the chest radiograph, the opacified hemithorax may have decreased, normal, or increased volume. The change in volume is easily determined by assessing the position of the trachea and mediastinum. Air bronchograms are typically present in patients with extensive consolidation or compressive atelectasis and absent in patients with obstructive atelectasis due to endobronchial tumor, mucus, or foreign body and in massive pleural effusion.

Less Common Radiologic Manifestations

Opacified hemithorax due to massive pleural effusion may result in inversion of the hemidiaphragm. The endobronchial tumor may be visible on the radiograph.

Differential Diagnosis

- Whole-lung consolidation
- Large pleural effusion
- Pneumonectomy
- Massive diaphragmatic hernia
- Pulmonary aplasia or agenesis

Discussion

In many patients, opacification has a combination of causes, most commonly atelectasis, consolidation, and pleural effusion. An important consideration is assessment of the position of the trachea and mediastinum, which show an ipsilateral shift in patients with atelectasis and contralateral shift in patients with massive pleural effusion. Pleural malignancy may be associated with ipsilateral or contralateral shift of the mediastinum. Whole-lung atelectasis results from obstruction of the main bronchus, most commonly by an endotracheal tube, mucus, tumor, blood clot, or foreign body.

Pleural effusions in opacified hemithorax may be a minor or major component of the opacification. The effusion may represent a hydrothorax, chylothorax, hemothorax, or empyema. It may be benign or malignant, and it may be associated or not with benign or malignant pleural disease (e.g., tuberculous empyema, fibrothorax, mesothelioma, metastatic carcinoma). Massive pleural effusions usually are caused by malignancy or bacterial or mycobacterial infection.

Congenital or post-traumatic diaphragmatic hernias are most common on the left side and may result in partial or complete opacification of the hemithorax with contralateral shift of the mediastinum. The cause of the opacified hemithorax can usually be readily identified on contrast-enhanced CT.

Diagnosis

Atelectasis of the whole lung (opacified hemithorax)

Suggested Readings

Molina PL, Hiken JN, Glazer HS: Imaging evaluation of obstructive atelectasis. J Thorac Imaging 11:176-186, 1966.
Porcel JM, Vives M: Etiology and pleural fluid characteristics of large and massive effusions. Chest 124:978-983, 2003.

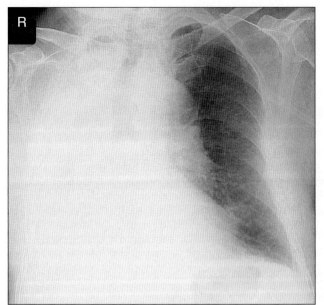

Figure 1. In a 79-year-old man with acute shortness of breath, the chest radiograph shows opacification and decreased volume of the right hemithorax. The trachea and mediastinum are shifted to the right. The lack of air bronchograms within the opacified atelectatic right lung is consistent with obstructive atelectasis. Bronchoscopy showed complete obstruction by mucus.

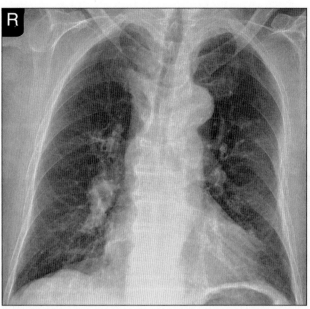

Figure 2. In the same patient after bronchoscopy and physiotherapy, the chest radiograph 2 days later shows complete re-expansion of the right lung.

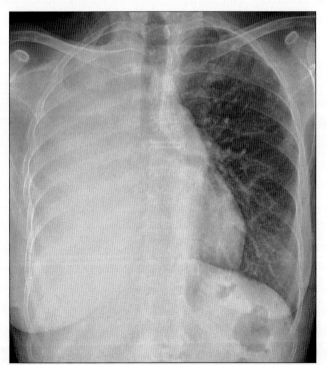

Figure 3. In a 73-year-old woman with shortness of breath, the chest radiograph shows complete opacification of the right hemithorax with only mild volume loss, as denoted by a slight ipsilateral shift of the trachea. Notice the abrupt termination of the right main bronchus. The patient had a combination of large right pleural effusion, obstructive pneumonitis, and atelectasis of the right lung due to bronchogenic carcinoma.

Case 36

DEMOGRAPHICS/CLINICAL HISTORY

A 75-year-old woman, undergoing computed tomography (CT).

FINDINGS

CT shows a cardiac bronchus originating from the medial wall of the bronchus intermedius (Fig. 1).

DISCUSSION

Definition/Background

Accessory cardiac bronchus is a supernumerary bronchus that arises from the medial wall of the right main or intermediate bronchus opposite to the origin of the right upper lobe bronchus and that courses medially and caudally for 1 to 5 cm. It is lined by bronchial mucosa and has cartilage within its wall, which distinguishes it from a diverticulum; the anomaly occurs in approximately 0.1% of the general population.

Characteristic Clinical Features

Most patients are asymptomatic, and the abnormal bronchus is found incidentally on CT. The most common complications are cough and hemoptysis due to infection or carcinoma.

Characteristic Radiologic Findings

CT demonstrates the anomalous bronchus originating in the medial wall of the main bronchus or bronchus intermedius cephalad to the origin of the middle lobe bronchus and ending blindly 1 to 2 cm distally (Fig. 2). The course of the cardiac bronchus is best depicted using reformation techniques, such as multiplanar reconstruction, volume rendering, or virtual bronchoscopy (Figs. 2 and 3).

Less Common Radiologic Manifestations

The accessory cardiac bronchus usually ends blindly but occasionally may be associated with small amounts of abnormal pulmonary parenchyma.

Differential Diagnosis

The CT features are diagnostic.

Diagnosis

Accessory cardiac bronchus

Suggested Readings

Ghaye B, Kos X, Dondelinger RF: Accessory cardiac bronchus: 3D CT demonstration in nine cases. Eur Radiol 9:45-48, 1999.

McGuinness G, Naidich DP, Garay SM, et al: Accessory cardiac bronchus: Computed tomographic features and clinical significance. Radiology 189:563-566, 1993.

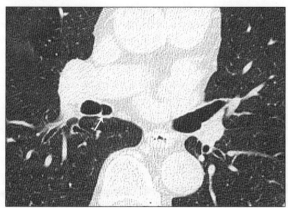

Figure 1. CT image shows a cardiac bronchus *(arrow)* originating from the medial wall of the bronchus intermedius.

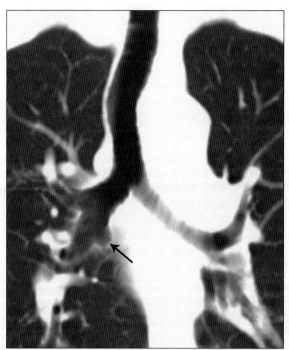

Figure 2. Coronal reformation image shows the medial and inferior course of the cardiac bronchus *(arrow)*.

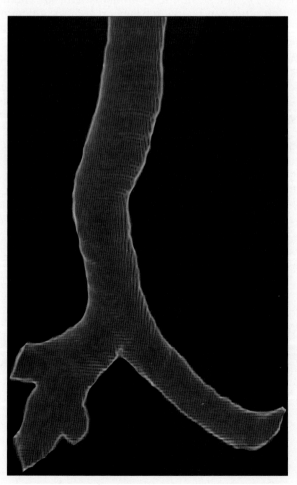

Figure 3. Anterior view of a three-dimensional, external, volume-rendering image of the central airways shows the medial and inferior course of the cardiac bronchus. It ends blindly, resembling a diverticulum.

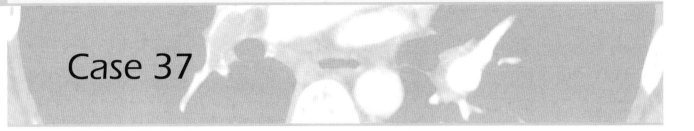

Case 37

DEMOGRAPHICS/CLINICAL HISTORY

A 45-year-old man, asymptomatic, undergoing computed tomography (CT).

FINDINGS

High-resolution CT images (Figs. 1 and 2) show decreased attenuation and vascularity in the anterior portion of the left upper lobe. Notice the dilated airway with mucus corresponding to the superior lingular bronchus (Fig. 2).

DISCUSSION

Definition/Background

The patient has a rare congenital anomaly characterized by short-segment obliteration of the lobar, segmental, or subsegmental bronchus at its origin. Bronchial atresia can affect any bronchus, but it most commonly involves apicoposterior segmental bronchus of the left upper lobe.

Characteristic Clinical Features

Most patients are asymptomatic. Some present with recurrent pneumonia.

Characteristic Radiologic Findings

The chest radiograph typically shows an area of pulmonary hyperlucency (90% of cases) and hilar nodule or mass (80%). CT shows decreased vascularity and attenuation and an increased volume of the affected segment; bronchial occlusion; and mucoid impaction with bronchial dilatation (i.e., bronchocele) immediately distal to atretic bronchus.

Less Common Radiologic Manifestations

Radiology may show bronchiectasis or findings suggesting emphysema within the atretic segment.

Differential Diagnosis

- Endobronchial tumor
- Endobronchial foreign body
- Congenital lobar emphysema

Discussion

The main differential diagnosis is partial airway obstruction due to endobronchial tumor or foreign body. Similar to those conditions, the lung distal to bronchial atresia is hyperlucent and shows air trapping. However, endobronchial lesions are not associated with overinflation of affected bronchopulmonary segments at total lung capacity, a typical finding in bronchial atresia. The distinction often can be made based on a chest radiograph performed at maximal inspiration. The confident diagnosis of mucoid impaction distal to bronchial atresia usually can be based on CT. However, bronchoscopy may be required to rule out other causes of obstruction such as foreign body or endobronchial tumor. Congenital lobar emphysema involves a whole lobe rather than a segment and is associated with a patent bronchus.

Diagnosis

Bronchial atresia

Suggested Readings

Berrocal T, Madrid C, Novo S, et al: Congenital anomalies of the tracheobronchial tree, lung, and mediastinum: Embryology, radiology, and pathology. Radiographics 24:e17, 2004.

Ghaye B, Szapiro D, Fanchamps JM, Dondelinger RF: Congenital bronchial abnormalities revisited. Radiographics 21:105-119, 2001.

Kinsella D, Sissons G, Williams MP: The radiological imaging of bronchial atresia. Br J Radiol 65:681-685, 1992.

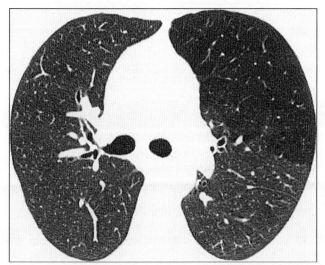

Figure 1. High-resolution CT image shows a decrease in attenuation and vascularity in the anterior portion of the left upper lobe in a 45-year-old man with bronchial atresia.

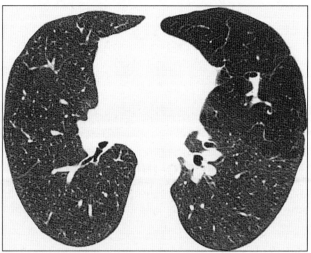

Figure 2. High-resolution CT image shows a dilated airway with mucus corresponding to the superior lingular bronchus in a 45-year-old man with bronchial atresia.

Case 38

DEMOGRAPHICS/CLINICAL HISTORY

A 55-year-old woman with an incidental finding on the chest radiograph, undergoing computed tomography (CT).

FINDINGS

Contrast-enhanced CT image shows a smoothly margined, homogeneous water-density mass in the right paratracheal region (Fig. 1).

DISCUSSION

Definition/Background

Bronchogenic cyst is a congenital cyst lined by respiratory epithelium that contains cartilage in its wall. It contains mucoid or serous fluid unless it communicates with an airway, in which case it contains air.

Characteristic Clinical Features

Most patients are asymptomatic. Mediastinal bronchogenic cysts may result in cough, wheezing, stridor, or pneumonia due to compression of trachea or bronchi; dysphagia due to compression of esophagus; or occasionally, localized pulmonary edema due to compression of adjacent pulmonary vein. Approximately 20% of patients with intraparenchymal cysts present with pneumonia.

Characteristic Radiologic Findings

Radiographically, mediastinal bronchogenic cysts usually manifest as round or oval masses in the right paratracheal or subcarinal region (Fig. 2) and pulmonary bronchogenic cysts as sharply circumscribed, solitary, round or oval masses usually occurring in the medial third of a lower lobe. Approximately 50% have homogeneous attenuation at or near water density (-10 to $+10$ HU) on CT, and 50% have soft tissue attenuation from the presence of protein (Fig. 3), hemorrhage, or less commonly, calcium oxalate within the mucoid cyst contents. The cysts do not enhance with intravenous contrast, and virtually all have homogeneous high signal intensity on T2-weighted MRI (Fig. 4).

Less Common Radiologic Manifestations

The cyst may contain air because of a communication with an airway, which usually results from cyst infection.

Differential Diagnosis

- Lung cancer
- Abscess
- Congenital cystic adenomatoid malformation
- Lymphangioma
- Echinococcosis (hydatid disease)

Discussion

Bronchogenic cysts usually can be distinguished from lung cancer by the characteristic water density on CT, homogeneous high signal intensity on T2-weighted MRI (Fig. 4), and lack of enhancement after intravenous administration of contrast for CT (Fig. 1) and MRI. In most cases, these findings together with the presence of a thin, smooth wall allow distinction of bronchogenic cysts from lung abscess. However, infected or hemorrhagic cysts may have heterogeneous attenuation values on CT and heterogeneous signal intensity on MRI and therefore may resemble lung abscesses. Pulmonary bronchogenic cysts can usually be distinguished from congenital cystic adenomatoid malformation because they consist of a single cystic mass, whereas the latter usually consist of multiple cystic lesions.

Diagnosis

Bronchogenic cyst

Suggested Readings

Berrocal T, Madrid C, Novo S, et al: Congenital anomalies of the tracheobronchial tree, lung, and mediastinum: Embryology, radiology, and pathology. Radiographics 24:e17, 2004.

Yoon YC, Lee KS, Kim TS, et al: Intrapulmonary bronchogenic cyst: CT and pathologic findings in five adult patients. AJR Am J Roentgenol 179:167-170, 2002.

Nakata H, Egashira K, Watanabe H, et al: MRI of bronchogenic cysts. J Comput Assist Tomogr 17:267-270, 1993.

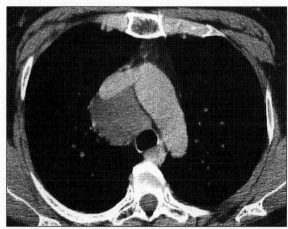

Figure 1. Contrast-enhanced CT image shows a smoothly margin-ated, homogeneous water density mass in the right paratracheal region in a 55-year-old woman with a bronchogenic cyst.

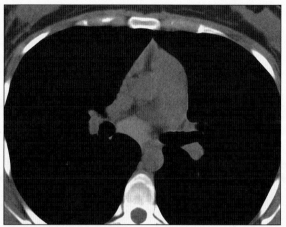

Figure 3. Non-enhanced CT image shows a mass in the subcarinal region with increased attenuation in a 32-year-old woman with a bronchogenic cyst.

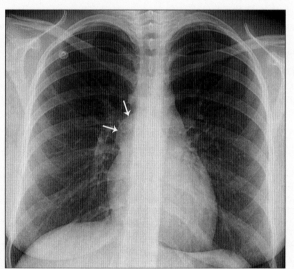

Figure 2. Posteroanterior chest radiograph shows increased focal opacity in the subcarinal region *(arrows)* displacing the bronchus intermedius in a 32-year-old woman with a bronchogenic cyst presenting with cough.

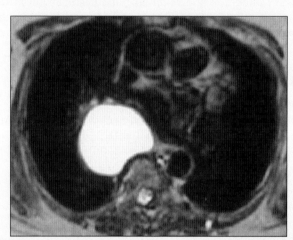

Figure 4. T2-weighted MRI shows a subcarinal mass with homogeneous high signal intensity, similar to that of cerebrospi-nal fluid, in a 70-year-old woman with a bronchogenic cyst.

Case 39

DEMOGRAPHICS/CLINICAL HISTORY

A 36-year-old woman with an incidental finding on a chest radiograph, undergoing computed tomography (CT).

FINDINGS

Chest radiograph shows an air-filled cystic lesion in the left lower lung zone (Fig. 1). CT demonstrates a left lower lobe cystic lesion (Fig. 2).

DISCUSSION

Definition/Background

Congenital cystic adenomatoid malformation (CCAM), also known as congenital pulmonary airway malformation (CPAM), is an uncommon abnormality characterized by a multicystic mass of pulmonary tissue with an abnormal proliferation of bronchial structures. Most cases are diagnosed in the first 5 years of life, but the abnormality may be first recognized in adults.

Characteristic Clinical Features

CCAM in adults may be asymptomatic or result in symptoms related to recurrent respiratory infections. Less common complications include pneumothorax and, occasionally, development of bronchioloalveolar carcinoma, adenocarcinoma, or squamous cell carcinoma.

Characteristic Radiologic Findings

In older children and adults, CCAMs usually appear radiologically as a unilocular or multiloculated cyst or complex soft tissue and cystic mass. The CT manifestations in adults typically consist of a unilocular or multiloculated cyst or complex soft tissue and cystic mass ranging from 4 to 12 cm in diameter and most commonly located in the lower lobe.

Less Common Radiologic Manifestations

CT may show consolidation in the surrounding parenchyma and air-fluid levels due to superimposed infection (Fig. 3).

Differential Diagnosis

- Bronchogenic cyst
- Lung abscess
- Echinococcosis (hydatid disease)

Discussion

Cystic adenomatoid malformation must be differentiated from lung abscess and bronchogenic cyst. Many thin-walled, complex cystic masses usually allow the distinction from bronchogenic cysts, which typically are isolated. The findings, however, may mimic those of lung abscess radiologically. The distinction often can be made by the lack of clinical symptoms of fever and productive cough and the lack of change over several weeks, but infected congenital pulmonary airway malformations may be indistinguishable from lung abscess.

Diagnosis

Congenital cystic adenomatoid malformation (congenital pulmonary airway malformation)

Suggested Readings

Berrocal T, Madrid C, Novo S, et al: Congenital anomalies of the tracheobronchial tree, lung, and mediastinum: Embryology, radiology, and pathology. Radiographics 24:e17, 2004.

Oh BJ, Lee JS, Kim JS, et al: Congenital cystic adenomatoid malformation of the lung in adults: Clinical and CT evaluation of seven patients. Respirology 11:496-501, 2006.

Patz EF Jr, Müller NL, Swensen SJ, Dodd LG: Congenital cystic adenomatoid malformation in adults: CT findings. J Comput Assist Tomogr 19:361-364, 1995.

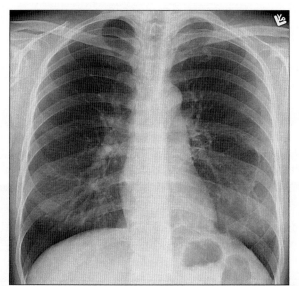

Figure 1. Posteroanterior chest radiograph shows a thin-walled cyst in left lower lung zone. The patient was a 36-year-old woman with congenital cystic adenomatoid malformation.

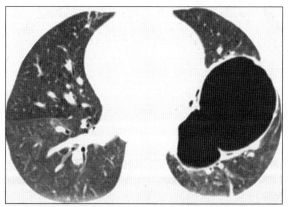

Figure 2. CT image shows a left lower lobe cystic lesion in a 36-year-old woman with a congenital cystic adenomatoid malformation.

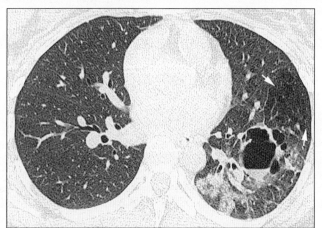

Figure 3. CT image shows a large, cystic mass with a fluid level and adjacent smaller cysts in the left lower lobe in a 33-year-old woman with an infected congenital cystic adenomatoid malformation. Notice the focal ground-glass opacities and consolidation due to pneumonia and focal emphysematous changes *(arrows)*.

Case 40

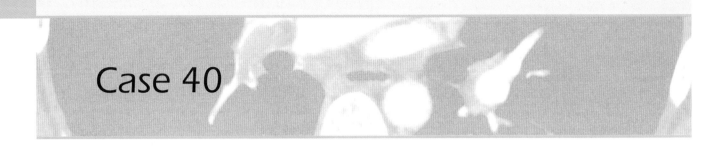

DEMOGRAPHICS/CLINICAL HISTORY

An 88-year-old woman with recurrent pneumonia, undergoing chest radiography and computed tomography (CT).

FINDINGS

Posteroanterior (Fig. 1) and lateral (Fig. 2) chest radiographs show consolidation in the posterior basal region of the left lower lobe, contiguous with the hemidiaphragm. Coronal CT image (Fig. 3) shows an artery originating from the descending thoracic aorta and extending into the consolidation.

DISCUSSION

Definition/Background

Pulmonary sequestration is a malformation in which a portion of lung is detached from the remaining normal lung and receives its blood supply through a systemic artery; the anomaly may be intralobar or extralobar. In intralobar sequestration, the detached portion of lung is contiguous with normal lung parenchyma and within the same visceral pleural envelope. Extralobar sequestration is separate from normal lung and is enclosed within its own pleural membrane.

Characteristic Clinical Features

Pulmonary sequestrations in adults are usually asymptomatic, with the abnormality being found incidentally on a chest radiograph or CT scan. The most common clinical manifestations are related to superimposed infection, when the signs and symptoms are those of acute lower lobe pneumonia.

Characteristic Radiologic Findings

The radiographic presentation of intralobar sequestration is as a homogeneous opacity or as a focal area of lucency in the posterior basal segment of a lower lobe and almost invariably is contiguous with the hemidiaphragm (Figs. 1 and 2). The most common CT findings of intralobar pulmonary sequestration consist of focal areas of consolidation (Fig. 3) or focal areas of lucency with or without irregular cystic spaces and emphysematous changes (Fig. 4) in the posterior basal segment of a lower lobe. The diagnostic feature on CT (Fig. 3) or magnetic resonance imaging (MRI) is the presence of an anomalous systemic vessel, typically coursing from the lower thoracic or upper abdominal aorta into the sequestered lung.

Less Common Radiologic Manifestations

Air-fluid levels result from superimposed infection.

Differential Diagnosis

- Bronchogenic cyst
- Congenital cystic adenomatoid malformation
- Lung abscess
- Pneumonia
- Extralobar pulmonary sequestration

Discussion

The essential feature in the differential diagnosis from other causes of focal lucency or consolidation in the region of the basal segments of a lower lobe is the demonstration of the systemic arterial supply to the abnormal lung. Extralobar sequestration usually manifests as a homogeneous opacity or well-circumscribed mass on CT; cystic areas are seen occasionally. Extralobar sequestrations are frequently associated with diaphragmatic anomalies and therefore most commonly diagnosed in the neonatal period. Venous drainage occurs through systemic veins in extralobar sequestration and through pulmonary veins in intralobar sequestration.

Diagnosis

Intralobar pulmonary sequestration

Suggested Readings

Bolca N, Topal U, Bayram S: Bronchopulmonary sequestration: Radiologic findings. Eur J Radiol 52:185-191, 2004.

Frazier AA, Rosado de Christenson ML, Stocker JT: Templeton PA: Intralobar sequestration: Radiologic-pathologic correlation. Radiographics 17:725-745, 1997.

Rosado-de-Christenson ML, Frazier AA, Stocker JT, Templeton PA: From the archives of the AFIP. Extralobar sequestration: Radiologic-pathologic correlation. Radiographics 13:425-441, 1993.

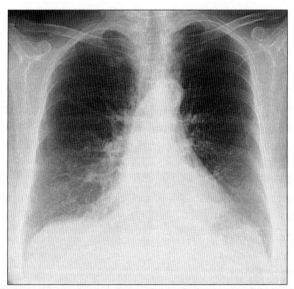

Figure 1. Posteroanterior chest radiograph shows consolidation in the retrocardiac regions of the left lower lobe contiguous with the hemidiaphragm in an 88-year-old woman with intralobar pulmonary sequestration.

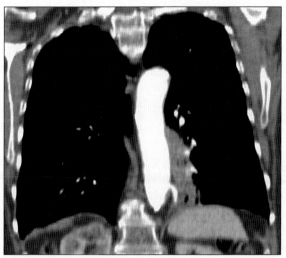

Figure 3. Coronal reformation CT image shows an artery originating from the descending thoracic aorta and extending into the consolidation in an 88-year-old woman with intralobar pulmonary sequestration.

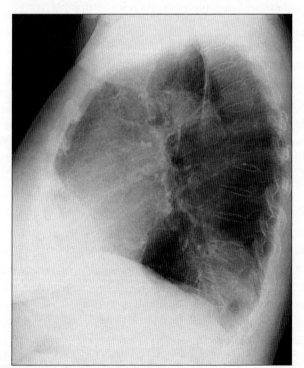

Figure 2. Lateral chest radiograph shows consolidation in the posterior basal region of the left lower lobe contiguous with the hemidiaphragm in an 88-year-old woman with intralobar pulmonary sequestration.

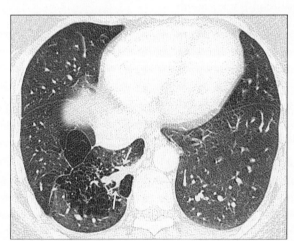

Figure 4. CT image shows a localized area of abnormal lung with emphysematous changes in the posteromedial region of the right lung base. The area is supplied by vessels (arrows) originating from the descending thoracic aorta in a 34-year-old man with asymptomatic intralobar pulmonary sequestration.

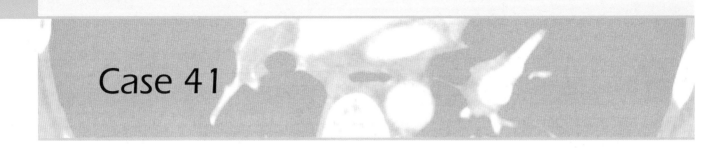

Case 41

DEMOGRAPHICS/CLINICAL HISTORY

A 24-year-old woman, exertional dyspnea, cyanosis.

FINDINGS

Posteroanterior chest radiograph (Fig. 1) and magnified view of the right lower lung zone (Fig. 2) show enlarged and tortuous vessels that extend to nodular opacities.

DISCUSSION

Definition/Background

Pulmonary arteriovenous malformations (PAVM) are congenital direct communications between the branches of pulmonary artery and pulmonary veins. They may be single or multiple. The majority of patients have Osler-Weber-Rendu syndrome (hereditary hemorrhagic telangiectasia), which is associated with autosomal-dominant transmission. PAVMs are classified into simple (supplied by a single afferent vascular pedicle) and complex (supplied by more than one vascular pedicle).

Characteristic Clinical Features

The patients may be asymptomatic or may present with symptoms related to right-to-left shunt with orthopnea resulting from the predominantly basal location of most PAVMs, hypoxia, cyanosis, or paradoxical septic or thrombotic emboli.

Characteristic Radiologic Findings

Large PAVMs can be detected and diagnosed on the chest radiograph by the presence of a nodule and identification of the feeding and draining vessels, resulting in a "comet-tail" appearance that is virtually diagnostic (Figs. 1 and 2). Small PAVMs are usually missed on the radiograph. CT is far more sensitive and specific than the chest radiograph in the detection of PAVMs, allowing identification of the malformation and its feeding and draining vessels even when less than a millimeter in size (Fig. 3). CT is currently considered the most diagnostically accurate and least invasive examination for detection of PAVMs. The majority of PAVMs can also be diagnosed on MR imaging. Although angiography is diagnostic, it is only required immediately prior to treatment by endovascular embolotherapy (Fig. 4).

Less Common Radiologic Manifestations

Ground-glass opacities may occasionally be present around the PAVM as the result of pulmonary hemorrhage.

Differential Diagnosis

- Lung nodule
- Aberrant intrapulmonary venous pathways
- Shunts between pulmonary arteries or veins and systemic arteries

Discussion

CT is currently considered the most diagnostically accurate examination for detection and diagnosis of PAVMs allowing identification of the malformation and its feeding and draining vessels. CT is ideally performed on a multidetector scanner with thin sections (1 mm or less) and viewed on a workstation. In the vast majority of cases a diagnosis can be readily made without intravenous contrast.

Diagnosis

Pulmonary arteriovenous malformations

Suggested Readings

Ohno Y, Hatabu H, Takenaka D, Adachi S, Hirota S, Sugimura K: Contrast-enhanced MR perfusion imaging and MR angiography/ utility for management of pulmonary arteriovenous malformations for embolotherapy. Eur J Radiol 41:36-46, 2002.

Remy J, Remy-Jardin M, Wattinne L, Deffontaines C: Pulmonary arteriovenous malformations: Evaluation with CT of the chest before and after treatment. Radiology 182:809-16, 1992.

Remy-Jardin M, Dumont P, Brillet PY, Dupuis P, Duhamel A, Remy J: Pulmonary arteriovenous malformations treated with embolotherapy: Helical CT evaluation of long-term effectiveness after 2-21-year follow-up. Radiology 239:576-85, 2006.

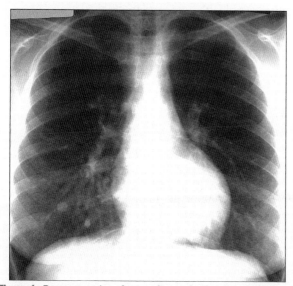

Figure 1. Posteroanterior chest radiograph shows enlarged and tortuous vessels that extend to nodular opacities. The patient was a 24-year-old woman with multiple pulmonary arteriovenous malformations in the right lower lobe.

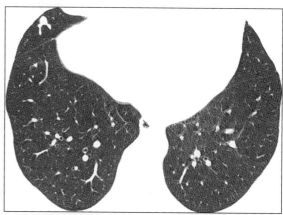

Figure 3. CT scan image demonstrates arteriovenous malformation and feeding artery and draining vein in the right middle lobe. The patient was a 57-year-old man with pulmonary arteriovenous malformation.

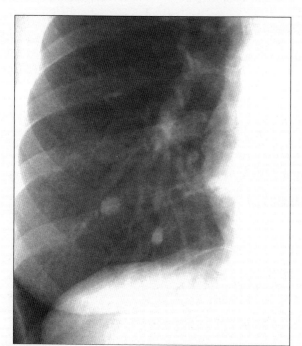

Figure 2. Magnified view of the right lower lung zone from a chest radiograph shows enlarged and tortuous vessels that extend to nodular opacities. The patient was a 24-year-old woman with multiple pulmonary arteriovenous malformations in the right lower lobe.

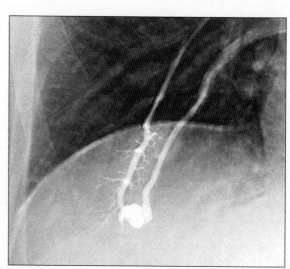

Figure 4. Selective pulmonary angiogram demonstrates arteriovenous malformation and feeding artery and draining vein in the right middle lobe. The patient was a 57-year-old man with pulmonary arteriovenous malformation.

Case 42

DEMOGRAPHICS/CLINICAL HISTORY

A 62-year-old woman with an incidental radiographic finding, undergoing radiography and computed tomography (CT)

FINDINGS

Posteroanterior chest radiograph shows a vertically oriented curvilinear vessel coursing toward the region of the right cardiophrenic angle (Fig. 1). Coronal, reformatted, contrast-enhanced CT shows a vertically oriented pulmonary vein draining into the inferior vena cava (Fig. 2).

DISCUSSION

Definition/Background

Partial anomalous pulmonary venous return from the right lung is a congenital abnormality characterized by venous drainage of the right lung to a systemic vein, most commonly the inferior vena cava, and, in other cases, drainage to a suprahepatic vein, the superior vena cava, or the right atrium. In its classic configuration, it takes the form of a Turkish sword (i.e., scimitar vein). It is often associated with malformations of the right lung, most commonly hypoplasia, in which case it is referred to as hypogenetic lung syndrome.

Characteristic Clinical Features

Partial anomalous pulmonary venous return may be asymptomatic or result in symptoms related to associated congenital pulmonary or cardiac malformations or in pulmonary arterial hypertension. In order of decreasing frequency, clinical symptoms include recurrent respiratory tract infections, dyspnea on effort, chronic cough, chest pain, wheezing, and recurrent hemoptysis.

Characteristic Radiologic Findings

The characteristic appearance on radiography is a vertically oriented curvilinear vein (i.e., scimitar vein) that is convex inferolaterally and increases in diameter from superior to inferior. In most cases, the right lung is hypoplastic, resulting in deviation of the mediastinum to the right and cardiac dextroposition. The diagnosis can be confirmed with CT or magnetic resonance imaging.

Less Common Radiologic Manifestations

Associated anomalies can include the absence of interlobar fissures, lobar agenesis, absent right pulmonary artery, systemic arterial supply to the right lung, and atrial septal defect. Occasionally, a portion of the right lung herniates into the left hemithorax behind the heart and comes into contact with the mediastinal aspect of the left lower lobe; this is known as a horseshoe lung.

Differential Diagnosis

- Hypoplastic right lung with normal venous drainage
- Scimitar vein draining into the left atrium

Discussion

The scimitar vein most commonly drains into the inferior vena cava. This course should be differentiated from a scimitar vein draining into the left atrium and from anomalous, simultaneous drainage into the left atrium and the inferior vena cava. The pseudoscimitar syndrome specifically corresponds to an abnormal pathway of a scimitar-like vein that terminates in the left atrium. This latter anomaly may be associated with azygous continuation of the inferior vena cava, systemic arterial supply to the right lung, and a hypogenetic right lung.

Diagnosis

Partial anomalous pulmonary venous return

Suggested Readings

Konen E, Raviv-Zilka L, Cohen RA, et al: Congenital pulmonary venolobar syndrome: Spectrum of helical CT findings with emphasis on computed reformatting. Radiographics 23:1175-1184, 2003.

Kramer U, Dörnberger V, Fenchel M, et al: Scimitar syndrome: Morphological diagnosis and assessment of hemodynamic significance by magnetic resonance imaging. Eur Radiol 13:L147-L150, 2003.

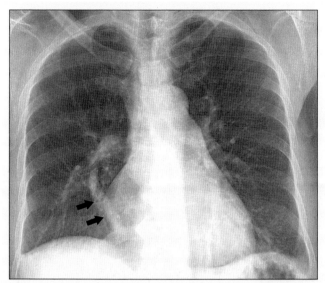

Figure 1. Posteroanterior chest radiograph shows a vertically oriented curvilinear vessel *(arrows)* coursing toward the region of the right cardiophrenic angle. This vessel is commonly known as the scimitar vein. The patient was a 62-year-old woman.

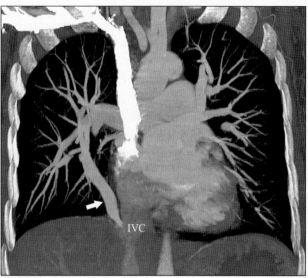

Figure 2. In the same patient, coronal, reformatted, contrast-enhanced CT shows a vertically oriented pulmonary vein *(arrow)* draining into the inferior vena cava (IVC).

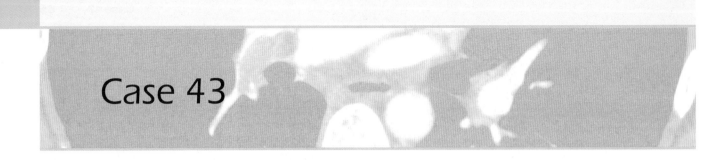

Case 43

DEMOGRAPHICS/CLINICAL HISTORY

A 66-year-old, female smoker, undergoing computed tomography (CT).

FINDINGS

View of the right upper lung from a chest radiograph (Fig. 1) shows a poorly defined, 2.2-cm nodule in the right upper lobe. High-resolution CT image (Fig. 2) shows a nodule with soft tissue and ground-glass components. The nodule has spiculated margins and pleural tags. Surgical resection identified pulmonary adenocarcinoma. In another patient, CT image (Fig. 3) shows a smoothly marginated nodule in the right lower lobe, and CT using soft tissue windows (Fig. 4) shows diffuse calcification of the right lower lobe nodule consistent with calcified tuberculous granuloma.

DISCUSSION

Definition/Background

Pulmonary nodule is defined as pulmonary lesion that is a well-defined, discrete, approximately circular opacity that is 3 cm in diameter or smaller. Lesions larger than 3 cm in diameter are referred to as masses. Most solitary nodules in adults are granulomas (e.g., tuberculoma, histoplasmoma, coccidioidomycosis) or neoplasms (e.g., carcinoma, carcinoid tumor, hamartoma, solitary metastasis).

Characteristic Clinical Features

Patients with solitary lung nodules usually have no associated symptoms, and the nodule is found incidentally on chest radiography or CT. Patients with pulmonary carcinoma usually have a history of cigarette smoking.

Characteristic Radiologic Findings

Features that favor carcinoma include a diameter greater than 2 cm, spiculated margins, and absence of calcification on CT.

Less Common Radiologic Manifestations

Imaging may show hilar and mediastinal lymphadenopathy and extrathoracic metastases to the liver, adrenals, or brain.

Differential Diagnosis

- Granuloma
- Carcinoma
- Bronchogenic cyst
- Hamartoma
- Carcinoid tumor
- Metastasis

Discussion

Features suggesting a benign nodule include calcification, homogeneous water-density signal, or fat. Diffuse and concentric (i.e., laminated) calcification or central calcification in a nodule less than 2 cm in diameter is virtually diagnostic of a granuloma. Demonstration of fat (i.e., −30 to −120 HU attenuation values on thin-section CT) within a smoothly marginated lung nodule is virtually diagnostic of hamartoma. Water-density signal (0 HU) on CT and a thin or invisible wall are diagnostic of a cystic lesion. Benign nodules tend to have smooth margins, and carcinoma usually has spiculated margins. The estimated likelihood ratio for malignancy of a nodule that has irregular or spiculated margins is approximately 5.5; the corresponding figures for lobulated and smoothly marginated nodules are about 0.75 and 0.30.

Diagnosis

Solitary lung nodule

Suggested Readings

Erasmus JJ, Connolly JE, McAdams HP, Roggli VL: Solitary pulmonary nodules. Part I. Morphologic evaluation for differentiation of benign and malignant lesions. Radiographics 20:43-58, 2000.

Erasmus JJ, McAdams HP, Connolly JE: Solitary pulmonary nodules. Part II. Evaluation of the indeterminate nodule. Radiographics 20:59-66, 2000.

Kim SK, Allen-Auerbach M, Goldin J, et al: Accuracy of PET/CT in characterization of solitary pulmonary lesions. J Nucl Med 48:214-220, 2007.

Rosado-de-Christenson ML, Templeton PA, Moran CA: Bronchogenic carcinoma: Radiologic-pathologic correlation. Radiographics 14:429-446, 1994.

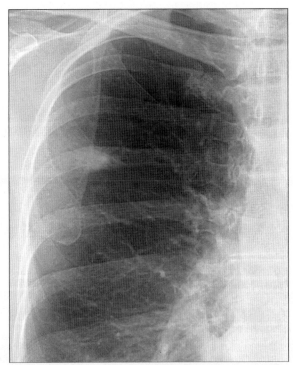

Figure 1. Chest radiograph of the right lung shows a poorly defined, 2.2-cm nodule in the right upper lobe. The patient was a 66-year-old woman with a surgically proven pulmonary adenocarcinoma.

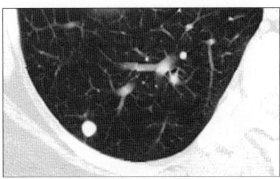

Figure 3. CT shows a smoothly marginated nodule in the right lower lobe. The patient was a 52-year-old woman with a calcified tuberculous granuloma.

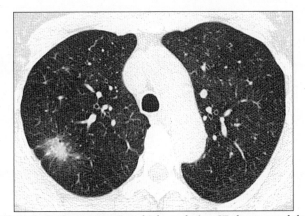

Figure 2. In the same patient, high-resolution CT shows a nodule with soft tissue and ground-glass components. The nodule has spiculated margins and pleural tags.

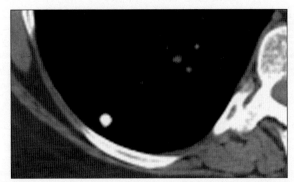

Figure 4. CT using soft tissue windows shows diffuse calcification of the right lower lobe nodule in a 52-year-old woman with a calcified tuberculous granuloma.

Case 44

DEMOGRAPHICS/CLINICAL HISTORY

A 53-year-old man, shoulder pain.

FINDINGS

Contrast-enhanced CT images (Figs. 1 and 2) show left apical mass. T1-weighted coronal MR images (Figs. 3 and 4) demonstrate left apical mass with focal extension into the chest wall.

DISCUSSION

Definition/Background
Superior sulcus (Pancoast) tumor is a pulmonary carcinoma that arises in apical region of lung and frequently invades the thoracic inlet. The most common cell types are adenocarcinoma and squamous cell carcinoma. Superior sulcus tumors account for less than 5% of pulmonary carcinomas.

Characteristic Clinical Features
Horner syndrome (triad of miosis, partial ptosis, and hemifacial anhidrosis) from sympathetic chain involvement. Shoulder pain and brachial plexopathy.

Characteristic Radiologic Findings
Asymmetric apical opacity with convex inferior margin on chest radiograph. Apical mass, commonly with chest wall invasion, best seen on MR imaging or coronal and sagittal reformations on contrast-enhanced CT (Figs. 1, 2, 3, and 4).

Less Common Radiologic Manifestations
Destruction of adjacent rib or vertebra, local invasion of subclavian artery or brachial plexus.

Differential Diagnosis
- Nonspecific apical pleural thickening
- Primary chest wall tumor

Discussion
Presence of chest wall invasion with mass extending through intercostal space or associated bone destruction distinguishes superior sulcus tumor from benign apical pleural thickening. Chest wall invasive mass is radiographically difficult to distinguish from primary chest wall lesions; biopsy is necessary for diagnosis.

Diagnosis
Superior sulcus (Pancoast) tumor

Suggested Readings
Rosado-de-Christenson ML, Templeton PA, Moran CA: Bronchogenic carcinoma: Radiologic-pathologic correlation. Radiographics 14:429-446, 1994.
Rusch VW: Management of Pancoast tumours. Lancet Oncology 7:997-1005, 2006.

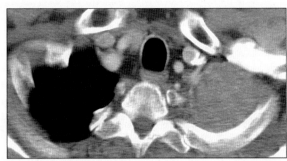

Figure 1. Contrast-enhanced CT image at the level of the thoracic inlet shows left apical mass. The patient was a 53-year-old man with Pancoast tumor.

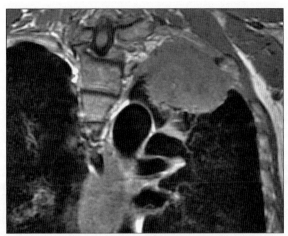

Figure 3. T1-weighted coronal MR image demonstrates left apical mass with focal extension into the chest wall. The patient was a 53-year-old man with Pancoast tumor.

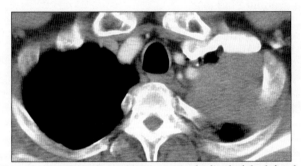

Figure 2. Contrast-enhanced CT image at the level of the left sub-clavian vein shows left apical mass. The patient was a 53-year-old man with Pancoast tumor.

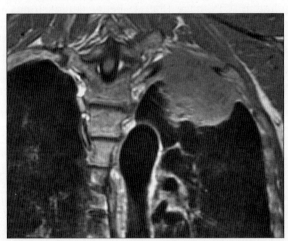

Figure 4. T1-weighted coronal MR image demonstrates left apical mass with focal extension into the chest wall. The patient was a 53-year-old man with Pancoast tumor.

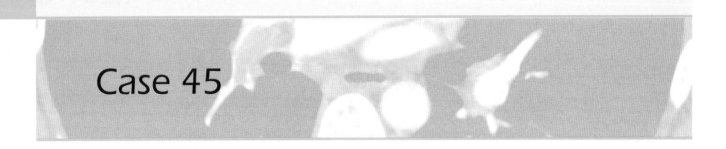

Case 45

DEMOGRAPHICS/CLINICAL HISTORY

An 83-year-old woman, cough, hemoptysis, exertional dyspnea.

FINDINGS

Posteroanterior chest radiograph (Fig. 1) shows cavitating left upper lobe mass and elevation of the left hemidiaphragm. CT image (Fig. 2) better demonstrates the left upper lobe cavitating mass. Contrast-enhanced CT photographed at soft tissue windows (Fig. 3) demonstrates cavitating mass and soft tissue infiltration into the mediastinum.

DISCUSSION

Definition/Background

Squamous cell carcinoma accounts for approximately 20–30% of all lung cancers and is closely associated with cigarette smoking. Approximately 50–70% occur centrally and 30–50% peripherally. Central tumors most often arise from a central (i.e., main, lobar or segmental) bronchus with early spread to regional hilar and mediastinal lymph nodes.

Characteristic Clinical Features

Peripheral tumors are commonly asymptomatic. Central tumors result in symptoms related to airway involvement, including cough, shortness of breath, hemoptysis, and postobstructive pneumonia or abscess formation.

Characteristic Radiologic Findings

Peripheral tumors frequently cavitate (Figs. 1, 2, and 3). Central squamous cell carcinomas (Fig. 4) frequently result in bronchial obstruction, distal atelectasis and obstructive pneumonitis, and hilar and mediastinal lymphadenopathy. Squamous cell carcinomas show increased uptake on Fluoro-2-deoxy-D-glucose (FDG) positron emission tomography (PET) imaging.

Less Common Radiologic Manifestations

Partial bronchial obstruction with decreased attenuation and vascularity distal to the obstruction and air trapping on expiration. Abscess formation. Pleural effusion.

Differential Diagnosis

- Benign nodule or mass
- Carcinoid tumor
- Adenocarcinoma
- Small cell carcinoma
- Abscess

Discussion

Benign nodules tend to have smooth margins and tend to be small. Larger nodules having spiculated margins are much more likely to be malignant.

Carcinoid tumors, which can also be endobronchial, resemble squamous cell carcinomas.

Small cell carcinomas usually are central and are associated with extensive lymphadenopathy.

Biopsy is required for a definitive diagnosis of squamous cell carcinoma and for distinction from other benign and malignant tumors.

Diagnosis

Pulmonary squamous cell carcinoma

Suggested Readings

Beadsmoore CJ, Screaton NJ: Classification, staging and prognosis of lung cancer. Eur J Radiol 45:8-17, 2003.

Collins LG, Haines C, Perkel R, Enck RE: Lung cancer: Diagnosis and management. Am Fam Physician 75:56-63, 2007.

Hollings N, Shaw P: Diagnostic imaging of lung cancer. Eur Respir J 19:722-742, 2002.

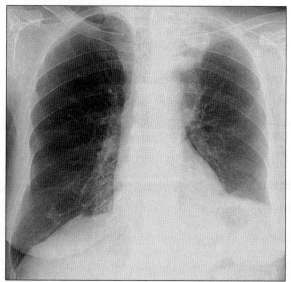

Figure 1. Posteroanterior chest radiograph shows cavitating left upper lobe mass and elevation of the left hemidiaphragm. The patient was an 83-year-old woman with pulmonary squamous cell carcinoma with invasion of the phrenic nerve and mediastinum.

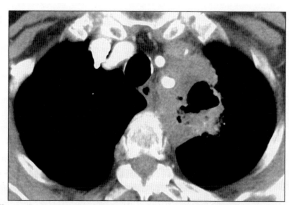

Figure 3. Contrast-enhanced CT photographed at soft tissue windows demonstrates cavitating mass and soft tissue infiltration into the mediastinum. The patient was an 83-year-old woman with pulmonary squamous cell carcinoma with invasion of the phrenic nerve and mediastinum.

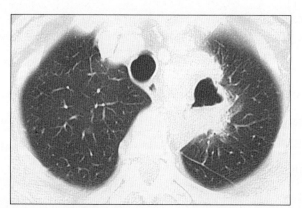

Figure 2. CT image shows the left upper lobe cavitating mass. The patient was an 83-year-old woman with pulmonary squamous cell carcinoma with invasion of the phrenic nerve and mediastinum.

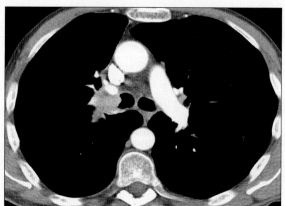

Figure 4. Contrast-enhanced CT image reveals endobronchial tumor within the right main and upper lobe bronchi. The patient was a 54-year-old man with pulmonary squamous cell carcinoma.

Case 46

DEMOGRAPHICS/CLINICAL HISTORY

A 76-year-old male smoker with an incidental finding on chest radiography, undergoing computed tomography (CT).

FINDINGS

CT shows a 2-cm, solitary, spiculated nodule in the right upper lobe (Fig. 1).

DISCUSSION

Definition/Background

Adenocarcinoma is the most common type of lung cancer, accounting for approximately one third of cases. It is often histologically heterogeneous and is classified as five subtypes: acinar (gland forming), papillary, bronchioloalveolar, solid with mucous formation, and mixed; most occur in the lung periphery.

Characteristic Clinical Features

Patients often are asymptomatic. Clinical symptoms include cough, dyspnea, hemoptysis, weight loss, and paraneoplastic syndromes.

Characteristic Radiologic Findings

Adenocarcinomas usually manifest as solitary, spiculated nodules or masses that are less than 4 cm in diameter. They may be solid (Fig. 1) or have mixed solid and ground-glass components (i.e., CT halo sign) (Fig. 2) on CT. Bubble-like lucencies may be seen and represent patent, small bronchi or small cystic spaces within the tumor (Fig. 3). Masses typically show increased uptake on ^{18}F-fluorodeoxyglucose positron emission tomography (FDG-PET).

Less Common Radiologic Manifestations

Less common findings include a cavitated nodule, hilar and mediastinal lymphadenopathy, and liver and adrenal metastases.

Differential Diagnosis

- Squamous cell carcinoma
- Large cell carcinoma
- Small cell carcinoma
- Granuloma
- Inflammatory pseudotumor
- Organizing pneumonia (i.e., focal bronchiolitis obliterans organizing pneumonia)
- Lipoid pneumonia

Discussion

Benign nodules tend to have smooth margins and to be small. Larger nodules that have spiculated margins are much more likely to be malignant. Biopsy is required for a definitive diagnosis of adenocarcinoma and for differentiation from other benign and malignant tumors.

Diagnosis

Pulmonary adenocarcinoma

Suggested Readings

Collins LG, Haines C, Perkel R, Enck RE: Lung cancer: Diagnosis and management. Am Fam Physician 75:56-63, 2007.
Beadsmoore CJ, Screaton NJ: Classification, staging and prognosis of lung cancer. Eur J Radiol 45:8-17, 2003.
Hollings N, Shaw P: Diagnostic imaging of lung cancer. Eur Respir J 19:722-742, 2002.
Shiau MC, Bonavita J, Naidich DP: Adenocarcinoma of the lung: Current concepts in radiologic diagnosis and management. Curr Opin Pulm Med 13:261-266, 2007.

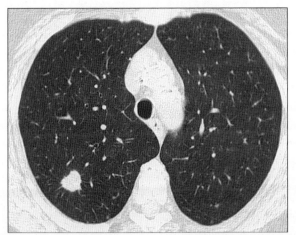

Figure 1. CT shows a 2-cm, solitary, spiculated nodule in the right upper lobe of a 76-year-old male smoker with pulmonary adenocarcinoma.

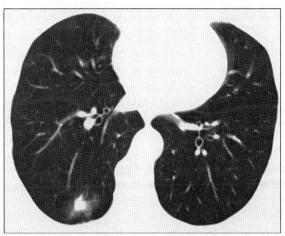

Figure 2. CT shows a mixed-attenuation lesion with a central solid component and peripheral ground-glass attenuation (i.e., CT halo sign) in the right lower lobe of a 75-year-old man with pulmonary adenocarcinoma.

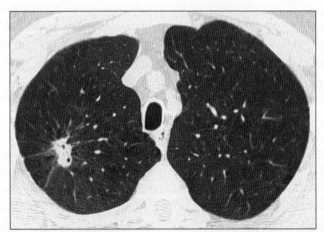

Figure 3. CT shows a spiculated nodule containing small, round lucencies (i.e., bubble lucencies) in a 57-year-old man with pulmonary adenocarcinoma.

Case 47

DEMOGRAPHICS/CLINICAL HISTORY

A 69-year-old man who is asymptomatic, undergoing computed tomography (CT).

FINDINGS

CT shows a 2.5-cm, focal, round area of ground-glass opacity in the left upper lobe (Figs. 1 and 2)

DISCUSSION

Definition/Background

Bronchioloalveolar cell carcinoma (BAC) accounts for less than 4% of pulmonary carcinomas. BAC is a subtype of adenocarcinoma that is characterized by lepidic growth along alveolar septa without vascular, stromal, or pleural invasion. It may be associated with mucin production.

Characteristic Clinical Features

Patients usually are asymptomatic, although they occasionally may have cough and dyspnea.

Characteristic Radiologic Findings

The most common presentation is as a focal, round area of ground-glass opacity on CT.

Less Common Radiologic Manifestations

CT may show multiple foci of ground-glass opacity (Fig. 3) and extensive, unilateral or bilateral ground-glass opacities progressing to consolidation.

Differential Diagnosis

- Benign nodule
- Atypical adenomatous hyperplasia (AAH)
- Focal pneumonia
- Hemorrhage

Discussion

Benign nodules tend to have soft tissue rather than ground-glass opacity and to have smooth margins. AAH is a preinvasive lesion for lung adenocarcinoma, consisting of bronchioloalveolar proliferation of a few millimeters. Similar to bronchioloalveolar carcinoma, it manifests as a focal, round ground-glass opacity, and lesions may be single or multiple. AAH typically is less than 5 mm in diameter, whereas BAC tends to be larger than 10 mm in diameter. Focal pneumonia and hemorrhage tend to have a lobular distribution, seldom manifesting as a focal, round ground-glass opacity. The lesions resolve on follow-up, whereas BAC grows slowly over several months or years. Biopsy is required for a definitive diagnosis of BAC and differentiation from other benign and malignant tumors.

Diagnosis

Focal bronchioloalveolar cell carcinoma

Suggested Readings

Gandara DR, Aberle D, Lau D, et al: Radiographic imaging of bronchioloalveolar carcinoma: Screening, patterns of presentation and response assessment. J Thorac Oncol 1(Suppl):S20-S26, 2006.

Raz DJ, Kim JY, Jablons DM: Diagnosis and treatment of bronchioloalveolar carcinoma. Curr Opin Pulm Med 13:290-296, 2007.

Yousem SA, Beasley MB: Bronchioloalveolar carcinoma: A review of current concepts and evolving issues. Arch Pathol Lab Med 131:1027-1032, 2007.

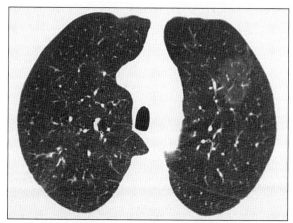

Figure 1. CT shows a 2.5-cm, focal, round area of ground-glass opacity in the left upper lobe of a 69-year-old man with bronchioloalveolar cell carcinoma.

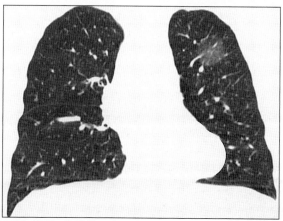

Figure 2. Coronal CT shows a 2.5-cm, focal, round area of ground-glass opacity in the left upper lobe of a 69-year-old man with bronchioloalveolar cell carcinoma.

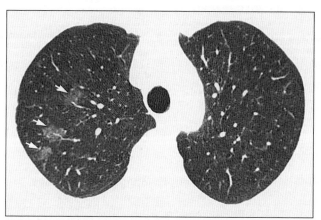

Figure 3. CT shows several focal, round areas of ground-glass opacity *(arrows)* in the right upper lobe of a 73-year-old woman with bronchioloalveolar carcinoma.

Case 48

DEMOGRAPHICS/CLINICAL HISTORY

A 73-year-old man with nonresolving consolidation undergoing computed tomography (CT).

FINDINGS

CT image shows focal consolidation surrounded by areas of ground-glass attenuation and small nodules in the right lower lobe (Fig. 1). The CT image obtained 2 years later (Fig. 2) shows persistent abnormalities in the right lower lobe and new areas of consolidation, ground-glass opacities, and centrilobular nodules bilaterally.

DISCUSSION

Definition/Background
Bronchioloalveolar cell carcinoma (BAC) accounts for less than 4% of pulmonary carcinomas. BAC is a subtype of adenocarcinoma characterized by lepidic growth along alveolar septa without vascular, stromal, or pleural invasion. It may be associated with mucin production.

Characteristic Clinical Features
Patients with BAC usually are asymptomatic. Extensive BAC may result in cough and progressive dyspnea.

Characteristic Radiologic Findings
The most common manifestation is a focal, round area of ground-glass opacity on CT.

Less Common Radiologic Manifestations
Less common features include multiple foci of ground-glass opacity and extensive, unilateral or bilateral ground-glass opacities progressing to consolidation.

Differential Diagnosis
- Pneumonia
- Hemorrhage
- Lymphoma

Discussion
BAC presenting with extensive, unilateral or bilateral ground-glass opacities with or without associated consolidation may mimic pneumonia or hemorrhage. BAC typically grows over several months, and pneumonia and hemorrhage usually resolve. Definitive diagnosis requires lung biopsy.

Diagnosis
Diffuse bronchioloalveolar cell carcinoma

Suggested Readings
Gandara DR, Aberle D, Lau D, et al: Radiographic imaging of bronchioloalveolar carcinoma: Screening, patterns of presentation and response assessment. J Thorac Oncol 1(Suppl):S20-S26, 2006.

Raz DJ, Kim JY, Jablons DM: Diagnosis and treatment of bronchioloalveolar carcinoma. Curr Opin Pulm Med 13:290-296, 2007.

Yousem SA, Beasley MB: Bronchioloalveolar carcinoma: A review of current concepts and evolving issues. Arch Pathol Lab Med 131:1027-1032, 2007.

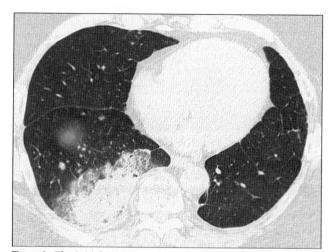

Figure 1. The initial CT image shows focal consolidation surrounded by ground-glass opacities and small nodules in the right lower lobe. The patient was a 73-year-old man with bronchioloalveolar cell carcinoma.

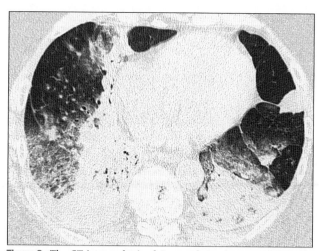

Figure 2. The CT image obtained 2 years later shows persistent abnormalities in the right lower lobe and new areas of consolidation, ground-glass opacities. and centrilobular nodules bilaterally in a 73-year-old man with bronchioloalveolar carcinoma.

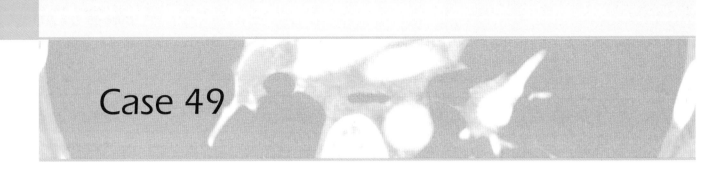

Case 49

DEMOGRAPHICS/CLINICAL HISTORY

A 63-year-old man with weight loss and superior vena cava syndrome, undergoing radiography and computed tomography (CT).

FINDINGS

Posteroanterior chest radiograph shows a right paratracheal and hilar increased opacity consistent with lymphadenopathy (Fig. 1). Contrast-enhanced CT scan shows a large, infiltrative, right hilar and mediastinal mass invading and compressing the superior vena cava (Fig. 2).

DISCUSSION

Definition/Background

Small cell carcinoma accounts for approximately 20% of all lung cancers. The highly aggressive tumor is closely associated with cigarette smoking. Because of the usual peribronchial location, the tumor infiltrates the bronchial submucosa and peribronchial tissue, often causing circumferential compression and bronchial obstruction. Extensive hilar and mediastinal lymph node metastases are common.

Characteristic Clinical Features

Patients have weight loss, malaise, and symptoms related to central airway involvement, including cough, hemoptysis, and shortness of breath. Small cell carcinoma is the most common cause of superior vena cava syndrome, and symptoms often are related to distal metastases, including headache, seizures, and bone pain.

Characteristic Radiologic Findings

Characteristic features include a hilar and mediastinal mass and findings of central airway obstruction, including complete lung or lobar obstructive pneumonitis and atelectasis (Figs. 3 and 4).

Less Common Radiologic Manifestations

Less common features include superior vena cava obstruction (Figs. 2 and 4), pleural effusion, and liver, adrenal, and brain metastases.

Differential Diagnosis

- Large cell carcinoma
- Lymphoma
- Tuberculosis
- Histoplasmosis

Discussion

The presence of massive unilateral hilar or mediastinal lymphadenopathy in a smoker older than 50 years strongly suggests small cell carcinoma. Occasionally, large cell carcinoma, lymphoma, tuberculosis, and histoplasmosis may cause similar findings, and definitive diagnosis requires a biopsy.

Diagnosis

Pulmonary small cell carcinoma

Suggested Readings

Ginsberg MS, Grewal RK, Heelan RT: Lung cancer. Radiol Clin North Am 45:21-43, 2007.

Jackman DM, Johnson BE: Small-cell lung cancer. Lancet 366:1385-1396, 2005.

Rosado-de-Christenson ML, Templeton PA, Moran CA: Bronchogenic carcinoma: Radiologic-pathologic correlation. Radiographics 14:429-446, 1994.

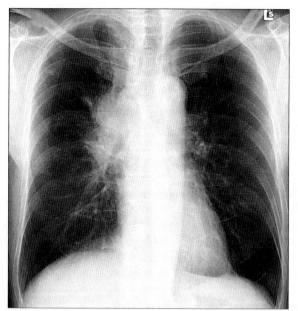

Figure 1. Posteroanterior chest radiograph shows right paratracheal and hilar increased opacity that is consistent with extensive lymphadenopathy. The patient was a 63-year-old man with pulmonary small cell carcinoma who presented with weight loss and superior vena cava syndrome.

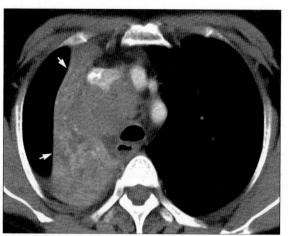

Figure 3. CT shows a large, infiltrative, right paratracheal lymphadenopathy and complete atelectasis of the right upper lobe *(arrows)* in a 56-year-old woman with pulmonary small cell carcinoma.

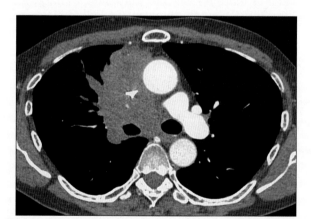

Figure 2. Contrast-enhanced CT scan shows a large, infiltrative, right hilar and mediastinal mass invading and compressing the superior vena cava. The patient was a 63-year-old man with pulmonary small cell carcinoma who presented with weight loss and superior vena cava syndrome.

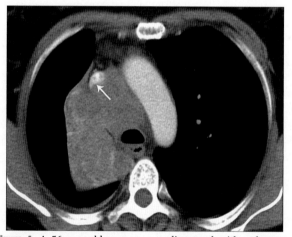

Figure 4. A 56-year-old woman was diagnosed with pulmonary small cell carcinoma. CT shows infiltrative, right paratracheal lymphadenopathy invading the superior vena cava *(arrow)* and right upper lobe atelectasis.

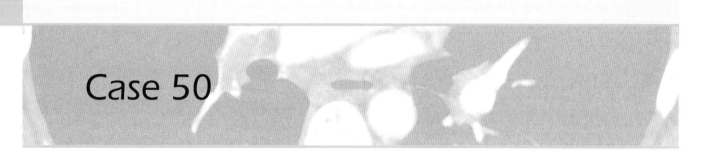

Case 50

DEMOGRAPHICS/CLINICAL HISTORY

A 42-year-old man with wheezing and progressive short-ness of breat, undergoing computed tomography (CT).

FINDINGS

CT image shows a polypoid endotracheal mass with associated focal thickening of the lateral tracheal wall (Fig. 1).

DISCUSSION

Definition/Background

Adenoid cystic carcinoma is a low-grade malignancy that usually grows into the lumen of the trachea or bronchus, forming a smooth-surfaced, polypoid mass. It is the second most common primary malignant tumor of the trachea (after squamous cell carcinoma). It is not associated with cigarette smoking. The mean age at diagnosis is 45 to 50 years.

Characteristic Clinical Features

The most common symptoms are stridor, wheezing, and progressive shortness of breath. Symptoms of dyspnea and wheeze frequently lead to an initial misdiagnosis of asthma. Hemoptysis may occur.

Characteristic Radiologic Findings

A lobulated, polypoid endoluminal mass with associated focal thickening of airway wall involves the trachea (Figs. 1 and 2)or, less commonly, the main or lobar bronchus.

Less Common Radiologic Manifestations

Less common manifestations include extensive thickening of the tracheal (Fig. 2) or bronchial wall, obstructive atelectasis, or pneumonitis distal to endobronchial adenoid cystic carcinoma. Lung metastases typically are slow growing.

Differential Diagnosis

- Squamous cell carcinoma
- Carcinoid tumor
- Papilloma
- Metastases
- Amyloidosis

Discussion

Adenoid cystic carcinoma of the trachea must be differentiated from other polypoid intratracheal or intra-bronchial lesions, such as squamous cell carcinoma, metastases, and papilloma. These tumors cannot be reliably distinguished radiologically; definitive diagnosis requires biopsy. Extensive thickening of the tracheal wall is an uncommon manifestation of adenoid cystic carcinoma and may involve the posterior portion of the tracheal wall, mimicking tracheal amyloidosis. In relapsing polychondritis, the posterior wall of the trachea is typically spared.

Diagnosis

Adenoid cystic carcinoma of the trachea

Suggested Readings

Jeong SY, Lee KS, Han J, et al: Integrated PET/CT of salivary gland type carcinoma of the lung in 12 patients. AJR Am J Roentgenol 189:1407-1413, 2007.

Kwak SH, Lee KS, Chung MJ, et al: Adenoid cystic carcinoma of the airways: Helical CT and histopathologic correlation. AJR Am J Roentgenol 183:277-281, 2004.

Kwong JS, Müller NL, Miller RR: Diseases of the trachea and main-stem bronchi: Correlation of CT with pathologic findings. Radiographics 12:645-657, 1992.

McCarthy MJ, Rosado-de-Christenson ML: Tumors of the trachea. J Thorac Imaging 10:180-198, 1995.

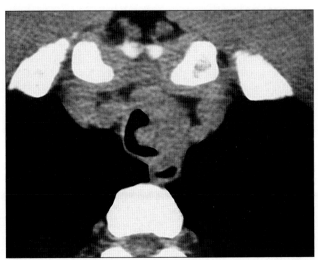

Figure 1. CT image shows a polypoid endotracheal mass with associated focal thickening of the lateral tracheal wall. Adenoid cystic carcinoma of the trachea was diagnosed in a 42-year-old man who presented with wheezing and progressive shortness of breath.

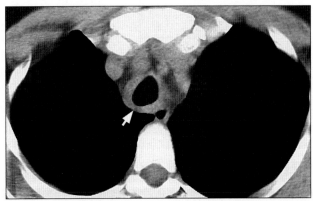

Figure 2. CT image shows extensive thickening of the tracheal wall, including the posterior portion *(arrow)*, in a 53-year old woman diagnosed with adenoid cystic carcinoma of the trachea.

Case 51

DEMOGRAPHICS/CLINICAL HISTORY

A 27-year-old woman with hemoptysis, undergoing computed tomography (CT).

FINDINGS

Contrast-enhanced CT shows a smooth, homogenous, endotracheal, soft tissue nodule (Fig. 1).

DISCUSSION

Definition/Background

Mucoepidermoid carcinoma is an uncommon tracheobronchial gland tumor, accounting for less than 0.2% of pulmonary carcinomas. It is usually located in a segmental bronchus; less commonly, it arises within a lobar or main bronchus or the trachea. Patients are between 3 months and 78 years old, but almost one half are younger than 30 years.

Characteristic Clinical Features

Symptoms are related predominantly to growth in the airway wall and lumen, and they include cough, hemoptysis, recurrent pneumonia, and dyspnea.

Characteristic Radiologic Findings

A mucoepidermoid carcinoma of the bronchus usually manifests as a smoothly oval or lobulated, soft tissue nodule or mass measuring 1 to 4 cm in diameter. Endobronchial tumors may be associated with distal obstructive pneumonitis and atelectasis. Punctate calcification within the tumor is evident on CT in 50% of cases. The tumors are homogeneous and show slight enhancement after the administration of contrast but usually show marked uptake on ^{18}F-fluorodeoxyglucose positron emission tomography (FDG-PET).

Less Common Radiologic Manifestations

A mucoepidermoid carcinoma can manifest as a polypoid endotracheal tumor and as hilar or mediastinal lymphadenopathy.

Differential Diagnosis

- Lung cancer
- Carcinoid tumor
- Granuloma
- Adenoid cystic carcinoma
- Endotracheal metastasis

Discussion

The differential diagnosis of mucoepidermoid carcinoma presenting as a solitary nodule is broad and includes pulmonary carcinoma, carcinoid tumor, and granuloma. The differential diagnosis of tumors presenting as polypoid intratracheal or intrabronchial lesions includes squamous cell carcinoma, adenoid cystic carcinoma, metastases, and benign lesions such as papilloma. These tumors cannot be reliably distinguished radiologically. Definitive diagnosis or mucoepidermoid carcinoma usually requires biopsy or surgical resection.

Diagnosis

Mucoepidermoid carcinoma of the trachea

Suggested Readings

Kim TS, Lee KS, Han J, et al: Mucoepidermoid carcinoma of the tracheobronchial tree: Radiographic and CT findings in 12 patients. Radiology 212:643-648, 1999.

Kwong JS, Müller NL, Miller RR: Diseases of the trachea and mainstem bronchi: Correlation of CT with pathologic findings. Radiographics 12:645-657, 1992.

McCarthy MJ, Rosado-de-Christenson ML: Tumors of the trachea. J Thorac Imaging 10:180-198, 1995.

Vadasz P, Egervary M: Mucoepidermoid bronchial tumors: A review of 34 operated cases. Eur J Cardiothorac Surg 17:566-569, 2000.

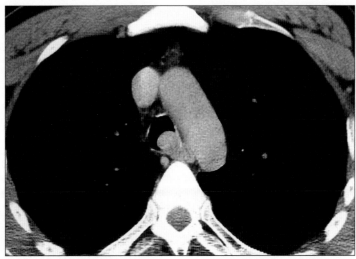

Figure 1. Contrast-enhanced CT shows a smooth, homogeneous, endotracheal, soft tissue nodule diagnosed as mucoepidermoid carcinoma of the trachea in a 27-year-old woman.

Case 52

DEMOGRAPHICS/CLINICAL HISTORY

A 41-year-old woman with hemoptysis, undergoing computed tomography (CT).

FINDINGS

Contrast-enhanced CT image using lung (Fig. 1) and soft tissue (Fig. 2) windows shows an enhancing, polypoid endobronchial lesion in the right main and upper lobe bronchus. Notice the associated mild, distal pneumonitis and volume loss. Bronchoscopic biopsy revealed a typical carcinoid tumor. In another patient with carcinoid tumor, CT image at the level of the lung bases shows a left lower lobe nodule with slightly lobulated margins (Fig. 3), and CT at the level of the lung bases using soft tissue windows shows homogeneous attenuation of a left lower lobe nodule (Fig. 4).

DISCUSSION

Definition/Background

Pulmonary carcinoid tumors are neuroendocrine neoplasms with immunohistochemical features similar to the neuroendocrine (Kulchitsky) cells normally present in the tracheobronchial epithelium. They are uncommon, accounting for only about 1% to 2% of all pulmonary neoplasms. Carcinoid tumors range from low-grade, typical carcinoids, which account for 80% to 90% of cases, and more aggressive, atypical carcinoids, which account for 10% to 20% of cases. Typical carcinoid tumors are the most common primary pulmonary neoplasm in children and adolescents, but they may occur at any age.

Characteristic Clinical Features

The most common symptoms are cough and hemoptysis. Some patients have symptoms simulating asthma.

Characteristic Radiologic Findings

Most carcinoid tumors arise centrally in the main, lobar, or segmental bronchi. CT usually shows a smooth endobronchial lesion with or without distal obstructive pneumonitis or atelectasis. Less commonly, carcinoid may manifest as a smoothly marginated or lobulated, peripheral nodule that is 1 to 3 cm in diameter. Homogeneous enhancement on CT after intravenous administration of contrast may be seen in carcinoid tumors because they have a rich vascular stroma. Because carcinoid tumors usually do not show increased metabolic activity on ^{18}F-fluorodeoxyglucose positron emission tomography (FDG-PET), they cannot be differentiated from benign lesions by this technique.

Less Common Radiologic Manifestations

Imaging may show recurrent pneumonia, bronchiectasis distal to the endobronchial carcinoid, and hilar and mediastinal lymphadenopathy. Approximately 30% of tumors have foci of calcification evident on CT.

Differential Diagnosis

- Pulmonary carcinoma
- Benign endobronchial tumor
- Benign lung nodule

Discussion

The differential diagnosis for endobronchial carcinoid tumors includes pulmonary carcinoma and benign lesions such as papilloma. The distinction cannot be reliably made radiologically. The diagnosis of carcinoid tumor often can be confirmed by bronchoscopic biopsy. Bronchial carcinoids have a characteristic bronchoscopic appearance of smooth, cherry red, polypoid, endobronchial nodules.

Diagnosis

Pulmonary carcinoid tumor

Suggested Readings

Chong S, Lee KS, Chung MJ, et al: Neuroendocrine tumors of the lung: Clinical, pathologic, and imaging findings. Radiographics 26:41-57, 2006.

Jeung MY, Gasser B, Gangi A, et al: Bronchial carcinoid tumors of the thorax: Spectrum of radiologic findings. Radiographics 22:351-365, 2002.

Rosado de Christenson ML, Abbott GF, Kirejczyk WM, et al: Thoracic carcinoids: Radiologic-pathologic correlation. Radiographics 19:707-736, 1999.

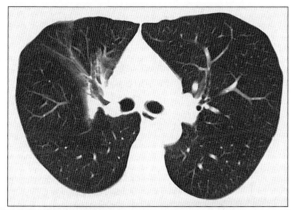

Figure 1. CT image using lung windows shows a polypoid endobronchial lesion in the right main and upper lobe bronchus. Notice the associated mild, distal pneumonitis, and volume loss. The patient was a 41-year-old woman with an endobronchial typical carcinoid tumor.

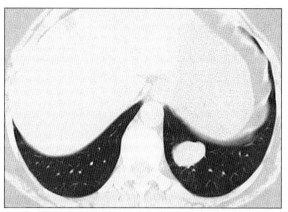

Figure 3. CT image at the level of the lung bases shows a left lower lobe nodule with slightly lobulated margins. The patient was a 67-year-old woman with a typical carcinoid tumor.

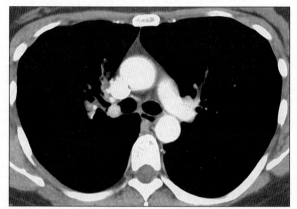

Figure 2. In the same patient, contrast-enhanced CT image using soft tissue windows shows an enhancing, polypoid, endobronchial lesion in the right main and upper lobe bronchus.

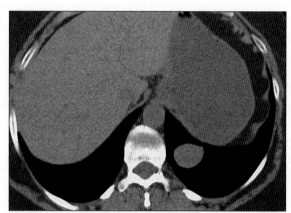

Figure 4. CT image at the level of the lung bases using soft tissue windows shows homogeneous attenuation of a left lower lobe nodule in a 67-year-old woman with a typical carcinoid tumor.

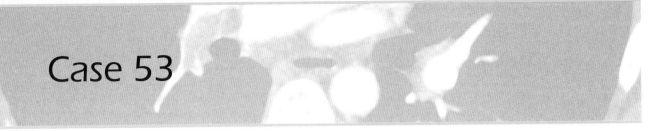

Case 53

DEMOGRAPHICS/CLINICAL HISTORY

A 41-year-old woman with hemoptysis, undergoing computed tomography (CT) and compared with radiography.

FINDINGS

Contrast-enhanced CT shows an enhancing, 4-cm-diameter mass with small foci of calcification in the left lower lobe (Fig. 1). In another patient with an atypical carcinoid tumor, a chest radiograph shows a 6-cm-diameter mass in the right lower lobe (Fig. 2).

DISCUSSION

Definition/Background

Pulmonary carcinoid tumors are neuroendocrine neoplasms with immunohistochemical features similar to the neuroendocrine (Kulchitsky) cells normally present in the tracheobronchial epithelium. They are uncommon, accounting for only about 1% to 2% of all pulmonary neoplasms. Carcinoid tumors range from low-grade, typical carcinoids, which account for 80% to 90% of cases, to more aggressive, atypical carcinoids, which account for 10% to 20% of cases. Atypical carcinoids are more common in males, and the typical age of presentation is between 50 and 70 years.

Characteristic Clinical Features

The most common symptoms are cough and hemoptysis.

Characteristic Radiologic Findings

Most tumors arise centrally in the main, lobar, or segmental bronchi. CT most commonly shows a central nodule or mass with associated obstructive pneumonitis or atelectasis. Atypical carcinoids usually are 2 to 5 cm in diameter, and they often have irregular margins. Approximately 50% are associated with hilar and mediastinal lymph node enlargement. Atypical carcinoids tend to show less uniform contrast enhancement on CT than typical carcinoids. Atypical carcinoids have increased activity on ^{18}F-fluorodeoxyglucose positron emission tomography (FDG-PET).

Less Common Radiologic Manifestations

Imaging may show recurrent pneumonia, bronchiectasis distal to the endobronchial tumor, and extensive mediastinal invasion.

Differential Diagnosis

- Typical carcinoid tumor
- Pulmonary carcinoma
- Benign lung nodule

Discussion

Radiologically, atypical carcinoid tumors are indistinguishable from pulmonary carcinoma. Like carcinoma, they tend to occur in older patients, particularly smokers, and they have positive radiotracer uptake on FDG-PET. Typical carcinoids tend to occur in young adults or adolescents, are more common in women, have no association with cigarette smoking, and usually have negative results on FDG-PET. Definitive diagnosis requires biopsy.

Diagnosis

Pulmonary atypical carcinoid tumor

Suggested Readings

Chong S, Lee KS, Chung MJ, et al: Neuroendocrine tumors of the lung: Clinical, pathologic, and imaging findings. Radiographics 26:41-57, 2006.

Jeung MY, Gasser B, Gangi A, et al: Bronchial carcinoid tumors of the thorax: Spectrum of radiologic findings. Radiographics 22:351-365, 2002.

Rosado de Christenson ML, Abbott GF, Kirejczyk WM, et al: Thoracic carcinoids: Radiologic-pathologic correlation. Radiographics 19:707-736, 1999.

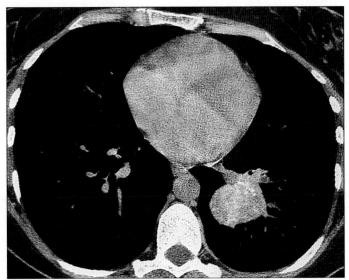

Figure 1. Contrast-enhanced CT shows an enhancing, 4-cm-diameter mass with foci of calcification in the left lower lobe. Several small areas of calcification can be seen within the tumor. The patient was a 41-year-old woman with an atypical carcinoid tumor.

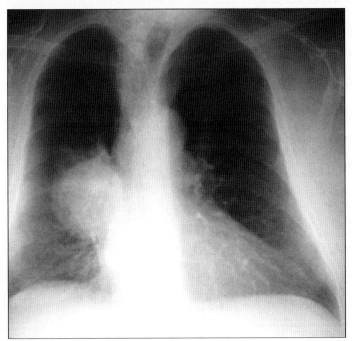

Figure 2. Chest radiograph shows a 6-cm-diameter mass in the right lower lobe. The patient was a 64-year-old man with an atypical carcinoid tumor.

Case 54

DEMOGRAPHICS/CLINICAL HISTORY

A 72-year-old woman with progressive shortness of breath over several months, undergoing computed tomography (CT).

FINDINGS

High-resolution CT images at the level of the upper lung zones (Fig. 1) and lung bases (Fig. 2) show several small nodules and areas of decreased attenuation and vascularity adjacent to areas of increased attenuation and vascularity, resulting in a mosaic perfusion (attenuation) pattern.

DISCUSSION

Definition/Background

Diffuse idiopathic pulmonary neuroendocrine cell hyperplasia (DIPNECH) is a rare condition characterized by extensive proliferation of neuroendocrine cells seen as clusters of cells or as linear arrays along the basement membrane. The main manifestation is progressive airway obstruction due to a combination of intraluminal obstruction by hyperplastic neuroendocrine cells and peribronchiolar fibrosis resulting in obliterative bronchiolitis. The latter presumably results from peptide secretory products released by the proliferating neuroendocrine cells.

Characteristic Clinical Features

The most common symptoms are dry cough and progressive shortness of breath. Most patients are women between the ages of 45 and 65 years.

Characteristic Radiologic Findings

The chest radiograph often shows normal anatomy or may show a reticulonodular pattern. CT shows typical findings of bronchiolitis obliterans with areas of decreased attenuation and vascularity on inspiratory CT and air trapping on expiratory CT. Small nodules (1 to 5 mm in diameter) consistent with carcinoid tumorlets are seen in most patients.

Less Common Radiologic Manifestations

Imaging may show a large nodule (1 to 3 cm in diameter) representing a carcinoid tumor, associated carcinoid tumorlets, and findings of bronchiolitis obliterans.

Differential Diagnosis

- Bronchiolitis obliterans
- Pulmonary metastases
- Previous granulomatous infection

Discussion

The main differential diagnosis for DIPNECH is bronchiolitis obliterans from other causes. The combination of bronchiolitis obliterans and several noncalcified pulmonary nodules in a middle-aged woman with progressive shortness of breath suggests the diagnosis. Similar findings may be seen in patients with postinfectious bronchiolitis obliterans caused by prior granulomatous infection. Definitive diagnosis requires lung biopsy.

Diagnosis

Diffuse idiopathic pulmonary neuroendocrine cell hyperplasia

Suggested Readings

Brown MJ, English J, Müller NL: Bronchiolitis obliterans due to neuroendocrine hyperplasia: High-resolution CT-pathologic correlation. AJR Am J Roentgenol 168:1561-1562, 1997.

Davies SJ, Gosney JR, Hansell DM, et al: Diffuse idiopathic pulmonary neuroendocrine cell hyperplasia: An under-recognised spectrum of disease. Thorax 6:248-252, 2007.

Lee JS, Brown KK, Cool C, et al: Diffuse pulmonary neuroendocrine cell hyperplasia: Radiologic and clinical features. J Comput Assist Tomogr 26:180-184, 2002.

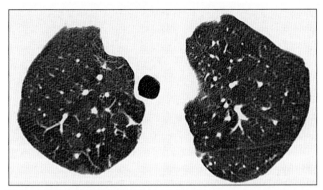

Figure 1. High-resolution CT at the level of the upper lung zones shows several small nodules and areas of decreased attenuation and vascularity adjacent to areas of increased attenuation and vascularity, resulting in a mosaic perfusion (attenuation) pattern. The patient was a 72-year-old woman with DIPNECH and carcinoid tumorlets.

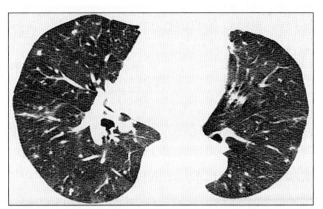

Figure 2. In the same patient, high-resolution CT at the level of the lung bases shows several small nodules and areas of decreased attenuation and vascularity adjacent to areas of increased attenuation and vascularity, resulting in a mosaic perfusion (attenuation) pattern.

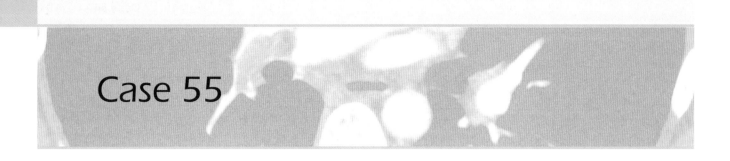

Case 55

DEMOGRAPHICS/CLINICAL HISTORY

A 78-year-old woman who is asymptomatic, undergoing computed tomography (CT) and radiography.

FINDINGS

CT images show a 1.5-cm, well-circumscribed, solitary nodule (Fig. 1) in the left upper lobe with focal areas of fat density on soft tissue windows (Fig. 2).

DISCUSSION

Definition/Background
Pulmonary hamartomas are benign neoplasms that probably are derived from bronchial wall mesenchymal cells. Hamartomas are the most common benign pulmonary neoplasm, and they account for approximately 8% of primary lung tumors. Although they may be seen in adolescents and young adults, most occur in patients older than 40 years.

Characteristic Clinical Features
Pulmonary hamartomas usually do not cause symptoms.

Characteristic Radiologic Findings
Imaging shows solitary, well-circumscribed, slightly lobulated nodules, usually 1 to 4 cm in diameter and located within the parenchyma and in a peripheral location. Approximately 60% of cases have focal areas of fat density (between -40 and -120 HU) on thin-section CT. No uptake is seen on ^{18}F-fluorodeoxyglucose positron emission tomography (FDG-PET).

Less Common Radiologic Manifestations
Imaging shows coarse foci of calcification (i.e., popcorn calcification) (Fig. 3). Occasionally, lesions are seen in an endobronchial location (Fig. 4). Endotracheal and endobronchial hamartomas may appear on CT to be composed entirely of fat or a mixture of fat and soft tissue or calcification, or they may have soft tissue attenuation with or without foci of calcification. Multiple pulmonary hamartomas are uncommon but may occur as an isolated abnormality or may be part of Carney's syndrome (i.e., young women with multiple pulmonary hamartomas, gastric leiomyosarcoma, and functioning extra-adrenal paraganglioma).

Differential Diagnosis
- Lung cancer
- Carcinoid tumor
- Granuloma

Discussion
The presence of local areas of fat density (-40 to -120 HU) in a smoothly marginated lung nodule is considered a reliable indicator of a hamartoma. In the absence of evidence of focal areas of fat attenuation on CT, the differential diagnosis of pulmonary hamartomas must include all other solitary pulmonary nodules, particularly carcinoma. Core-needle biopsy often is required for a definitive diagnosis.

Diagnosis
Pulmonary hamartoma

Suggested Readings
Erasmus JJ, Connolly JE, McAdams HP, Roggli VL: Solitary pulmonary nodules. Part I. Morphologic evaluation for differentiation of benign and malignant lesions. Radiographics 20:43-58, 2000.
Gaerte SC, Meyer CA, Winer-Muram HT, et al: Fat-containing lesions of the chest. Radiographics 22:S61-S78, 2002.

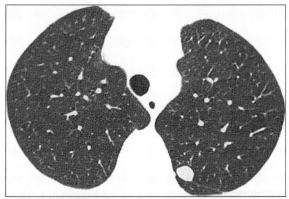

Figure 1. CT image shows a 1.5-cm, well-circumscribed, solitary nodule in the left upper lobe of a 78-year-old woman who was diagnosed with pulmonary hamartoma.

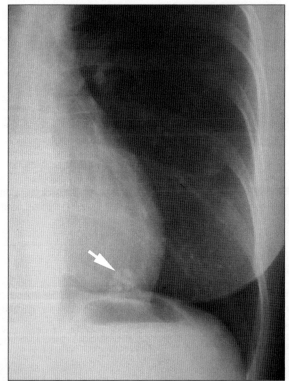

Figure 3. Magnified view of a frontal chest radiograph shows a nodule with typical popcorn calcification *(arrow)* in the left lower lobe of a 49-year-old woman with pulmonary hamartoma.

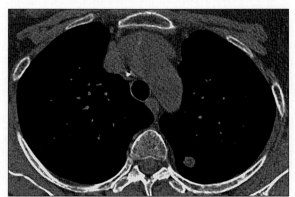

Figure 2. In the same patient CT image using soft tissue windows shows a 1.5-cm, well-circumscribed, solitary nodule in the left upper lobe with focal areas of fat density consistent with pulmonary hamartoma.

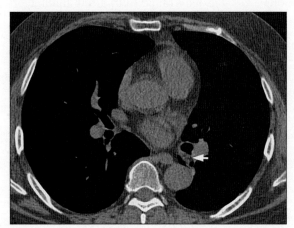

Figure 4. CT image using soft tissue windows shows an endobronchial tumor with focal areas of fat density *(arrow)* in a 49-year-old woman with endobronchial hamartoma.

Case 56

DEMOGRAPHICS/CLINICAL HISTORY

A 79-year-old man who is asymptomatic and has a history of primary adenocarcinoma of the rectum, undergoing radiography and computed tomography (CT).

FINDINGS

Chest radiograph shows many nodules that are most numerous in the lower lung zones (Fig. 1). CT shows smooth lung nodules of various sizes (Fig. 2).

DISCUSSION

Definition/Background
The most common manifestation of metastatic disease to the lungs consists of multiple nodules that tend to be most numerous in the lower lobes. The nodules are of various sizes and may range from a few millimeters to several centimeters in diameter.

Characteristic Clinical Features
Most patients are asymptomatic. When present, symptoms are nonspecific and include cough, hemoptysis, and shortness of breath.

Characteristic Radiologic Findings
Multiple pulmonary nodules of various sizes involve mainly the peripheral regions of the lower lobes. The nodules may have smooth or, less commonly, irregular margins.

Less Common Radiologic Manifestations
Thickening of the interlobular septa results from lymphangitic carcinomatosis, hilar and mediastinal lymphadenopathy, and pleural effusion. Approximately 4% of pulmonary metastases cavitate. Calcification of metastatic lesions is uncommon but may occur in patients with osteosarcoma, chondrosarcoma, synovial sarcoma, or carcinoma of the colon, ovary, thyroid, or breast.

Differential Diagnosis
- Fungal infections
- Tuberculosis, post-primary
- Septic embolism
- Wegener granulomatosis
- Arteriovenous malformations
- Lymphoma

Discussion
The differential diagnosis for multiple nodules larger than 1 cm in diameter is broad and includes congenital abnormalities (e.g., arteriovenous malformations), infection (e.g., multiple granulomas, septic embolism), inflammatory processes (e.g., Wegener granulomatosis), and pulmonary metastases. However, more than 95% of cases represent pulmonary metastases or infection. Multiple pulmonary nodules of various sizes in a patient with known extrathoracic malignancy strongly suggest the diagnosis, but cytologic or histologic proof is required for definitive diagnosis.

Diagnosis
Pulmonary metastases manifesting as multiple lung nodules

Suggested Readings
Hirakata K, Nakata H, Nakagawa T: CT of pulmonary metastases with pathological correlation. Semin Ultrasound CT MR 16:379-394, 1995.
Seo JB, Im JG, Goo JM, et al: Atypical pulmonary metastases: spectrum of radiologic findings. Radiographics 21:403-417, 2001.

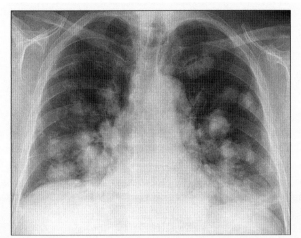

Figure 1. Chest radiograph shows many nodules that are most numerous in the lower lung zones of a 79-year-old man with metastatic adenocarcinoma of the rectum.

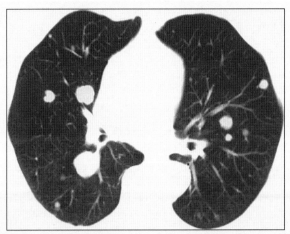

Figure 2. CT shows multiple, smooth lung nodules of various sizes in a 79-year-old man with metastatic adenocarcinoma of the rectum.

Case 57

DEMOGRAPHICS/CLINICAL HISTORY

A 50-year-old man with dyspnea and a history of adenocarcinoma of the colon, undergoing computed tomography (CT).

FINDINGS

High-resolution CT shows smooth and nodular, interlobular septal thickening and bilateral small nodules, some of which are located along the interlobar fissures and in the subpleural lung regions, and shows peribronchial interstitial thickening and subcarinal lymph node enlargement (Figs. 1 and 2). Mediastinal window settings show mediastinal lymphadenopathy (Fig. 3).

DISCUSSION

Definition/Background

Lymphangitic carcinomatosis refers to tumor spread along the pulmonary lymphatics. Most cases result from hematogenous dissemination to small pulmonary arteries and arterioles, followed by invasion of the adjacent interstitial space and lymphatics. Less commonly, extrathoracic tumors metastasize to mediastinal or hilar lymph nodes and then spread retrogradely along the lymphatic channels into the lungs. Although virtually any metastatic neoplasm can result in lymphatic spread, the most common primary sites are breast, lung, stomach, pancreas, and prostate.

Characteristic Clinical Features

The most common clinical manifestation of lymphatic spread of tumor is dyspnea. The dyspnea is typically insidious in onset but tends to progress rapidly.

Characteristic Radiologic Findings

Smooth or nodular thickening of the interlobular septa and peribronchovascular interstitium with preservation of normal lung architecture are best seen on high-resolution CT. The thickened interlobular septa may be seen as peripheral lines extending to the pleural surface or centrally as polygonal arcades, frequently with a nodular or beaded appearance. The abnormalities may be focal or asymmetric (Fig. 4), but they tend to progress to extensive bilateral disease with associated ground-glass opacities because of pulmonary edema.

Less Common Radiologic Manifestations

Pleural effusion is seen on the CT scan in approximately 30% of cases, and hilar or mediastinal lymph node enlargement is seen in approximately 40%.

Differential Diagnosis

- Interstitial pulmonary edema
- Lymphoma
- Pulmonary sarcoidosis
- Churg-Strauss syndrome
- Niemann-Pick disease

Discussion

The presence of septal lines, particularly when nodular or associated with nodules in a patient with history of carcinoma of the breast, lung, stomach, pancreas, or prostate, suggests the diagnosis of lymphangitic carcinomatosis. However, biopsy is required for definitive diagnosis.

Diagnosis

Lymphangitic carcinomatosis

Suggested Readings

Johkoh T, Ikezoe J, Tomiyama N, et al: CT findings in lymphangitic carcinomatosis of the lung: Correlation with histologic findings and pulmonary function tests. AJR Am J Roentgenol 158:1217-1222, 1992.

Seo JB, Im JG, Goo JM, et al: Atypical pulmonary metastases: Spectrum of radiologic findings. Radiographics 21:403-417, 2001.

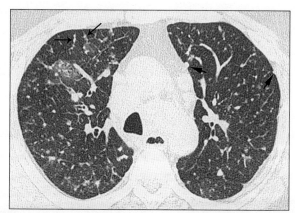

Figure 1. High-resolution CT image at the level of the upper lobes shows smooth and nodular *(arrows)*, interlobular septal thickening and bilateral, small nodules, some of which are located in the subpleural lung regions *(short arrows)*. Focal areas of ground-glass opacities can be seen in the right upper lobe and are consistent with pulmonary edema. The patient was a 50-year-old man with known metastatic adenocarcinoma of the colon and lymphangitic carcinomatosis.

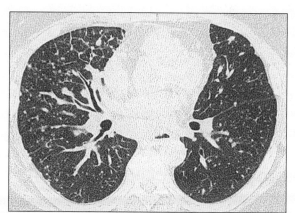

Figure 2. High-resolution CT image at the level of the middle lobe in the same patient shows smooth and nodular interlobular septal thickening and bilateral, small nodules, some of which are located along the interlobar fissures and in the subpleural lung regions. Peribronchial interstitial thickening and subcarinal lymph node enlargement can be seen.

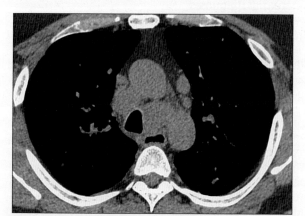

Figure 3. Mediastinal window settings show mediastinal lymphadenopathy. The patient was a 50-year-old man with metastatic adenocarcinoma of the colon.

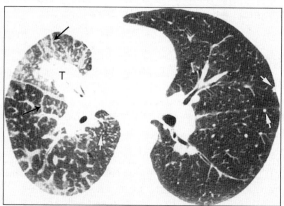

Figure 4. Asymmetric lymphangitic carcinomatosis was diagnosed in a 43-year-old woman with primary pulmonary adenocarcinoma. CT shows extensive, interlobular septal thickening *(arrow)* in the right lung and small, bilateral nodules *(short arrows)* that are consistent with pulmonary metastases. Thickening of the interlobar fissures, peribronchovascular thickening, and prominent intralobular vessels caused by centrilobular interstitial thickening can be seen. T, tumor.

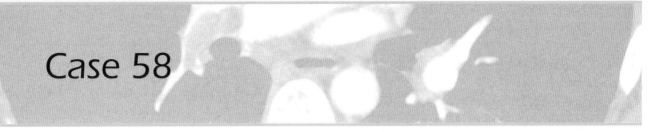

Case 58

DEMOGRAPHICS/CLINICAL HISTORY

A 70-year-old man with dyspnea and a history of renal cell carcinoma, undergoing computed tomography (CT).

FINDINGS

Axial and coronal CT images show enlarged segmental and subsegmental pulmonary arteries with a nodular or beaded appearance and branching centrilobular opacities representing enlarged centrilobular arteries, mainly in the right upper lobe (Figs. 1 and 2). Right paratracheal lymph node enlargement can be seen (Fig. 2).

DISCUSSION

Definition/Background

Occasionally, hematogenous metastases to the lungs may result in tumor growth only in the vessel lumen and wall, without extension into the extravascular tissue. This condition, also known as tumor embolism, most commonly occurs in patients with metastatic renal cell carcinoma, hepatocellular carcinoma, or carcinoma of the breast, stomach, or prostate. Usually, tumor is identified only histologically in small to medium-sized muscular arteries and arterioles. Occasionally, emboli occur in segmental and larger arteries.

Characteristic Clinical Features

The patients may be asymptomatic or present with non-specific symptoms of cough and dyspnea. Occasionally, large tumor emboli may mimic acute pulmonary thromboembolism.

Characteristic Radiologic Findings

Large tumor emboli may result in filling defects in the central pulmonary arteries on contrast-enhanced CT, resembling pulmonary thromboembolism. Tumor emboli to peripheral pulmonary arteries may manifest as nodular or beaded thickening of the peripheral pulmonary arteries or as nodular and branching centrilobular opacities (i.e., tree-in-bud pattern), representing enlarged centrilobular arteries.

Less Common Radiologic Manifestations

Patients may have pleural effusions and hilar or mediastinal lymphadenopathy. Calcification of intravascular metastases is uncommon, but it may occur, particularly in patients with osteogenic sarcoma (Fig. 3).

Differential Diagnosis

- Pulmonary thromboembolism
- Infectious bronchiolitis

Discussion

Large tumor emboli can mimic acute pulmonary thromboembolism. The tumor enhances on delayed images and shows increased uptake on ^{18}F-fluorodeoxyglucose positron emission tomography (FDG-PET). Peripheral tumor emboli may result in centrilobular nodules and a tree-in-bud pattern, mimicking infectious bronchiolitis. Presumed diagnosis can sometimes be made based on the CT findings and history of a primary tumor with a propensity for intravascular metastases, such as breast, kidney, or liver carcinoma. Definitive diagnosis requires biopsy.

Diagnosis

Intravascular pulmonary metastases

Suggested Readings

Han D, Lee KS, Franquet T, et al: Thrombotic and nonthrombotic pulmonary arterial embolism: Spectrum of imaging findings. Radiographics 23:1521-1539, 2003.

Seo JB, Im JG, Goo JM, et al: Atypical pulmonary metastases: Spectrum of radiologic findings. Radiographics 21:403-417, 2001.

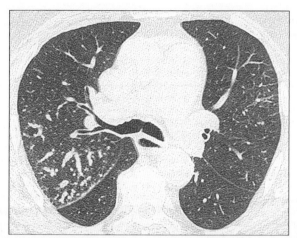

Figure 1. Intravascular pulmonary metastases were diagnosed in a 70-year-old man with a history of renal cell carcinoma. Axial CT image shows enlarged, segmental and subsegmental pulmonary arteries with a nodular or beaded appearance and branching centrilobular opacities, representing enlarged centrilobular arteries.

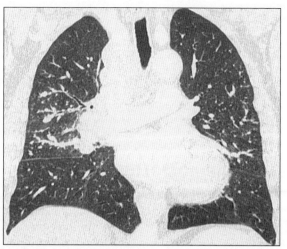

Figure 2. Coronal CT shows enlarged, segmental and subsegmental pulmonary arteries with a nodular or beaded appearance and branching centrilobular opacities, representing enlarged centrilobular arteries. Right paratracheal lymph node enlargement can be seen.

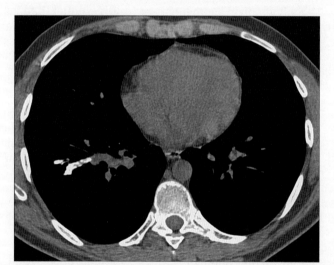

Figure 3. Calcified intravascular pulmonary metastases were diagnosed in a 26-year-old man with osteosarcoma of the fibula. CT shows calcified intravascular pulmonary metastases in the right lower lobe.

Case 59

DEMOGRAPHICS/CLINICAL HISTORY

A 53-year-old woman with dyspnea and a history of primary carcinoma of the cervix, undergoing computed tomography (CT).

FINDINGS

CT shows an endoluminal polypoid lesion within the bronchus intermedius (Fig. 1). CT in another patient shows complete obstruction of the left main bronchus by tumor and associated obstructive pneumonitis and mucoid impaction (Fig. 2). Radiograph in another patient shows a smoothly marginated, round nodule within the tracheal lumen (Fig. 3). Coronal, reformatted CT in another patient shows an endoluminal polypoid lesion in the right lower lobe bronchus and distal opacities caused by partial bronchial obstruction (Fig. 4).

DISCUSSION

Definition/Background

Secondary malignant neoplasms of the airways may result from hematogenous metastases or, more commonly, direct invasion from the thyroid, esophagus, mediastinum, or lung. Endobronchial and endotracheal metastases usually are caused by carcinoma of the breast, colorectum, kidney, or cervix or to melanoma or sarcoma. Most cases are incidental findings seen by the pathologist at autopsy. Endobronchial metastases may manifest as intraluminal lesions and may be associated with partial (causing oligemia and expiratory air trapping) or complete (with atelectasis and obstructive pneumonitis) bronchial obstruction.

Characteristic Clinical Features

The most common symptom of endobronchial and endotracheal metastases is dyspnea. Other common symptoms include cough and hemoptysis.

Characteristic Radiologic Findings

Endobronchial and endotracheal metastases manifest as single or multiple, endoluminal, soft tissue lesions. The lesions, particularly endobronchial ones, are better seen on CT. The tumors may be polypoid or have a glove-in-finger appearance with bronchial dilatation. The tumors enhance after intravenous administration of contrast. Bronchial obstruction may result in distal atelectasis or pneumonitis.

Less Common Radiologic Manifestations

Some patients have mediastinal lymphadenopathy.

Differential Diagnosis

- Tracheobronchial papillomatosis
- Squamous cell carcinoma
- Adenoid cystic carcinoma
- Carcinoid tumor

Discussion

The main differential diagnosis for multiple tracheal and bronchial nodules includes metastases and tracheobronchial papillomatosis. The differential diagnosis for a single endotracheal or endobronchial lesion includes mainly squamous cell carcinoma, adenoid cystic carcinoma, carcinoid tumor, and solitary metastasis. These various lesions are indistinguishable radiologically, and definitive diagnosis requires biopsy.

Diagnosis

Endobronchial and endotracheal metastases

Suggested Readings

Hirakata K, Nakata H, Nakagawa T: CT of pulmonary metastases with pathological correlation. Semin Ultrasound CT MR 16:379-394, 1995.

Seo JB, Im JG, Goo JM, et al: Atypical pulmonary metastases: Spectrum of radiologic findings. Radiographics 21:403-417, 2001.

Sorensen JB: Endobronchial metastases from extrapulmonary solid tumors. Acta Oncol 43:73-79, 2004.

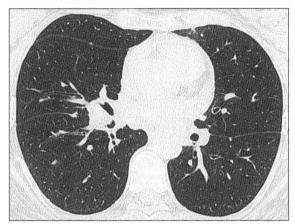

Figure 1. Endobronchial metastasis was diagnosed in a 53-year-old woman with known primary carcinoma of the cervix. CT shows an endoluminal polypoid lesion within the bronchus intermedius.

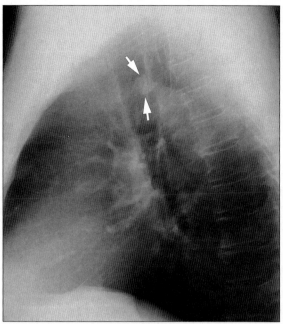

Figure 3. Endotracheal metastasis was diagnosed in a 57-year-old patient. Lateral chest radiograph shows a smoothly marginated, round nodule *(arrows)* within the tracheal lumen. The final diagnosis was metastatic melanoma of an unknown site.

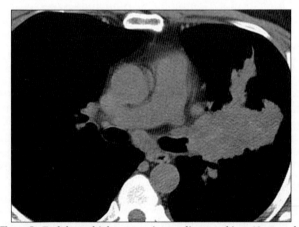

Figure 2. Endobronchial metastasis was diagnosed in a 43-year-old man with primary carcinoma of the colon. CT shows complete obstruction of the left main bronchus by tumor and associated obstructive pneumonitis and mucoid impaction. Bronchial biopsy showed metastatic adenocarcinoma of the colon.

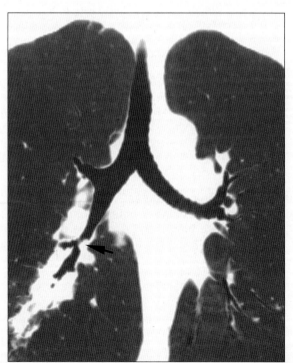

Figure 4. Endobronchial metastasis was diagnosed in a 53-year-old woman with known primary carcinoma of the cervix. Coronal, reformatted CT shows an endoluminal polypoid lesion in the right lower lobe bronchus and distal opacities due to obstructive pneumonitis and atelectasis.

Case 60

DEMOGRAPHICS/CLINICAL HISTORY

A 40-year-old woman who is asymptomatic and has a history of scleroderma, undergoing computed tomography (CT)

FINDINGS

CT image shows poorly defined, centrilobular, ground-glass nodules (Fig. 1).

DISCUSSION

Definition/Background

Pulmonary lymphoid hyperplasia, also known as follicular bronchiolitis, is an uncommon, benign condition characterized histologically by the presence of polyclonal lymphoid aggregates along the bifurcation of the bronchioles and along the pulmonary lymphatics. It is commonly associated with collagen vascular diseases, particularly rheumatoid arthritis and scleroderma; immunodeficiency, particularly acquired immunodeficiency syndrome (AIDS); hypersensitivity disorders; and as a nonspecific response in patients with airway infection, airway obstruction, or bronchiectasis. Pulmonary lymphoid hyperplasia may occur in children and adults (age range, 1.5 to 77 years).

Characteristic Clinical Features

Usually asymptomatic. The most common presenting symptoms are progressive shortness of breath and cough. Other manifestations include fever and recurrent pneumonia.

Characteristic Radiologic Findings

The chest radiograph may be normal or show bilateral reticular or reticulonodular opacities. The main high-resolution CT findings consist of bilateral centrilobular (Fig. 1, Fig. 2) and peribronchial nodules. Most nodules measure less than 3 mm in diameter. Nodules 3 to 12 mm in diameter are present in approximately 50% of patients and patchy ground-glass opacities in approximately 75% of patients.

Less Common Radiologic Manifestations

CT may show foci of consolidation.

Differential Diagnosis

- Infectious bronchiolitis
- Respiratory bronchiolitis
- Hypersensitivity pneumonitis
- Lymphoid interstitial pneumonia (LIP)

Discussion

Centrilobular nodules are seen in a variety of diseases that affect predominantly the bronchioles or peribronchiolar interstitium. Common causes include hypersensitivity pneumonitis, respiratory bronchiolitis, and infectious bronchiolitis. The diagnosis of pulmonary lymphoid hyperplasia requires a lung biopsy. The main differential diagnosis is LIP, which shows several histologic features that are similar to those seen in lymphoid hyperplasia and is seen with increased frequency in patients with autoimmune disorders, particularly Sjögren syndrome and immunodeficiency states. The two conditions can usually be distinguished histologically by the predominantly peribronchial and peribronchiolar infiltration in lymphoid hyperplasia as compared with the diffuse interstitial lymphocytic infiltration seen in LIP.

Diagnosis

Lymphoid hyperplasia (follicular bronchiolitis)

Suggested Readings

Do KH, Lee JS, Seo JB, et al: Pulmonary parenchymal involvement of low-grade lymphoproliferative disorders. J Comput Assist Tomogr 29:825-830, 2005.

Howling SJ, Hansell DM, Wells AU, et al: Follicular bronchiolitis: Thin-section CT and histologic findings. Radiology 212:637-642, 1999.

Travis WD, Galvin JR: Non-neoplastic pulmonary lymphoid lesions. Thorax 56:964-971, 2001.

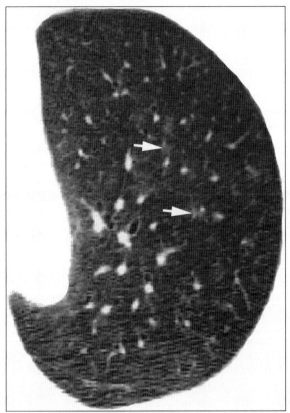

Figure 1. Lymphoid hyperplasia was diagnosed in a 40-year-old woman with scleroderma. CT image of the left upper lobe shows a few poorly defined, centrilobular nodules *(arrows)*.

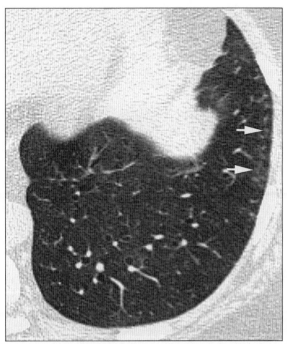

Figure 2. Lymphoid hyperplasia was diagnosed in a 63-year-old woman with scleroderma. CT image of the left lung base shows poorly defined, centrilobular nodules *(arrows)* located in the subpleural regions.

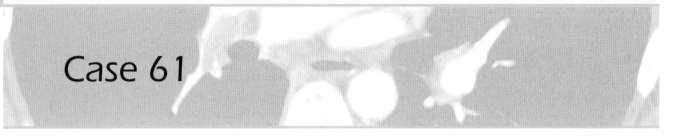

Case 61

DEMOGRAPHICS/CLINICAL HISTORY

A 42-year-old woman with a dry cough, dyspnea, and history of Sjögren syndrome, undergoing computed tomography (CT).

FINDINGS

CT image shows diffuse, ground-glass opacities associated with a few thin-walled cysts of various sizes (Fig. 1) and poorly defined centrilobular nodules (Fig. 2).

DISCUSSION

Definition/Background

Lymphoid interstitial pneumonia (i.e., lymphocytic interstitial pneumonia [LIP]) is an interstitial lung disease characterized by diffuse infiltration of alveolar septa by polyclonal lymphocytes. It is uncommon and usually occurs in patients (particularly in children) with underlying immunodeficiency such as acquired immunodeficiency syndrome (AIDS) or autoimmune disease, most commonly Sjögren syndrome. Idiopathic LIP is rare. Approximately 80% of patients have serum dysproteinemia, typically polyclonal hypergammaglobulinemia.

Characteristic Clinical Features

LIP has an insidious onset occurring over several years. Patients have cough and progressive dyspnea.

Characteristic Radiologic Findings

The radiographic findings are nonspecific. Typical CT manifestations include extensive, bilateral, ground-glass opacities that are associated with a few thin-walled cystic air spaces. Poorly defined centrilobular nodules and subpleural nodules may be seen. Slightly enlarged mediastinal lymph nodes are often present, particularly in patients with LIP associated with multicentric Castleman disease.

Less Common Radiologic Manifestations

CT may show large nodules, consolidation, reticulation, or honeycombing (i.e., end-stage disease with fibrosis). Patients may present with isolated ground-glass opacities or isolated cystic changes.

Differential Diagnosis

- Nonspecific interstitial pneumonia (NSIP)
- Hypersensitivity pneumonitis
- *Pneumocystis* pneumonia
- Lymphoma

Discussion

The main differential diagnosis of LIP histologically is lymphoma. This distinction usually requires immunohistochemical analysis to determine the presence of polyclonal lymphocytes. High-resolution CT findings that favor LIP over lymphoma include the presence of cysts and the lack of pleural effusion.

In patients with Sjögren syndrome, the main differential diagnosis of bilateral, ground-glass opacities includes NSIP, LIP, and opportunistic infection. Cystic air spaces in association with ground-glass opacities may be seen in LIP, hypersensitivity pneumonitis, Langerhans cell histiocytosis, and *Pneumocystis* pneumonia. Definitive diagnosis of LIP requires surgical biopsy.

Diagnosis

Lymphoid interstitial pneumonia

Suggested Readings

Cha SI, Fessler MB, Cool CD, et al: Lymphoid interstitial pneumonia: Clinical features, associations and prognosis. Eur Respir J 28: 364-369, 2006.

Johkoh T, Müller NL, Pickford HA, et al: Lymphocytic interstitial pneumonia: Thin-section CT findings in 22 patients. Radiology 212: 567-572, 1999.

Silva CI, Flint JD, Levy RD, Muller NL: Diffuse lung cysts in lymphoid interstitial pneumonia: High-resolution CT and pathologic findings. J Thorac Imaging 21:241-244, 2006.

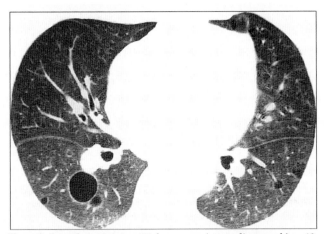

Figure 1. Lymphocytic interstitial pneumonia was diagnosed in a 42-year-old woman with Sjögren syndrome. CT image shows diffuse, ground-glass opacities associated with a few, thin-walled cysts of various sizes.

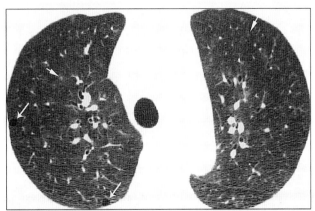

Figure 2. In the same patient, CT image shows patchy, ground-glass opacities; a few, thin-walled cysts *(long arrows)*, and poorly defined centrilobular nodules *(short arrows)*.

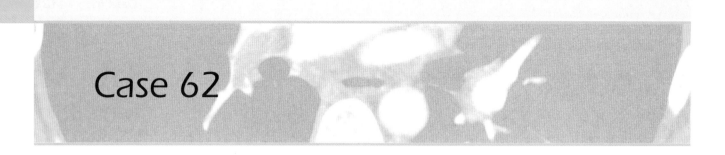

Case 62

DEMOGRAPHICS/CLINICAL HISTORY

A 58-year-old woman with a chronic cough, undergoing computed tomography (CT) for chronic consolidation.

FINDINGS

CT image shows left lower lobe consolidation with an air bronchogram and associated lung volume loss (Fig. 1). Contrast-enhanced CT (Fig. 2) image shows normal parenchymal enhancement within the area of consolidation and air bronchograms.

DISCUSSION

Definition/Background

Pulmonary mucosa-associated lymphoid tissue lymphoma (MALToma) is a low-grade, primary non-Hodgkin lymphoma that arises from bronchus-associated lymphoid tissue (BALT). Primary pulmonary lymphoma is defined as a clonal lymphoid proliferation affecting the lungs or bronchi in a patient with no detectable extrapulmonary involvement at diagnosis or in the subsequent 3 months. They are low-grade, B-cell lymphomas and typically grow very slowly over several years. The overall 5-year survival rate is 80% to 90%.

Characteristic Clinical Features

Patients with a solitary nodule or mass are usually asymptomatic. A large consolidation or diffuse lung involvement may lead to cough, dyspnea, or chest pain.

Characteristic Radiologic Findings

CT may show single or multiple nodules (Fig. 3) usually with spiculated margins, an air bronchogram, or an adjacent ground-glass opacity. Focal areas of consolidation can be seen (Figs. 1 and 2).

The diagnosis of primary pulmonary lymphoma should be considered in patients with single or multiple nodules or areas of consolidation that grow slowly over several months or years.

Less Common Radiologic Manifestations

Thickening of the interlobular septa and interlobar fissures.

Differential Diagnosis

- Adenocarcinoma
- Bronchiolitis obliterans organizing pneumonia (BOOP)
- Pneumonia
- Bronchioloalveolar carcinoma

Discussion

The main imaging differential diagnosis for primary pulmonary MALToma includes adenocarcinoma, indolent granulomatous infection, bacterial pneumonia, and BOOP, especially when abnormalities are bilateral. The definitive diagnosis requires surgical biopsy or resection.

Diagnosis

Pulmonary MALToma

Suggested Readings

Bae YA, Lee KS, Han J, et al: Marginal zone B-cell lymphoma of bronchus-associated lymphoid tissue: Imaging findings in 21 patients. Chest 133:433-440, 2008.

King LJ, Padley SP, Wotherspoon AC, Nicholson AG: Pulmonary MALT lymphoma: Imaging findings in 24 cases. Eur Radiol 10:1932-1938, 2000.

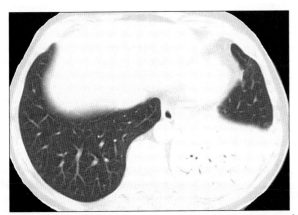

Figure 1. Pulmonary MALToma was diagnosed in a 58-year-old woman with chronic cough. CT shows left lower lobe consolidation with air bronchograms and associated lung volume loss.

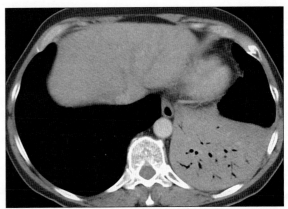

Figure 2. In the same patient, contrast-enhanced CT shows normal parenchymal enhancement within the area of consolidation and air bronchograms.

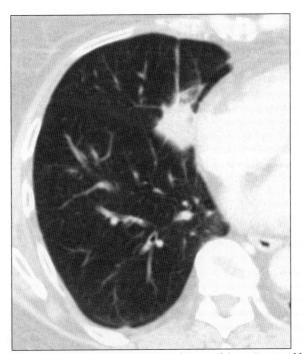

Figure 3. Pulmonary MALToma was diagnosed in a 53-year-old woman. CT targeted to the right lung shows a spiculated nodule in the right middle lobe.

Case 63

DEMOGRAPHICS/CLINICAL HISTORY

A 53-year-old man with cough, fever, and malaise, undergoing radiography and computed tomography (CT).

FINDINGS

Posteroanterior chest radiograph shows increased density and convexity in the right and left paratracheal regions that is consistent with lymphadenopathy and asymmetric bilateral hilar lymphadenopathy (Fig. 1). Contrast-enhanced CT at the level of the aortic arch shows enlarged, right and left paratracheal, right internal mammary, and bilateral axillary lymph nodes (Fig. 2). Contrast-enhanced CT at the level of the lower lobe bronchi shows enlarged, right internal mammary, subcarinal, and right and left hilar lymph nodes (Fig. 3).

DISCUSSION

Definition/Background

Non-Hodgkin lymphoma accounts for 70% to 75% of all cases of lymphoma, and approximately 40% to 50% of these patients have intrathoracic disease at initial presentation, compared with approximately 80% with Hodgkin lymphoma. Lymphoma constitutes about 20% of all mediastinal neoplasms in adults and 50% in children. Although lymphoma is one of the most common mediastinal tumors, it is uncommon for non-Hodgkin lymphoma or Hodgkin disease to be limited to the mediastinum at the time of diagnosis. Most are B-cell lymphomas. Non-Hodgkin lymphoma occurs most commonly in children and in middle-aged adults (median age, 55 years).

Characteristic Clinical Features

Patients may have systemic symptoms, including fever, night sweats, and weight loss, or have more localized complaints, such as cough and chest pain.

Characteristic Radiologic Findings

The characteristic manifestation is mediastinal lymphadenopathy, most commonly involving the prevascular and paratracheal nodes and typically associated with extrathoracic lymphadenopathy. Non-Hodgkin lymphoma tends to invade the pericardium, pleura, lungs, sternum, and chest wall.

Less Common Radiologic Manifestations

Primary mediastinal non-Hodgkin lymphoma occurs in some patients and may manifest as a large, anterior mediastinal mass.

Differential Diagnosis

- Hodgkin lymphoma
- Sarcoidosis
- Thymoma
- Germ cell tumor

Discussion

The differential diagnosis for an anterior mediastinal mass includes non-Hodgkin and Hodgkin lymphoma, thymic neoplasms, substernal thyroid mass, germ cell tumors, and mediastinal tuberculous lymphadenopathy. Findings that favor lymphoma include lobulation and involvement of contiguous lymph node groups in the paratracheal and hilar regions. Lymphoma may manifest with prevascular, paratracheal, and hilar lymphadenopathy and may resemble sarcoidosis. Unlike sarcoidosis, the hilar lymphadenopathy in lymphoma tends to be asymmetric, and the patients typically have systemic symptoms. Definitive diagnosis requires biopsy.

Diagnosis

Non-Hodgkin lymphoma

Suggested Readings

Ansell SM, Armitage J: Non-Hodgkin lymphoma: Diagnosis and treatment. Mayo Clin Proc 80:1087-1097, 2005.
Jhanwar YS, Straus DJ: The role of PET in lymphoma. J Nucl Med 47:1326-1334, 2006.
Brown LR, Aughenbaugh GL: Masses of the anterior mediastinum: CT and MR imaging. AJR Am J Roentgenol 157:1171-1180, 1991.

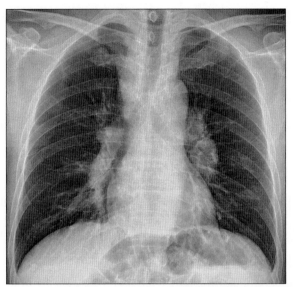

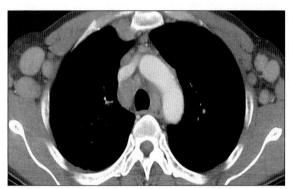

Figure 2. In the same patient, contrast-enhanced CT at the level of the aortic arch shows enlarged, right and left paratracheal, right internal mammary, and bilateral axillary lymph nodes.

Figure 1. Posteroanterior chest radiograph shows increased density and convexity in the right and left paratracheal regions consistent with lymphadenopathy and asymmetric bilateral hilar lymphadenopathy. The patient was a 53-year-old man with non-Hodgkin lymphoma.

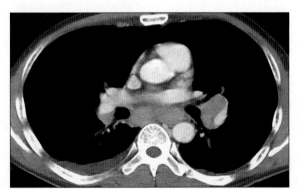

Figure 3. In the same patient, contrast-enhanced CT at the level of the lower lobe bronchi shows enlarged, right internal mammary, subcarinal, and right and left hilar lymph nodes. Small bilateral pleural effusions also can be seen.

Case 64

DEMOGRAPHICS/CLINICAL HISTORY

A 19-year-old woman with fever, night sweats, and chest pain, undergoing radiography and computed tomography (CT).

FINDINGS

Posteroanterior (Fig. 1) and lateral (Fig. 2) chest radiographs show a lobulated, anterior mediastinal mass. Contrast-enhanced CT images at the level of the bronchus intermedius (Fig. 3) and inferior pulmonary veins (Fig. 4) show large, lobulated, anterior mediastinal mass with heterogeneous enhancement and a cystic area.

DISCUSSION

Definition/Background

Hodgkin disease is a neoplasm of B lymphocytes characterized by the presence of Reed-Sternberg cells. The Reed-Sternberg cell is a large, bilobed cell with prominent eosinophilic nucleoli, perinucleolar clearing, a thickened nuclear membrane, and abundant cytoplasm. Hodgkin disease accounts for 25% to 30% of all lymphomas. It occurs in two main age groups: young adults and older adults, with a first peak in the third decade of life and a second peak after the age of 50. Unlike non-Hodgkin lymphoma, in which thoracic involvement is seen at presentation in only 40% to 50% of cases, thoracic involvement is common in Hodgkin lymphoma, occurring in approximately 80% of patients.

Characteristic Clinical Features

Patients may be asymptomatic or present with unexplained and persistent fever, night sweats, weight loss, cough, and chest pain.

Characteristic Radiologic Findings

Hodgkin lymphoma usually involves mainly the prevascular and paratracheal lymph nodes and may result in a discrete, anterosuperior mediastinal mass, which is usually lobulated and represents enlargement and coalescence of multiple lymph nodes. Paratracheal, subcarinal, and hilar lymphadenopathies usually are associated with enlarged anterior mediastinal nodes. Lymph nodes most commonly have homogeneous attenuation but may contain areas of low attenuation due to necrosis.

Less Common Radiologic Manifestations

Hodgkin disease may extend into the mediastimum and invade esophagus, superior vena cava, and pericardium. Pulmonary involvement results in multiple, irregularly marginated pulmonary nodules or masses. Imaging may show a pleural effusion.

Differential Diagnosis

- Non-Hodgkin lymphoma
- Thymoma
- Germ cell tumor
- Small cell carcinoma

Discussion

The differential diagnosis for an anterior mediastinal mass includes Hodgkin disease, non-Hodgkin lymphoma, thymic neoplasms, a substernal thyroid mass, germ cell tumors, and mediastinal tuberculous lymphadenopathy. Findings that favor Hodgkin disease include lobulation and involvement of contiguous lymph node groups in the paratracheal and hilar regions. Definitive diagnosis requires biopsy and histologic demonstration of characteristic Reed-Sternberg cells in association with an appropriate stromal or cellular background.

Diagnosis

Mediastinal Hodgkin lymphoma

Suggested Readings

Gossmann A, Eich HT, Engert A, et al: CT and MR imaging in Hodgkin's disease–present and future. Eur J Haematol Suppl 66:83-89, 2005.

Guermazi A, Brice P, de Kerviler EE, et al: Extranodal Hodgkin disease: Spectrum of disease. Radiographics 21:161-179, 2001.

Thomas RK, Re D, Zander T, et al: Epidemiology and etiology of Hodgkin's lymphoma. Ann Oncol 13(Suppl 4):147-152, 2002.

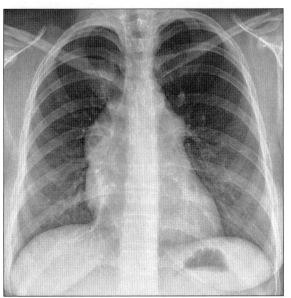

Figure 1. Posteroanterior chest radiograph shows widening of the mediastinum with a lobulated contour. The patient was a 19-year-old woman with primary mediastinal Hodgkin disease.

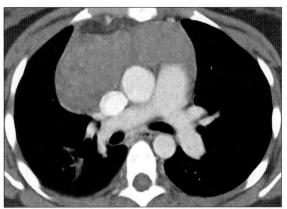

Figure 3. In the same patient, contrast-enhanced CT image at the level of the bronchus intermedius shows a large, lobulated, anterior mediastinal mass with heterogeneous enhancement.

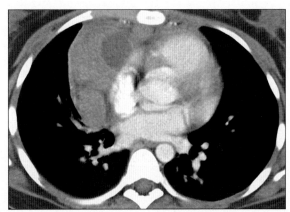

Figure 4. In the same patient, contrast-enhanced CT image at the level of the inferior pulmonary veins shows a large, lobulated, anterior mediastinal mass with heterogenous enhancement and a cystic area.

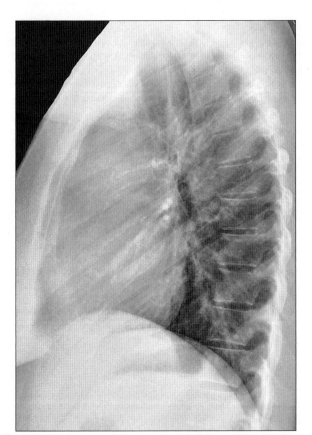

Figure 2. In the same patient, a lateral chest radiograph shows a poorly defined, anterior mediastinal mass and filling of the retrosternal air space.

Case 65

DEMOGRAPHICS/CLINICAL HISTORY

A 40-year-old man with AIDS, increasing cough, and low-grade fever, undergoing radiography and computed tomography (CT).

FINDINGS

Chest radiograph (Fig. 1) shows bilateral masses, one of which is cavitated. Notice the increased opacity in the right paratracheal region, which is consistent with lymph node enlargement. CT images (5-mm collimation) (Figs. 2 and 3) show bilateral nodules and masses of various sizes. The right upper lobe mass has cavitated.

DISCUSSION

Definition/Background

Lymphoma is the second most common malignancy in AIDS patients. AIDS-related lymphoma is typically a non-Hodgkin lymphoma that usually affects patients with CD4$^+$ levels of less than 100 cells/mm^3. It is most commonly extranodal, involving the lungs, central nervous system, gastrointestinal tract, liver, spleen, kidneys, and bone marrow.

Characteristic Clinical Features

The most common symptoms are cough, dyspnea, and pleuritic chest pain.

Characteristic Radiologic Findings

The most common findings on chest radiography consist of multiple pulmonary nodules or masses, areas of consolidation, and pleural effusions. CT usually shows well-circumscribed nodules or masses 0.5 to 5 cm in diameter. The nodules frequently contain air bronchograms and may be surrounded by a halo of ground-glass attenuation. Mediastinal or hilar lymphadenopathy is evident on CT in 30% to 50% of patients

Less Common Radiologic Manifestations

Imaging may show a mediastinal, chest wall, or pleural mass in the absence of pulmonary parenchymal disease. Patients may have a pleural effusion.

Differential Diagnosis

- Kaposi sarcoma
- Lung cancer
- Pulmonary infection

Discussion

Intrathoracic lymphoma in patients with AIDS is usually extranodal, manifesting most commonly as smoothly marginated nodules up to 5 cm in diameter. Lung cancer most commonly manifests as a focal nodule or mass that has irregular margins. The presence of septal lines and irregularly shaped nodules along the peribronchovascular bundles in patients with AIDS strongly suggests Kaposi sarcoma. A very helpful feature clinically is the presence of characteristic cutaneous lesions in patients with pulmonary Kaposi sarcoma.

Diagnosis

Lymphoma in an AIDS patient

Suggested Readings

Boiselle, PM, Aviram G, Fishman JE: Update on lung disease in AIDS. Semin Roentgenol 37:54-71, 2002.

Kanmogne GD: Noninfectious pulmonary complications of HIV/AIDS. Curr Opin Pulm Med 11:208-212, 2005.

Marchiori E, Müller NL, Soares Souza A Jr, et al: Pulmonary disease in patients with AIDS: High-resolution CT and pathologic findings. AJR Am J Roentgenol 184:757-764, 2005.

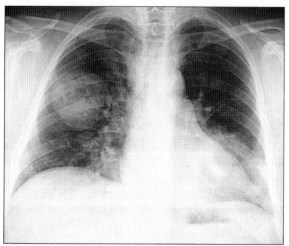

Figure 1. Chest radiograph shows bilateral masses, one of which is cavitated. Noticed the increased opacity in the right paratracheal region, which is consistent with lymph node enlargement. The patient was a 40-year-old man with AIDS-related lymphoma.

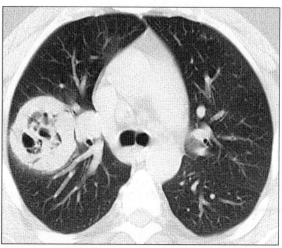

Figure 2. In the same patient, CT image (5-mm collimation) at the level of the main bronchi shows a cavitating, right upper lobe mass and adjacent nodule.

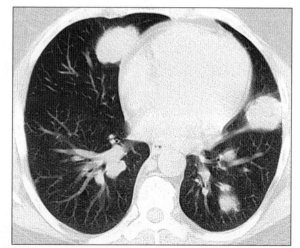

Figure 3. CT image (5-mm collimation) at the level of the lower lung zones shows several bilateral nodules of various sizes in a 40-year-old man with AIDS-related lymphoma.

Case 66

DEMOGRAPHICS/CLINICAL HISTORY

A 31-year-old man with acquired immunodeficiency syndrome (AIDS), progressive shortness of breath, and oral mucosal lesions, undergoing computed tomography (CT)

FINDINGS

CT images show poorly defined peribronchovascular nodules with spiculated margins (i.e., flamed-shaped lesions), few septal lines (Figs. 1 and 2), and perihilar ground-glass opacities (Fig. 2).

DISCUSSION

Definition/Background

Kaposi sarcoma (KS) is a mesenchymal tumor that involves the blood and lymphatic vessels and that affects mainly the skin, lymph nodes, gastrointestinal tract, and lungs. It is seen most commonly in homosexual men with AIDS, particularly patients with advanced immunosuppression whose CD4 cell count is below 100 cells/mm^3. Pulmonary KS usually is associated with cutaneous involvement.

Characteristic Clinical Features

The most common presenting symptoms of pulmonary KS are cough and dyspnea. Less commonly, patients may present with hemoptysis.

Characteristic Radiologic Findings

The chest radiographic manifestations of KS include thickening of the peribronchovascular bundles, peribronchial cuffing (typically in the perihilar regions), septal lines, and reticulonodular opacities. CT shows bilateral and symmetric, ill-defined nodules in a peribronchovascular distribution (i.e., flame-shaped lesions) and interlobular septal thickening. Other common findings include hilar or mediastinal lymphadenopathy and pleural effusion.

Less Common Radiologic Manifestations

Less common features include lytic lesions of the sternum and thoracic spine and soft tissue masses or infiltration of the skin and subcutaneous fat.

Differential Diagnosis

- Lymphoma
- Lymphangitic carcinomatosis

Discussion

The presence of septal lines and irregularly shaped nodules along the peribronchovascular bundles in patients with AIDS suggests KS. A clinically helpful feature is the presence of characteristic cutaneous lesions in patients with pulmonary KS. Intrathoracic lymphoma in patients with AIDS is usually extranodal, manifesting most commonly as smoothly marginated nodules up to 5 cm in diameter. Pulmonary carcinoma most commonly manifests as a focal nodule or mass.

Diagnosis

Kaposi sarcoma in an AIDS patient

Suggested Readings

Boiselle, PM, Aviram G, Fishman JE: Update on lung disease in AIDS. Semin Roentgenol 37:54-71, 2002.

Kanmogne GD: Noninfectious pulmonary complications of HIV/AIDS. Curr Opin Pulm Med 11:208-212, 2005.

Restrepo CS, Martínez S, Lemos JA, et al: Imaging manifestations of Kaposi sarcoma. Radiographics 26:1169-1185, 2006.

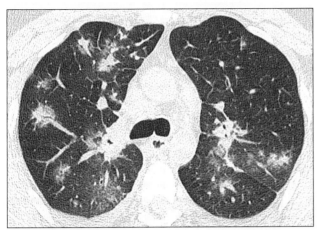

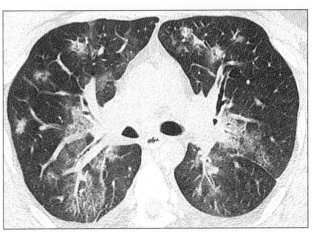

Figure 1. A 31-year-old man with AIDS, progressive shortness of breath, and oral mucosal lesions has Kaposi sarcoma. CT image shows poorly defined nodules (i.e., flamed-shaped lesions) in a peribronchovascular distribution and a few septal lines.

Figure 2. CT image at the level of the bronchus intermedius in the same patient shows poorly defined, spiculated, peribronchovascular nodules and perihilar ground-glass opacities.

Case 67

DEMOGRAPHICS/CLINICAL HISTORY

A 37-year-old man with acute-onset fever and cough, undergoing radiography.

FINDINGS

Posteroanterior (Fig. 1) and lateral (Fig. 2) chest radiographs show consolidation in the right middle lobe with associated obscuration of the right heart border. Notice that the consolidation is limited to one lobe and crosses segmental boundaries, a characteristic feature of lobar pneumonia.

DISCUSSION

Definition/Background

Lobar pneumonia is characterized histologically by filling of alveolar air spaces by an exudate of edema fluid and neutrophils. Radiologically, the consolidation tends to occur initially in the periphery of the lung beneath visceral pleura and usually abuts an interlobar fissure. The consolidation spreads centrally across segmental boundaries and may eventually involve the entire lobe. Most cases of lobar pneumonia are community acquired and caused by *Streptococcus pneumoniae*. Other causes include *Klebsiella pneumoniae, Legionella pneumophila, Haemophilus influenzae,* and *Mycobacterium tuberculosis.*

Characteristic Clinical Features

Patients may have fever, cough, and purulent sputum. Pleuritic chest pain is relatively common, and hemoptysis may occur. Signs and symptoms of pneumonia may be milder or even absent in the elderly.

Characteristic Radiologic Findings

Consolidation tends to occur initially in the periphery of the lung beneath visceral pleura and usually abuts an interlobar fissure. The consolidation is homogeneous, and as it progresses, it typically involves adjacent segments of the lobe. In severe cases, it may involve the entire lobe and spread to the remaining lungs. The bronchi usually remain patent, resulting in air bronchograms within areas of consolidation

Less Common Radiologic Manifestations

Cavitation may occur, particularly in *K. pneumoniae* pneumonia and in tuberculosis. A small pleural effusion is relatively common. Large effusions, empyema, and bronchopleural fistula may occur.

Differential Diagnosis

- Lobar atelectasis
- Obstructive pneumonitis

Discussion

The lung volume in lobar pneumonia is usually preserved, whereas in lobar atelectasis it is decreased. Obstructive pneumonitis distal to obstruction of a lobar bronchus by a tumor or foreign body may mimic lobar pneumonia. The main differentiating feature on the radiograph is the absence of air bronchograms in obstructive pneumonitis. The main role of imaging in the diagnosis of pneumonia is identification of parenchymal abnormalities consistent with the clinical diagnosis. The radiography and CT are of limited value in establishing the specific cause of bacterial pneumonias. The cause can be determined from sputum, bronchoscopy specimens, or blood culture.

Diagnosis

Lobar pneumonia

Suggested Readings

Marrie TJ: Pneumococcal pneumonia: Epidemiology and clinical features. Semin Respir Infect 14:227-236, 1999.

Waite S, Jeudy J, White CS: Acute lung infections in normal and immunocompromised hosts. Radiol Clin North Am 44:295-315, ix, 2006.

Washington L, Palacio D: Imaging of bacterial pulmonary infection in the immunocompetent patient. Semin Roentgenol 42:122-145, 2007.

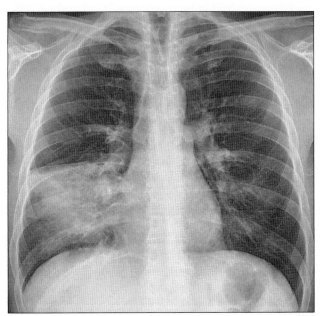

Figure 1. Posteroanterior chest radiograph shows a consolidation in the right lower lung zone associated with obscuration of the right heart border that is consistent with consolidation in the right middle lobe. The patient was a 37-year-old man with acute lobar pneumonia.

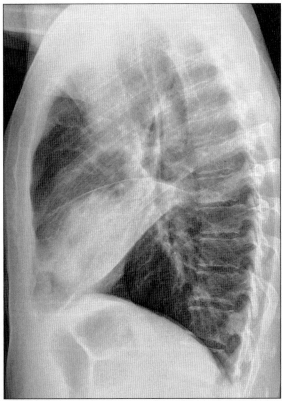

Figure 2. In the same patient, the lateral chest radiograph shows consolidation in the right middle lobe. Notice that the consolidation is limited to one lobe and crosses segmental boundaries, a characteristic feature of lobar pneumonia.

Case 68

DEMOGRAPHICS/CLINICAL HISTORY

A 35-year-old man who is an intravenous drug user with acute-onset fever, undergoing computed tomography (CT).

FINDINGS

Cross-sectional CT (Fig. 1) and coronal, reformatted, high-resolution CT images (Fig. 2) show several bilateral, 1- to 3-cm-diameter, cavitating nodules and peripheral, wedge-shaped areas of consolidation.

DISCUSSION

Definition/Background

Radiologically visible septic emboli represent lung abscesses from systemic spread of infection. The infection can originate in various sites, including cardiac valves (i.e., endocarditis), peripheral veins (i.e., thrombophlebitis), and infected venous catheters or pacemaker wires. Common organisms include *Staphylococcus aureus*, *Streptococcus viridans*, gram-negative bacteria, and *Aspergillus*.

Characteristic Clinical Features

Patients usually have fever, cough, and purulent sputum. Pleuritic chest pain may occur.

Characteristic Radiologic Findings

Septic embolism is characterized radiologically by the presence of nodules that usually are 1 to 3 cm in diameter and that are frequently cavitated. The nodules tend to be most numerous in the lower lobes. Occlusion of pulmonary arteries by septic emboli or thrombus may result in hemorrhage or infarction and result in pleural-based, wedge shaped consolidation and ground-glass opacities, which may also cavitate.

Less Common Radiologic Manifestations

Imaging may show pulmonary consolidation, pleural effusion, empyema, bronchopleural fistula, and hilar and mediastinal lymphadenopathy.

Differential Diagnosis

- Pulmonary metastases
- Wegener granulomatosis
- Rheumatoid nodules
- Angioinvasive aspergillosis
- Candidiasis

Discussion

The differential diagnosis of multiple nodules greater than 1 cm in diameter is broad and includes congenital abnormalities (e.g., arteriovenous malformations), infection (e.g., multiple granulomas, septic embolism), inflammatory processes (e.g., Wegener granulomatosis, rheumatoid nodules), and pulmonary metastases. However, more than 95% of cases represent pulmonary metastases or infection. In immunocompromised patients, multiple nodules due to infection may be seen in septic embolism, angioinvasive aspergillosis, candidiasis, and cytomegalovirus pneumonia. The differential diagnosis is based on the clinical and radiologic findings and on blood culture results.

Diagnosis

Septic embolism

Suggested Readings

Kwon WJ, Jeong YJ, Kim KI, et al: Computed tomographic features of pulmonary septic emboli: Comparison of causative microorganisms. J Comput Assist Tomogr 31:390-394, 2007.

Dodd JD, Souza CA, Müller NL: High-resolution MDCT of pulmonary septic embolism: Evaluation of the feeding vessel sign. AJR Am J Roentgenol 187:623-629, 2006.

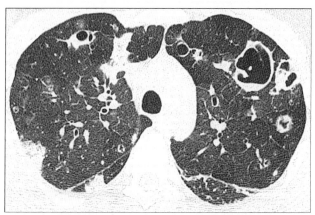

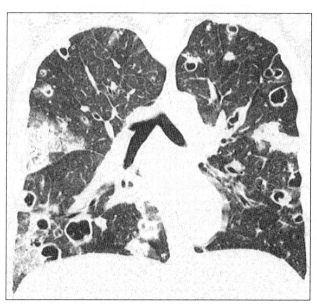

Figure 1. Axial, high-resolution CT shows several bilateral, 1- to 3-cm-diameter, cavitating nodules and peripheral, wedge-shaped areas of consolidation. The 35-year-old man was an intravenous drug abuser with septic embolism due to *Staphylococcus aureus*.

Figure 2. Coronal, reformatted CT image shows several 1- to 3-cm-diameter, cavitating nodules in all lobes and peripheral, wedge-shaped areas of consolidation in a 35-year-old, drug-abusing patient with septic embolism due to *Staphylococcus aureus*.

Case 69

DEMOGRAPHICS/CLINICAL HISTORY

A 36-year-old woman with acute-onset fever and productive cough, undergoing radiography.

FINDINGS

Posteroanterior chest radiograph shows a patchy consolidation in the left upper and lower lobes (Fig. 1). Notice the inhomogeneous increased opacity of the left heart as compared with the region of the right atrium, which is consistent with consolidation in the retrocardiac region of the left lower lobe. In another patient with acute myelogenous leukemia and *Streptococcus pneumoniae* bronchopneumonia, the chest radiograph shows poorly defined, nodular opacities and small foci of consolidation in the right lung (Fig 2), and coronal, reformatted CT shows centrilobular nodular opacities and small foci of consolidation in the right upper and middle lobes and, to a lesser extent, the left upper lobe (Fig. 3).

DISCUSSION

Definition/Background

Bronchopneumonia is characterized histologically by the production of a relatively small amount of fluid and the rapid exudation of numerous polymorphonuclear leukocytes, typically in relation to small membranous and respiratory bronchioles. The consolidation initially involves mainly the peribronchiolar region, but it gradually extends to involve entire lobules, subsegments, and segments. It usually involves several lobes. It may be caused by viral, bacterial, or fungal organisms.

Characteristic Clinical Features

Patients can have fever, cough, and purulent sputum. Pleuritic chest pain is relatively common, and hemoptysis may occur. Signs and symptoms of pneumonia may be milder or even absent in the elderly.

Characteristic Radiologic Findings

Bronchopneumonia (i.e., lobular pneumonia) typically manifests with poorly defined focal nodular opacities measuring 5 to 10 mm in diameter (air-space nodules) and patchy areas of consolidation involving one or more segments of a single lobe or multiple lobes. Confluence of pneumonia in adjacent lobules and segments may result in a pattern simulating lobar pneumonia; differentiation from the latter can be made in most cases by the presence of segmental or lobular distribution of the abnormalities in other areas.

Less Common Radiologic Manifestations

Imaging may show cavitation, pleural effusion, empyema, bronchopleural fistula, and hilar and mediastinal lymphadenopathy. Cavitation is common, particularly in patients with extensive consolidation.

Differential Diagnosis

- Aspiration
- Pulmonary hemorrhage
- Lung contusion

Discussion

A radiologic pattern identical to that of bronchopneumonia, with patchy distribution of consolidation, may be seen in aspiration, pulmonary hemorrhage, and lung contusion. The main role of imaging in the diagnosis of bronchopneumonia is to confirm the presence of parenchymal abnormalities consistent with the clinical diagnosis. The radiograph and CT scan are of limited value in establishing the specific cause of bronchopneumonia. The diagnosis is based on clinical features, and the specific cause can be determined from sputum, bronchoscopy specimens, blood culture, or serology.

Diagnosis

Bronchopneumonia

Suggested Readings

Waite S, Jeudy J, White CS: Acute lung infections in normal and immunocompromised hosts. Radiol Clin North Am 44:295-315, ix, 2006.

Washington L, Palacio D: Imaging of bacterial pulmonary infection in the immunocompetent patient. Semin Roentgenol 42:122-145, 2007.

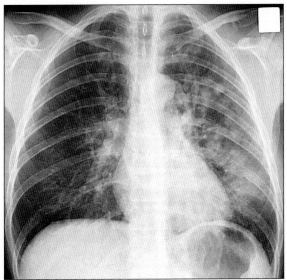

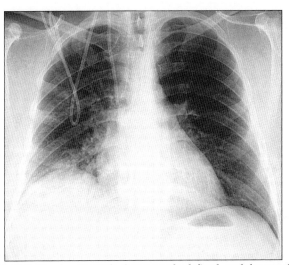

Figure 1. Posteroanterior chest radiograph shows patchy consolidation in the left upper and lower lobes. Notice the inhomogeneous increased opacity of the left heart compared with the region of the right atrium, which is consistent with consolidation in the retrocardiac region of the left lower lobe. The patient was a 36-year-old woman with bronchopneumonia.

Figure 2. Chest radiograph shows poorly defined, nodular opacities and small foci of consolidation in the right lung of a 29-year-old man with acute myelogenous leukemia and *S. pneumoniae* bronchopneumonia. A central venous line is in place.

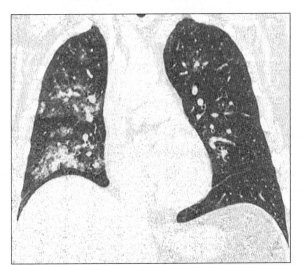

Figure 3. Coronal, reformatted CT shows centrilobular nodular opacities and small foci of consolidation in the right upper and middle lobes and, to a lesser extent, the left upper lobe of a 29-year-old man with acute myelogenous leukemia and *S. pneumoniae* bronchopneumonia.

Case 70

DEMOGRAPHICS/CLINICAL HISTORY

A 23-year-old man with low-grade fever, dry cough, and stridor, undergoing radiography and computed tomography (CT).

FINDINGS

Anteroposterior chest radiograph (Fig. 1) shows extensive right paratracheal lymphadenopathy and poorly defined right upper lobe consolidation. Contrast-enhanced CT (Fig. 2) shows markedly enlarged paratracheal lymph nodes with low-attenuation centers, which is consistent with necrosis and rim enhancement.

DISCUSSION

Definition/Background

Primary tuberculosis is characterized by a pulmonary parenchymal focus of infection that is typically associated with regional hilar or mediastinal lymphadenopathy and that develops after initial exposure to tuberculosis. Primary tuberculosis occurs mainly in children but is being seen with increasing frequency in adults. Tuberculosis is transmitted from person to person by droplet nuclei containing the organism, and it is spread mainly by coughing

Characteristic Clinical Features

Patients with primary pulmonary tuberculosis usually are asymptomatic. Symptoms can include mild or progressive dry cough, low-grade fever, fatigue, weight loss, and night sweats.

Characteristic Radiologic Findings

The most common manifestations of primary pulmonary tuberculosis in children consist of unilateral hilar or paratracheal lymph node enlargement, which is seen in 90% to 95% of cases, and focal air-space consolidation, which is evident radiographically in approximately 70% of cases. Compared with children, adults with primary tuberculosis are less likely to have lymph node enlargement (10% to 30% of patients) and more likely to have parenchymal consolidation (approximately 90% of patients). The consolidation shows no predilection for any particular lung zone. The enlarged lymph nodes in tuberculosis frequently have diffuse, low-attenuation areas or a central

area of low attenuation with rim enhancement on CT after intravenous administration of contrast.

Less Common Radiologic Manifestations

Unilateral pleural effusion is seen in 5% to 10% of children and 30% to 40% of adults with primary tuberculosis. Occasionally, patients develop disseminated disease (i.e., miliary tuberculosis), which manifests as 1- to 3-mm-diameter nodules that are diffusely distributed throughout the lungs. Miliary tuberculosis is much more common in immunocompromised patients than in normal hosts.

Differential Diagnosis

- Pneumonia due to other organisms
- Lung cancer
- Lymphoma

Discussion

The differential diagnosis of primary tuberculosis manifesting as focal consolidation includes bacterial and fungal pneumonia. In tuberculosis, the consolidation usually is associated with mediastinal or hilar lymph node enlargement. Mediastinal or hilar lymph node enlargement with a central area of low attenuation and peripheral rim enhancement after intravenous administration of contrast may also occur in lymphoma, metastases (particularly from testicular carcinoma), small cell lung cancer, and benign conditions such as Whipple and Crohn diseases. The differential diagnosis is based on the presence of a focal area of parenchymal consolidation in primary tuberculosis, history of exposure to tuberculosis, and a positive skin test result or culture.

Diagnosis

Primary tuberculosis

Suggested Readings

De Backer AI, Mortelé KJ, De Keulenaer BL, Parizel PM: Tuberculosis: Epidemiology, manifestations, and the value of medical imaging in diagnosis. JBR-BTR 89:243-250, 2006.

Lee KS, Song KS, Lim TH, et al: Adult-onset pulmonary tuberculosis: Findings on chest radiographs and CT scans. AJR Am J Roentgenol 160:753-758, 1993.

Leung AN: Pulmonary tuberculosis: The essentials. Radiology 210:307-322, 1999.

Leung AN, Müller NL, Pineda PR, FitzGerald JM: Primary tuberculosis in childhood: Radiographic manifestations. Radiology 182:87-89, 1992.

Powell DA, Hunt WG: Tuberculosis in children: An update. Adv Pediatr 53:279-322, 2006.

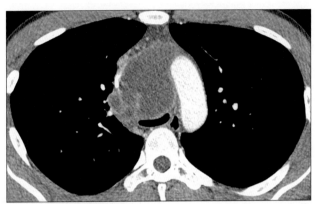

Figure 2. In the same patient, contrast-enhanced CT shows markedly enlarged paratracheal lymph nodes with low-attenuation centers, which is consistent with necrosis and rim enhancement.

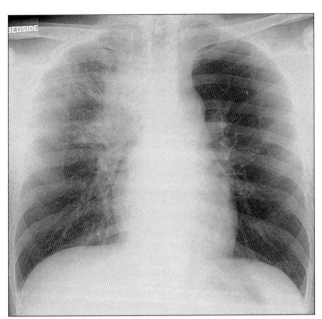

Figure 1. Anteroposterior chest radiograph shows extensive right paratracheal lymphadenopathy and poorly defined right upper lobe consolidation. The patient was a 23-year-old man with primary tuberculosis.

Case 71

DEMOGRAPHICS/CLINICAL HISTORY

An 82-year-old man with low-grade fever and cough, undergoing radiography and high-resolution computed tomography (CT).

FINDINGS

Posteroanterior chest radiograph shows an inhomogeneous, asymmetric, bilateral consolidation that is most severe in the right upper lobe and small, nodular opacities mainly in the right lower lung zone (Fig. 1). High-resolution CT at the level of the right upper lobe bronchus shows a large cavity in the superior segment of the right lower lobe, small nodules and a tree-in-bud pattern in the right upper lobe, and a lobular ground-glass opacity in the left upper lobe (Fig. 2). High-resolution CT at the level of the lower lung zones shows centrilobular nodules and a tree-in-bud pattern mainly in the right middle and lower lobes, bronchiectasis, and bronchial wall thickening (Fig. 3). In another patient, chest radiograph (Fig.2) shows an inhomogeneous consolidation; the small, nodular and linear opacities in the right upper lobe involve mainly the apical segment. Notice the focal lucency within the consolidation, which suggests cavitation.

DISCUSSION

Definition/Background

Tuberculosis is a chronic, contagious infection caused by Mycobacterium tuberculosis. Post-primary tuberculosis may result from reactivation of a previous focus of tuberculosis or from reinfection. Reactivation of dormant bacilli may result from malnutrition or impairment of immunity. It has been estimated that there were approximately 9 million new cases of tuberculosis worldwide and approximately 1.5 million deaths from tuberculosis in 2006.

Characteristic Clinical Features

Patients may be asymptomatic or present with mild or progressive dry or productive cough, fever, night sweats, fatigue, and weight loss.

Characteristic Radiologic Findings

The most common radiographic manifestation of post-primary tuberculosis is a focal or patchy, heterogeneous consolidation involving the apical and posterior segments of the upper lobes and the superior segments of the lower lobes. Other common findings are small nodules and linear opacities (i.e., fibronodular pattern of tuberculosis) and single or multiple cavities. The most common CT findings are centrilobular nodules and branching, linear and nodular opacities (i.e., tree-in-bud pattern, which is a characteristic finding of endobronchial spread); patchy or lobular areas of consolidation; and cavitation.

Less Common Radiologic Manifestations

Imaging may show a single nodule (i.e., tuberculoma), miliary nodules, hilar and mediastinal lymphadenopathy, or pleural effusion. Radiographic results may be normal, particularly for severely immunocompromised patients and for patients with miliary tuberculosis.

Differential Diagnosis

- Bacterial pneumonia
- Fungal infection, particularly histoplasmosis
- Carcinoma
- Nontuberculosis mycobacterial infection

Discussion

The differential diagnosis of tuberculosis manifesting as an upper lobe cavitary lesion includes nontuberculous mycobacterial infection, fungal infection, cavitary carcinoma, and bacterial pneumonia. Small (< 10 mm in diameter) centrilobular nodules or tree-in-bud opacities on CT may be observed in bacterial, fungal, or viral bronchiolitis and bronchopneumonia and nontuberculous mycobacterial infection. Miliary nodules may be seen in tuberculosis, miliary fungal infection, and miliary metastases. Definitive diagnosis requires culture of *M. tuberculosis*.

Diagnosis

Post-Primary tuberculosis

Suggested Readings

Kim HY, Song KS, Goo JM, et al: Thoracic sequelae and complications of tuberculosis. Radiographics 21:839-858, 2001:discussion 859-860, 2001.

Krysl J, Korzeniewska-Koesela M, Müller NL, FitzGerald JM: Radiologic features of pulmonary tuberculosis: An assessment of 188 cases. Can Assoc Radiol J 45:101-107, 1994.

Lee JY, Lee KS, Jung KJ, et al: Pulmonary tuberculosis: CT and pathologic correlation. J Comput Assist Tomogr 24:691-698, 2000.

Leung AN: Pulmonary tuberculosis: The essentials. Radiology 210:307-322, 1999.

Maartens G, Wilkinson RJ: Tuberculosis. Lancet 370:2030-2043, 2007.

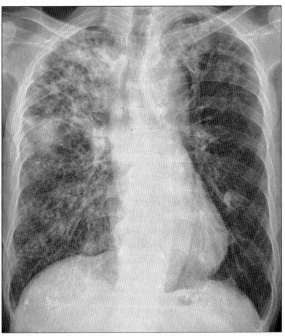

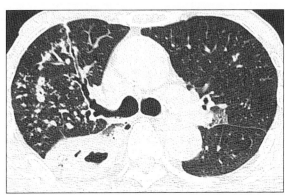

Figure 2. In an 82-year-old man with reactivation tuberculosis, high-resolution CT at the level of the right upper lobe bronchus shows a large cavity in the superior segment of the right lower lobe, small nodules and a tree-in-bud pattern in the right upper lobe, and a lobular ground-glass opacity in the left upper lobe.

Figure 1. Posteroanterior chest radiograph shows an inhomogeneous, asymmetric, bilateral consolidation that is most severe in the right upper lobe and shows small, nodular opacities mainly in the right lower lung zone. The patient was an 82-year-old man with reactivation tuberculosis.

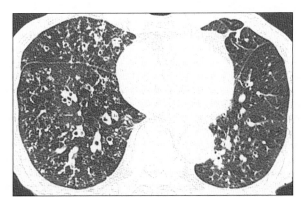

Figure 3. In the same 82-year-old patient, high-resolution CT at the level of the lower lung zones shows centrilobular nodules and a tree-in-bud pattern mainly in the right middle and lower lobes, bronchiectasis, and bronchial wall thickening.

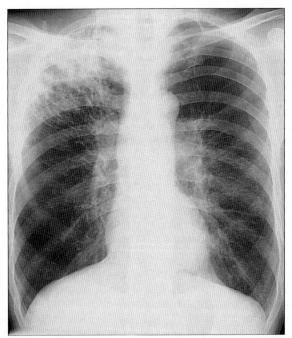

Figure 4. Chest radiograph shows an inhomogeneous consolidation and small nodular and linear opacities in the right upper lobe involving mainly the apical segment. Notice the focal lucency within the consolidation, which suggests of cavitation. The patient was a 52-year-old man with reactivation tuberculosis.

Case 72

DEMOGRAPHICS/CLINICAL HISTORY

A 39-year-old woman with AIDS, cough, and fever.

FINDINGS

Contrast-enhanced CT images at the level of great vessels (Fig. 1) and aortic arch (Fig. 2) demonstrate enlarged right paratracheal necrotic lymph nodes.

DISCUSSION

Definition/Background

HIV-infected individuals have 50- to 200-fold increased risk of tuberculosis compared to general population. Approximately one-third of nearly 40 million people living with HIV/AIDS worldwide are co-infected with TB. The diagnosis of TB in patients with AIDS can be difficult, requiring multiple sputum samples and polymerase-chain reaction testing to identify *Mycobacterium tuberculosis.*

Characteristic Clinical Features

Symptoms include cough, fever, hemoptysis, night sweats, and weight loss.

Characteristic Radiologic Findings

The radiologic findings are influenced by the degree of immune compromise. The pattern is typically that of postprimary TB (upper lobe consolidation, nodules, cavitation) in early HIV infection (moderate-to-good immune function) and that of primary TB (hilar and mediastinal lymphadenopathy, usually with decreased attenuation on CT) (Figs. 1 and 2), in markedly immunocompromised patients (CD 4 cell count < 200 cells/ mm^3). Immune reconstitution syndrome in patients with AIDS and tuberculosis is characterized by marked increase in the lymphadenopathy.

Less Common Radiologic Manifestations

Pleural effusion, miliary nodules. Severely immunocompromised patients with TB are more likely to have disseminated disease and miliary nodules or normal radiographs.

Differential Diagnosis

- Bacterial pneumonia
- Lymphoma
- Kaposi sarcoma
- Carcinoma
- Fungal infection

Discussion

TB presenting with focal upper lobe consolidation may mimic a bacterial or fungal pneumonia. In patients who present mainly with hilar or mediastinal lymphadenopathy, the differential diagnosis includes lymphoma, Kaposi sarcoma, and carcinoma. Although the presence of unilateral hilar or mediastinal nodes with decreased attenuation and rim enhancement on CT in patients with AIDS is suggestive of TB, definitive diagnosis requires identification or culture of *M. tuberculosis* from sputum, bronchoalveolar lavage, or biopsy specimens.

Diagnosis

Tuberculosis in patient with AIDS

Suggested Readings

Boiselle PM, Aviram G, Fishman JE: Update on lung disease in AIDS. Semin Roentgenol 37:54-71, 2002.

Castaner E, et al: Radiologic approach to the diagnosis of infectious pulmonary diseases in patients infected with the human immunodeficiency virus. Eur J Radiol 51:114-129, 2004.

Haramati LB, Jenny-Avital ER, Alterman DD: Thoracic manifestations of immune restoration syndromes in AIDS. Journal of Thoracic Imaging 22:213-220, 2007.

Lazarous DG, O'Donnell AE: Pulmonary infections in the HIV-infected patient in the era of highly active antiretroviral therapy: An update. Current Infectious Disease Reports 9:228-232, 2007.

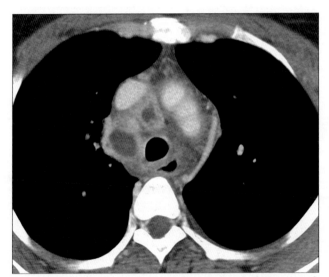

Figure 1. Contrast-enhanced CT image at the level of great vessels demonstrates enlarged right paratracheal necrotic lymph nodes. The patient was a 39-year-old woman with AIDS and tuberculosis.

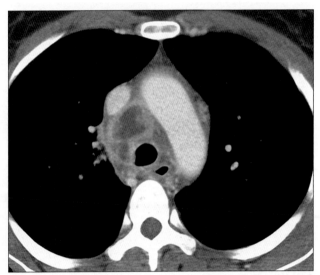

Figure 2. Contrast-enhanced CT image at the level of aortic arch demonstrates enlarged necrotic right paratracheal lymph node. The patient was a 39-year-old woman with AIDS and tuberculosis.

Case 73

DEMOGRAPHICS/CLINICAL HISTORY

A 41-year-old man with AIDS on highly active antiretroviral therapy (HAART) with cough, fever, and chills, undergoing computed tomography (CT).

FINDINGS

Contrast-enhanced CT images using lung (Fig. 1) and soft tissue (Fig. 2) windows show extensive consolidation in the left upper lobe; numerous bilateral, small nodular and linear opacities; and extensive mediastinal lymph node enlargement. The enlarged nodes have areas of low attenuation that suggest necrosis (Fig. 2).

DISCUSSION

Definition/Background

Immune restoration syndromes (IRS), also known as immune reconstitution inflammatory syndrome (IRIS), are a group of illnesses characterized by an exaggerated inflammatory response in patients with late-stage AIDS who start HAART. This response results in transient clinical worsening rather than improvement on therapy, which is associated with a recognized or occult infection. IRIS associated with tuberculosis typically manifests with marked mediastinal lymphadenopathy and worsening of pulmonary parenchymal abnormalities.

Characteristic Clinical Features

Patients may have fever, cough, malaise, and in severe cases, progressive shortness of breath.

Characteristic Radiologic Findings

Tuberculosis-related IRIS typically manifests with new or increased mediastinal lymph node enlargement and new or increased lung parenchymal abnormalities, including consolidation, nodules, or micronodules. The lymphadenopathy commonly has a low-attenuation center and rim enhancement on contrast-enhanced CT.

Less Common Radiologic Manifestations

Imaging may show pleural effusion. Occasionally, lymph node enlargement may be severe enough to result in narrowing of the trachea.

Differential Diagnosis

- Tuberculosis
- Nontuberculous mycobacterial infection
- Lymphoma

Discussion

The diagnosis of tuberculosis-related IRIS is based on the clinical history of recent-onset of treatment with HAART, clinical deterioration with new or worse symptoms, and identification or culture of *Mycobacterium tuberculosis* from sputum, bronchoalveolar lavage fluid, or biopsy specimens. IRIS usually begins within 6 weeks of HAART initiation.

Diagnosis

Immune reconstitution syndrome in a patient with tuberculosis and AIDS

Suggested Readings

Haramati LB, Jenny-Avital ER, Alterman DD: Thoracic manifestations of immune restoration syndromes in AIDS. J Thorac Imaging 22:213-220, 2007.
Hirsch HH, Kaufmann G, Sendi P, Battegay M: Immune reconstitution in HIV-infected patients. Clin Infect Dis 38:1159-1166, 2004.
Lazarous DG, O'donnell AE: Pulmonary infections in the HIV-infected patient in the era of highly active antiretroviral therapy: An update. Curr Infect Dis Rep 9:228-232, 2007.

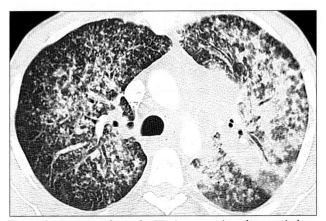

Figure 1. Contrast-enhanced CT image using lung windows shows extensive consolidation in the left upper lobe; numerous, bilateral, small nodular and linear opacities; and widening of the mediastinum due to lymph node enlargement. The patient was a 41-year-old man with AIDS, tuberculosis, and immune reconstitution syndrome.

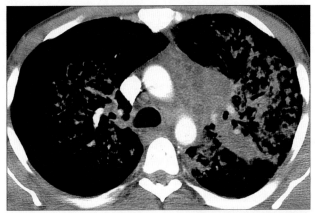

Figure 2. In the same patient, contrast-enhanced CT image using soft tissue windows shows extensive mediastinal lymph node enlargement. The enlarged nodes have areas of low attenuation that suggest necrosis

Case 74

DEMOGRAPHICS/CLINICAL HISTORY

A 67-year-old woman with chronic cough, undergoing computed tomography (CT).

FINDINGS

High-resolution CT (Fig. 1) at the level of the proximal right middle and lower lobe bronchi shows right middle lobe bronchiectasis, ground-glass opacities, centrilobular nodules, and branching opacities (i.e., tree-in-bud pattern). Notice the nodules and a few linear opacities in the left lower and upper lobes and the left lower lobe bronchiectasis. High-resolution CT (Fig. 2) at the level of the basal segmental bronchi shows bronchiectasis in the right middle lobe, lingula, and left lower lobe; nodules in the right middle lobe, lingula, and left lower lobe; and atelectasis and focal consolidation in the lingula.

DISCUSSION

Definition/Background

Pulmonary infection by *Mycobacterium avium-intracellulare* complex (MAC) is relatively common, and the clinical and radiological manifestations vary. Although there can be considerable overlap, the pulmonary manifestations are classified into two main types: cavitary and noncavitary (i.e., fibronodular bronchiectasis). The cavitary (Figs. 3 and 4) form resembles pulmonary tuberculosis and is seen mainly in patients with underlying lung disease, most commonly chronic obstructive pulmonary disease. The noncavitary form (Figs. 1 and 2) is seen mainly in previously healthy, elderly women and is therefore also known as the Lady Windermere syndrome.

Characteristic Clinical Features

The clinical manifestations of MAC are variable and nonspecific. Patients may be asymptomatic or present with chronic cough, low-grade fever, and weight loss.

Characteristic Radiologic Findings

The cavitary form of MAC usually manifests with a predominantly upper lobe cavitating nodule or nodules and areas of scarring (Figs. 3 and 4). Most patients have findings of underlying lung disease, most commonly chronic obstructive pulmonary disease (COPD). CT frequently shows multiple cavities. The noncavitary form (i.e., fibronodular bronchiectasis) usually has normal or nonspecific radiographic manifestations. High-resolution CT typically shows bronchiectasis involving the middle lobe or lingula, or both, and often shows extensive cylindrical bronchiectasis in the other lobes, centrilobular nodules, tree-in-bud pattern, noncavitary nodules, and foci of consolidation. The bronchiectasis frequently precedes the development of MAC infection but typically progresses with the disease.

Less Common Radiologic Manifestations

Imaging may show a single pulmonary nodule or mass. Rarely, patients have pleural effusion and hilar or mediastinal lymphadenopathy.

Differential Diagnosis

- Tuberculosis
- Fungal infection
- Bacterial pneumonia

Discussion

The clinical and radiologic manifestations of pulmonary MAC infection can mimic those of pulmonary tuberculosis and infectious bronchiolitis caused by viruses, bacteria, or fungi. Definitive diagnosis requires consistent clinical and radiologic findings and positive MAC cultures from sputum or bronchial washings.

Diagnosis

Mycobacterium avium-intracellulare complex pulmonary infection

Suggested Readings

Hartman TE, Swensen SJ, Williams DE: Mycobacterium avium-intracellulare complex: Evaluation with CT. Radiology 187:23-26, 1993.

Hollings NP, Wells AU, Wilson R, Hansell DM: Comparative appearances of non-tuberculous mycobacteria species: A CT study. Eur Radiol 12:2211-2217, 2002.

Jeong YJ, Lee KS, Koh WJ, et al: Nontuberculous mycobacterial pulmonary infection in immunocompetent patients: Comparison of thin-section CT and histopathologic findings. Radiology 231:880-886, 2004.

Swensen SJ, Hartman TE, Williams DE: Computed tomographic diagnosis of *Mycobacterium avium-intracellulare* complex in patients with bronchiectasis. Chest 105:49-52, 1994.

Waller EA, Roy A, Brumble L, et al: The expanding spectrum of *Mycobacterium avium complex*-associated pulmonary disease. Chest 130:1234-1241, 2006.

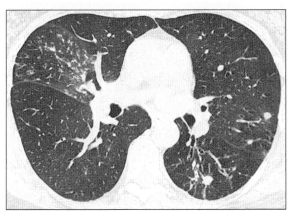

Figure 1. High-resolution CT at the level of the proximal right middle and lower lobe bronchi shows right middle lobe bronchiectasis, ground-glass opacities, centrilobular nodules, and branching opacities (i.e., tree-in-bud pattern). Notice the nodules and a few linear opacities in the left lower and upper lobes and left lower lobe bronchiectasis. The patient was a 67-year-old woman with *M. avium-intracellulare* pulmonary infection.

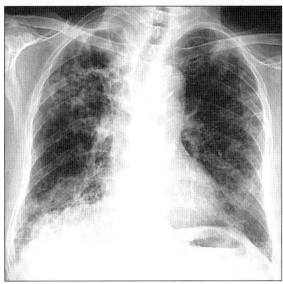

Figure 3. Chest radiograph shows large right upper lobe cavity, patchy areas of consolidation, and multiple, bilateral nodular opacities. The patient was a 74-year-old man with *M. avium-intracellulare* pulmonary infection.

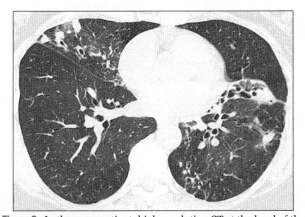

Figure 2. In the same patient, high-resolution CT at the level of the basal segmental bronchi shows bronchiectasis in the right middle lobe, lingula, and left lower lobe; nodules in the right middle lobe, lingula, and left lower lobe; and atelectasis and focal consolidation in the lingula.

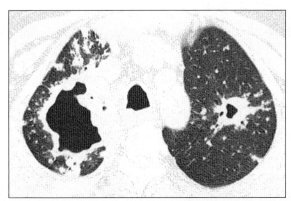

Figure 4. In the same patient, high-resolution CT shows large right upper and small left upper lobe cavity, bilateral small nodules, and peribronchial consolidation.

Case 75

DEMOGRAPHICS/CLINICAL HISTORY

A 35-year-old man with dry cough and mild shortness of breath who was a regular hot tub user, undergoing computed tomography (CT).

FINDINGS

High-resolution CT shows numerous bilateral, small centrilobular nodules and patchy ground-glass opacities (Fig. 1).

DISCUSSION

Definition/Background

Hot tub lung is an uncommon manifestation of *Mycobacterium avium-intracellulare* complex (MAC) pulmonary infection that occurs in users of hot tubs. There is controversy about whether hot tub lung represents a hypersensitive reaction or a granulomatous response to infection, or both. The high-resolution CT findings resemble those of subacute hypersensitivity pneumonitis.

Characteristic Clinical Features

The presentation is usually subacute, and patients have a dry cough and shortness of breath.

Characteristic Radiologic Findings

The chest radiograph shows poorly defined nodules and patchy ground-glass opacities. The high-resolution CT findings resemble those of subacute hypersensitivity pneumonitis and include poorly defined centrilobular nodules, patchy ground-glass opacities, areas of decreased attenuation and vascularity on inspiratory CT, and air trapping on expiratory CT.

Less Common Radiologic Manifestations

A tree-in-bud pattern may be seen, particularly in the lung periphery. This feature suggests the presence of active infection.

Occasionally, the nodules may have a random distribution.

Differential Diagnosis
- Hypersensitivity pneumonitis
- Viral infection
- Miliary tuberculosis
- Pneumoconiosis

Discussion

The clinical and radiologic manifestations of hot tub lung are similar to those of subacute hypersensitivity pneumonitis. The diagnosis of hot tub lung is based on clinical history and culture of MAC from the hot tub, bronchoalveolar lavage fluid, and bronchial or surgical biopsy specimens.

Diagnosis

Hot tub lung

Suggested Readings

Hanak V, Kalra S, Aksamit TR, et al: Hot tub lung: Presenting features and clinical course of 21 patients. Respir Med 100:610-615, 2006.

Hartman TE, Jensen E, Tazelaar HD, et al: CT findings of granulomatous pneumonitis secondary to *Mycobacterium avium-intracellulare* inhalation: "Hot tub lung." AJR Am J Roentgenol 188:1050-1053, 2007.

Sood A, Sreedhar R, Kulkarni P, Nawoor AR: Hypersensitivity pneumonitis-like granulomatous lung disease with nontuberculous mycobacteria from exposure to hot water aerosols. Environ Health Perspect 115:262-266, 2007.

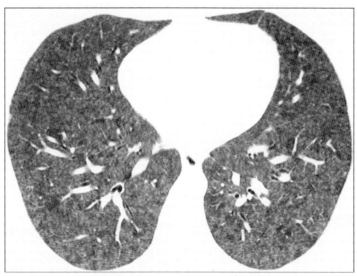

Figure 1. High-resolution CT shows numerous, bilateral, small centrilobular nodules and patchy ground-glass opacities. The patient was a 35-year-old man with biopsy-proven hot tub lung.

Case 76

DEMOGRAPHICS/CLINICAL HISTORY

A 46-year-old man with cough and shortness of breath after spelunking, undergoing radiography.

FINDINGS

Posteroanterior chest radiograph shows numerous, small nodules throughout both lungs (Fig. 1). In another patient, high-resolution CT shows areas of consolidation in the lower lobes, bilateral ground-glass opacities, and small nodules.

DISCUSSION

Definition/Background

Histoplasmosis is caused by inhalation of the dimorphic fungus *Histoplasma capsulatum*, which is endemic in central and eastern North America, especially in the Ohio, Mississippi, and St. Lawrence River valleys, and in South America. Bird and bat droppings enhance its growth by accelerating sporulation.

Characteristic Clinical Features

Patients may be asymptomatic or present with nonspecific symptoms of fever, cough, shortness of breath, and fatigue.

Characteristic Radiologic Findings

Acute histoplasmosis may manifest as a solitary or multiple nodules, single or patchy areas of consolidation, and hilar or mediastinal lymphadenopathy. Chronic histoplasmosis usually manifests as unilateral or bilateral upper lobe areas of consolidation. Patients with histoplasmosis commonly present with a solitary nodule that slowly enlarges over time (i.e., histoplasmoma).

The nodule may have a soft tissue density or central, diffuse, or laminated calcification. Imaging often shows associated satellite nodules and foci of calcification in the hilar and mediastinal nodes, liver, and spleen.

Less Common Radiologic Manifestations

Disseminated disease with miliary nodules (1 to 3 mm in diameter) occurs mainly in immunocompromised patients. Chronic complications include broncholithiasis, mediastinal granuloma, and fibrosing mediastinitis.

Differential Diagnosis

- Tuberculosis
- Lung cancer
- Pulmonary metastases

Discussion

CT without intravenous contrast is the imaging modality of choice for detection of central, diffuse, or laminated patterns of calcification in histoplasmomas, which is a helpful finding in differentiating histoplasmoma from lung cancer. The patterns of calcification are similar to those seen in tuberculomas. Noncalcified, single nodules are indistinguishable radiologically from carcinoma and may be positive findings on ^{18}F-fluorodeoxyglucose positron emission tomography (FDG-PET). Multiple nodules may resemble tuberculosis or pulmonary metastases.

Diagnosis

Pulmonary histoplasmosis.

Suggested Readings

Chong S, Lee KS, Yi CA, et al: Pulmonary fungal infection: Imaging findings in immunocompetent and immunocompromised patients. Eur J Radiol 59:371-383, 2006.

Waite S, Jeudy J, White CS: Acute lung infections in normal and immunocompromised hosts. Radiol Clin North Am 44:295-315, ix, 2006.

Wheat LJ, Goldman M, Sarosi G: State-of-the-art review of pulmonary fungal infections. Semin Respir Infect 17:158-181, 2002.

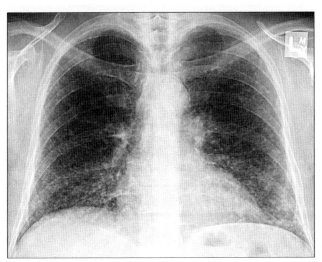

Figure 1. Posteroanterior chest radiograph shows numerous, small nodules throughout both lungs. The patient was a 46-year-old man who developed histoplasmosis after exposure while spelunking.

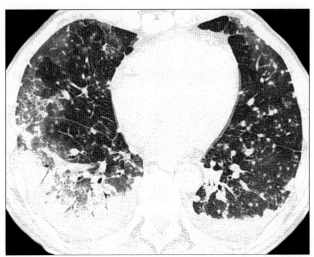

Figure 2. High-resolution CT shows areas of consolidation in the lower lobes, bilateral ground-glass opacities, and small nodules. The patient was a 60-year-old man with acute histoplasmosis.

Case 77

DEMOGRAPHICS/CLINICAL HISTORY

A 38-year-old man with cough and fever after travel to Arizona undergoing radiography and computed tomography (CT).

FINDINGS

Chest radiograph (Fig.1) and CT images using lung (Fig. 2) and soft tissue (Fig. 3) windows show focal consolidation in the right middle lobe (Figs. 1 and 2), a few centrilobular nodular opacities (Fig. 2), and paratracheal lymphadenopathy (Figs. 1 and 3).

DISCUSSION

Definition/Background

Coccidioidomycosis is caused by inhalation of the dimorphic fungus *Coccidioides immitis*, which is endemic in Arizona, southern California, and northern Mexico.

Characteristic Clinical Features

Patients may be asymptomatic or present with nonspecific symptoms of fever, cough, and fatigue.

Characteristic Radiologic Findings

The most common radiologic manifestations consist of single or multiple foci of air-space consolidation or single or multiple nodules that frequently cavitate (Fig. 4). The nodules may range from 0.5 to 5 cm in diameter.

Less Common Radiologic Manifestations

Disseminated disease with miliary nodules (1 to 3 mm in diameter) occurs mainly in immunocompromised patients. Hilar or mediastinal lymphadenopathy occurs in approximately 20% of cases, and small pleural effusions occur in 10% to 20% of cases (Figs. 1 to 3).

Differential Diagnosis

- Pneumonia due to other organisms
- Tuberculosis
- Lung cancer

Discussion

In acute coccidiodomycosis, the findings of single or multiple focal areas of consolidation in a patient with cough and fever resemble bacterial pneumonia. In patients presenting with a solitary soft tissue nodule or a thin-walled cavity, the features resemble those of tuberculosis and carcinoma. A history of travel to or residence in an endemic region is important in the diagnosis of coccidioidomycosis. Definitive diagnosis requires identification of the organisms in sputum, bronchoalveolar lavage fluid, or biopsy specimens.

Diagnosis

Pulmonary coccidioidomycosis

Suggested Readings

Chong S, Lee KS, Yi CA, et al: Pulmonary fungal infection: Imaging findings in immunocompetent and immunocompromised patients. Eur J Radiol 59:371-383, 2006.

Waite S, Jeudy J, White CS: Acute lung infections in normal and immunocompromised hosts. Radiol Clin North Am 44:295-315, ix, 2006.

Wheat LJ, Goldman M, Sarosi G: State-of-the-art review of pulmonary fungal infections. Semin Respir Infect 17:158-181, 2002.

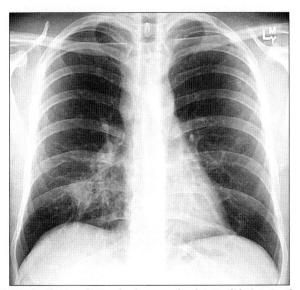

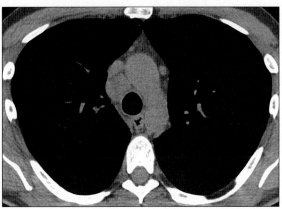

Figure 3. CT using soft tissue windows shows paratracheal lymphadenopathy in the 38-year-old patient with acute coccidioidomycosis.

Figure 1. Chest radiograph shows a focal consolidation in the right middle lobe and widening of the right paratracheal stripe with an associated lobulated contour characteristic of lymphadenopathy. The patient was a 38-year-old man with acute coccidioidomycosis.

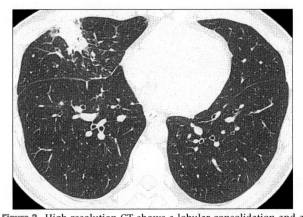

Figure 2. High-resolution CT shows a lobular consolidation and a few, small centrilobular, nodular opacities in the right middle lobe in a 38-year-old man with acute coccidioidomycosis.

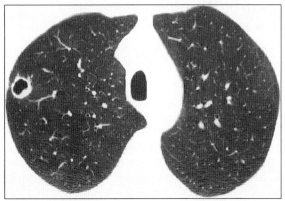

Figure 4. High-resolution CT shows a cavitating nodule in the right upper lobe. The patient was a 44-year-old man who frequently went on holidays in Arizona.

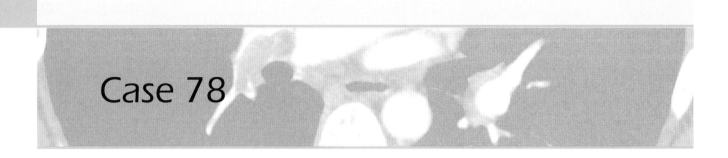

Case 78

DEMOGRAPHICS/CLINICAL HISTORY

A 31-year-old woman with asthma and increased cough and wheezing, undergoing radiography.

FINDINGS

Posteroanterior chest radiograph shows tubular and nodular opacities in the upper lobes and foci of consolidation in the right upper lobe (Fig. 1). Lateral chest radiograph shows a branching, tubular opacity characteristic of mucoid impaction in an ectatic bronchus (Fig. 2).

DISCUSSION

Definition/Background

Allergic bronchopulmonary aspergillosis (ABPA) is characterized by chronic airway inflammation, mucoid impaction, and airway damage resulting from persistent colonization and sensitization by *Aspergillus fumigatus* and related species. ABPA is seen almost exclusively in patients with asthma or cystic fibrosis.

Characteristic Clinical Features

The patients typically present with worsening of asthma, increased cough and wheezing, and expectoration of brown mucous plugs.

Characteristic Radiologic Findings

The characteristic radiologic manifestations of ABPA consist of bronchiectasis and mucoid impaction involving mainly the segmental and subsegmental bronchi of the upper lobes, resulting in branching opacities (Figs. 1 to 4). The bronchiectasis is most commonly varicose and tends to involve mainly the segmental and subsegmental upper

lobe bronchi. Other common findings include centrilobular nodules and a tree-in-bud pattern that reflects the presence of dilated bronchioles filled with mucus.

Less Common Radiologic Manifestations

In approximately 30% of patients, the mucous plugs have high signal attenuation, presumably because of the presence of calcium salts (Fig. 4).

Differential Diagnosis

- Bronchiectasis from other causes

Discussion

Because ABPA occurs almost exclusively in asthmatic patients, the presence of central bronchiectasis and mucoid impaction strongly suggests the diagnosis. However, patients with asthma have an increased prevalence of bronchiectasis and may have filling of the ectatic bronchi with secretions without having ABPA. Compared with asthmatics without ABPA, patients with ABPA typically have more extensive bronchiectasis (often affecting three or more lobes) and more severe bronchiectasis (typically varicose rather than the exclusively mild, cylindrical bronchiectasis that may be seen in other asthmatic patients).

Diagnosis

Allergic bronchopulmonary aspergillosis

Suggested Readings

Franquet T, Müller NL, Gimenez A, et al: Spectrum of pulmonary aspergillosis: Histologic, clinical, and radiologic findings. Radiographics 21:825-837, 2001.

Gibson PG: Allergic bronchopulmonary aspergillosis. Semin Respir Crit Care Med 27:185-191, 2006.

Virnig C, Bush RK: Allergic bronchopulmonary aspergillosis: A US perspective. Curr Opin Pulm Med 13:67-71, 2007.

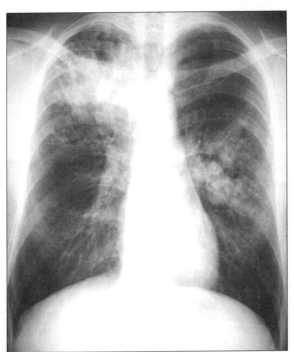

Figure 1. Posteroanterior chest radiograph shows tubular and nodular opacities in the upper lobes and foci of consolidation in the right upper lobe in a 31-year-old, asthmatic woman with ABPA.

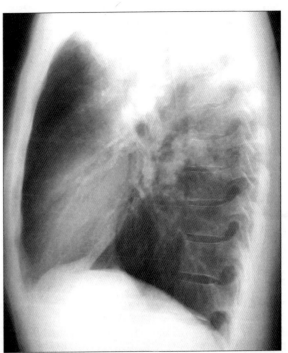

Figure 2. Lateral chest radiograph shows a branching, tubular opacity characteristic of mucoid impaction in an ectatic bronchus. The patient was a 31-year-old asthmatic woman with ABPA.

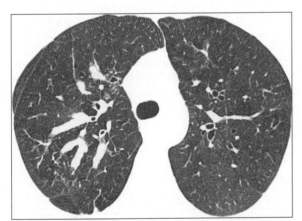

Figure 3. High-resolution CT shows branching, tubular opacities; focal areas of scarring; and bronchiectasis in the right upper lobe and shows mild bronchiectasis in the left upper lobe. The patient was a 32-year-old, asthmatic woman with ABPA.

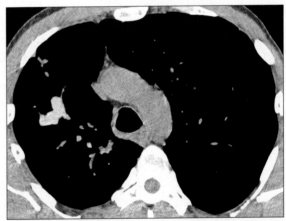

Figure 4. CT shows a branching, tubular opacity in the right upper lobe and volume loss of the right lung with ipsilateral shift of the mediastinum. The tubular opacity has increased signal attenuation, presumably caused by deposition of calcium salts within the mucoid impaction. The patient was a 54-year-old asthmatic man with ABPA.

Case 79

DEMOGRAPHICS/CLINICAL HISTORY

A 57-year-old man with fever and neutropenia after hematopoietic stem cell transplantation, undergoing radiography and computed tomography (CT).

FINDINGS

Chest radiograph (Fig. 1) shows a poorly defined, round opacity in the right lower lung zone. High-resolution CT (Fig. 2) shows a mass in the right lung and two nodules in the left lung surrounded by a rim of ground-glass opacity (i.e., CT halo sign).

DISCUSSION

Definition/Background

Aspergillus is a ubiquitous, opportunistic fungus that causes a wide range of pulmonary manifestations. The most common pathogen is *Aspergillus fumigatus*. The pulmonary manifestations can be classified as five main types: saprophytic aspergillosis (i.e., aspergilloma), allergic bronchopulmonary aspergillosis, semi-invasive aspergillosis, airway-invasive aspergillosis (i.e., *Aspergillus* bronchopneumonia), and angioinvasive aspergillosis.

Characteristic Clinical Features

Angioinvasive pulmonary aspergillosis occurs mainly in immunocompromised patients with severe neutropenia, as may be seen in hematologic malignancies, especially leukemia, and after stem cell transplantation. The clinical manifestations include fever, cough, dyspnea, and pleuritic chest pain.

Characteristic Radiologic Findings

Radiographic findings consist of multiple, ill-defined nodules and focal areas of consolidation. CT typically shows multiple nodules surrounded by a halo of ground-glass attenuation (i.e., CT halo sign). The halo sign is caused by hemorrhage surrounding the nodule or mass of necrotic fungal infected lung tissue. Another common finding is the presence of subpleural, wedge-shaped areas of consolidation.

Less Common Radiologic Manifestations

Imaging may show cavitation, an air crescent sign, a pleural effusion, and segmental or lobar consolidation.

Differential Diagnosis
- Candidiasis
- Mucormycosis
- Septic embolism
- Cytomagalovirus pneumonia
- Lung cancer (e.g., adenocarcinoma)
- Metastatic angiosarcoma
- Vasculitis (e.g., Wegener granulomatosis)

Discussion

The finding of multiple nodules surrounded by a rim of ground-glass attenuation (i.e., CT halo sign) in a neutropenic patient strongly suggests angioinvasive aspergillosis. Occasionally, immunocompromised patients with other fungal infections, particularly candidiasis and mucormycosis, and others with cytomegalovirus pneumonia may have identical findings. The differential diagnosis for non-immunocompromised patients is broad and includes neoplasms (e.g., adenocarcinoma, metastatic angiosarcoma), vasculitis (e.g., Wegener granulomatosis), and organizing pneumonia (i.e., bronchiolitis obliterans organizing pneumonia [BOOP]).

Diagnosis

Angioinvasive aspergillosis

Suggested Readings

Lee YR, Choi YW, Lee KJ, et al: CT halo sign: The spectrum of pulmonary diseases. Br J Radiol 78:862-865, 2005.

Primack SL, Hartman TE, Lee KS, Müller NL: Pulmonary nodules and the CT halo sign. Radiology 190:513-515, 1994.

Waite S, Jeudy J, White CS: Acute lung infections in normal and immunocompromised hosts. Radiol Clin North Am 44:295-315, ix, 2006.

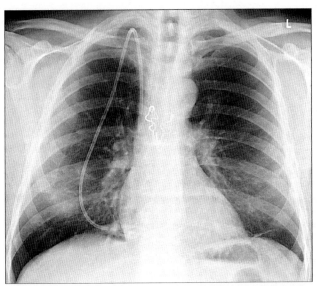

Figure 1. Chest radiograph shows a poorly defined, round opacity in the right lower lung zone. A double-lumen intravenous catheter is in place. The patient was a 57-year-old man with acute myelogenous leukemia, severe neutropenia, and angioinvasive aspergillosis.

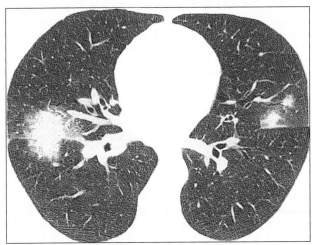

Figure 2. In the same patient, high-resolution CT shows a mass in the right lung and two nodules in the left lung surrounded by a ground-glass opacity (i.e. CT halo sign).

Case 80

DEMOGRAPHICS/CLINICAL HISTORY

A 23-year-old man with fever 2 months after hematopoietic stem cell transplantation for lymphoma, undergoing computed tomography (CT).

FINDINGS

High-resolution CT shows bilateral ground-glass opacities; poorly defined, small, centrilobular nodules; and small, focal areas of consolidation (Fig. 1).

DISCUSSION

Definition/Background

Cytomegalovirus (CMV) is a common human pathogen, but most infections are asymptomatic, with the only significant effect being the presence of latent virus as a potential source of reinfection. Pneumonia occurs almost exclusively in immunocompromised patients, particularly after transplantation. In the solid organ and hematopoietic stem cell transplantation populations, CMV pneumonia occurs most commonly between 30 and 100 days after transplantation.

Characteristic Clinical Features

The clinical manifestations of CMV pneumonia include cough, fever, and in severe cases, shortness of breath.

Characteristic Radiologic Findings

The radiographic manifestations of CMV pneumonia consist of a patchy, bilateral consolidation often associated with multiple, poorly defined, small pulmonary nodules. High-resolution CT findings include bilateral ground-glass opacities, focal areas of consolidation, and small nodules.

Less Common Radiologic Manifestations

The nodules may be surrounded by a halo pattern of ground-glass attenuation (i.e., CT halo sign).

Differential Diagnosis
- Fungal pneumonia
- Bacterial pneumonia
- Drug reaction

Discussion

The clinical and radiologic manifestations of CMV pneumonia are similar to those of other viral pneumonias, bacterial pneumonia, and opportunistic fungal infection. CMV should be considered, particularly in immunocompromised patients, 30 to 100 days after solid organ or hematopoietic stem cell transplantation.

Diagnosis

Cytomegalovirus pneumonia

Suggested Readings

Franquet T, Lee KS, Müller NL: Thin-section CT findings in 32 immunocompromised patients with cytomegalovirus pneumonia who do not have AIDS. AJR Am J Roentgenol 181:1059-1063, 2003.

Kanne JP, Godwin JD, Franquet T, et al: Viral pneumonia after hematopoietic stem cell transplantation: High-resolution CT findings. J Thorac Imaging 22:292-299, 2007.

Oh YW, Effman EL, Godwin JD: Pulmonary infections in immunocompromised hosts: The importance of correlating the conventional radiologic appearance with the clinical setting. Radiology 217:647-656, 2000.

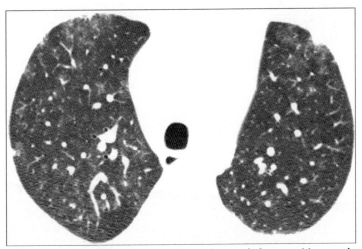

Figure 1. High-resolution CT shows bilateral ground-glass opacities; poorly defined, small, centrilobular nodules; and small, focal areas of consolidation. Notice the mediastinal widening due to residual lymphadenopathy. The patient was a 23-year-old man with cytomegalovirus pneumonia 2 months after stem cell transplantation for lymphoma.

Case 81

DEMOGRAPHICS/CLINICAL HISTORY

A 42-year-old woman with AIDS and progressive shortness of breath, undergoing radiography and computed tomography (CT).

FINDINGS

Chest radiograph (Fig. 1) shows bilateral, symmetric, poorly defined, hazy, increased densities (i.e., ground-glass opacities), mainly in the central lung regions. High-resolution CT (Fig. 2) shows extensive, bilateral ground-glass opacities and small foci of consolidation.

DISCUSSION

Definition/Background

Pneumocystis pneumonia (PCP) is caused by *P. jiroveci*, an opportunistic fungal pulmonary pathogen. PCP is the most common opportunistic pulmonary infection in human immunodeficiency virus (HIV)–infected patients in the United States and is responsible for approximately 25% of cases of pneumonia in patients with HIV infection. Patients who develop PCP almost always have fewer than 200 CD4$^+$ cells/mm^3.

Characteristic Clinical Features

Patients may have insidious and slowly progressive fever, dry cough, and dyspnea.

Characteristic Radiologic Findings

The characteristic radiographic presentation consists of a bilateral, perihilar or diffuse, symmetric interstitial pattern, which may have a finely granular, reticular, or ground-glass appearance. High-resolution CT typically shows extensive, bilateral ground-glass opacities that may have a geographic distribution, be diffuse, or have upper lobe predominance.

Less Common Radiologic Manifestations

Cystic lesions (Fig. 3) and reticulation may be superimposed on the ground-glass opacities. Severe pneumonia may result in areas of consolidation (Fig. 4). Pleural effusion and lymphadenopathy are uncommon.

Differential Diagnosis

- Bacterial pneumonia
- Drug-induced lung disease
- Pulmonary hemorrhage
- Cytomegalovirus pheumonia

Discussion

Extensive, bilateral ground-glass opacities in a patient with AIDS strongly suggest PCP. Bacterial pneumonia typically results in focal or multifocal areas of consolidation. The differential diagnosis of bilateral ground-glass opacities in immunocompromised, non-AIDS patients is more difficult and includes PCP, pneumonia due to cytomegalovirus, drug reaction, pulmonary hemorrhage, and pulmonary edema. Definitive diagnosis requires identification of the organism in sputum, bronchoalveolar lavage fluid, or lung biopsy specimens.

Diagnosis

Pneumocystis pneumonia in an AIDS patient

Suggested Readings

Boiselle PM, Aviram G, Fishman GE: Update on lung disease in AIDS. Semin Roentgenol 37:54-71, 2002.

Castaner E, Gallardo X, Mata JM, Esteba L: Radiologic approach to the diagnosis of infectious pulmonary diseases in patients infected with the human immunodeficiency virus. Eur J Radiol 51:114-129, 2004.

Maki DD: Pulmonary infections in HIV/AIDS. Semin Roentgenol 35:124-139, 2000.

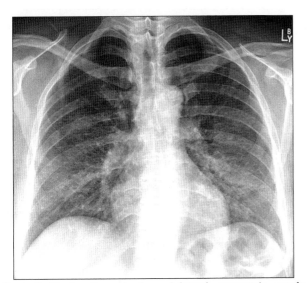

Figure 1. Chest radiograph shows bilateral, symmetric, poorly defined, hazy, increased densities (i.e., ground-glass opacities) mainly in the central lung regions. The patient was a 42-year-old woman with AIDS and *Pneumocystis* pneumonia.

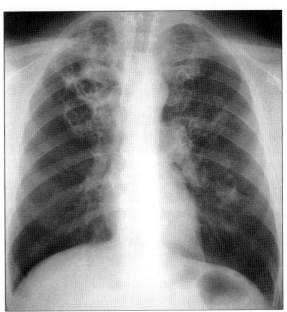

Figure 3. Chest radiograph shows bilateral cystic lesions mainly in the upper lobes. They were not present 3 months earlier, when the patient developed *Pneumocystis* pneumonia, and they were seen most clearly after resolution of the ground-glass opacities. The patient was a 53-year-old man with AIDS.

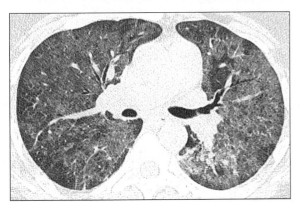

Figure 2. In the same 42-year-old patient, high-resolution CT shows extensive, bilateral ground-glass opacities and small foci of consolidation.

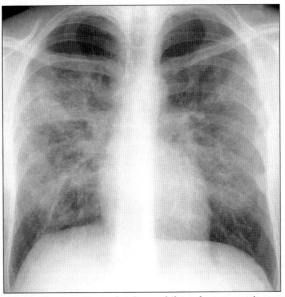

Figure 4. Chest radiograph shows bilateral, symmetric areas of consolidation and ground-glass opacities. The patient was a 32-year-old man with AIDS and *Pneumocystis* pneumonia

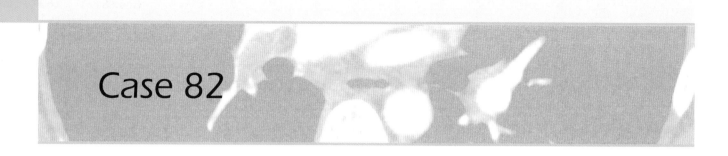

Case 82

DEMOGRAPHICS/CLINICAL HISTORY

A 27-year-old man with lower chest pain, undergoing computed tomography (CT)

FINDINGS

Contrast-enhanced CT at the level of the bronchus intermedius (Fig. 1) shows a cystic mass with homogeneous fluid density and adjacent compressive atelectasis in the right middle lobe. CT at the level of the upper abdomen (Fig. 2) shows a cystic mass with homogeneous fluid density in the right lobe of the liver.

DISCUSSION

Definition/Background

Hydatid disease is caused by larvae of *Echinococcus*, usually *E. granulosus*, also called the hydatid worm. It occurs in two forms: pastoral and sylvatic. The pastoral form is the more common and is seen mainly in the Mediterranean region, South America, the Middle East, Australia, and New Zealand. The intermediate hosts are usually sheep, cows, or pigs and the definite hosts are dogs. The sylvatic form is more common in Alaska and northern Canada. The intermediate hosts of the sylvatic variety are usually moose, deer, or caribou, and the definite hosts are dogs, wolves, and coyotes.

Characteristic Clinical Features

Most patients are asymptomatic. Cyst rupture that occurs spontaneously or as a result of secondary infection may result in abrupt onset of cough, expectoration, and fever.

Characteristic Radiologic Findings

Hydatid cysts manifest as sharply circumscribed, spherical or oval masses ranging from 1 to more than 20 cm in diameter. The cysts have water density on CT (about 0 Hounsfield units) and have homogeneous, high signal intensity on T2-weighted magnetic resonance imaging and thin, smooth walls. Pulmonary hydatid cysts may occur in isolation or in association with similar lesions in the liver.

Less Common Radiologic Manifestations

When communication develops between the cyst and the bronchial tree, air may enter the space between the pericyst and exocyst and produce a thin crescent around the periphery of the cyst (i.e., meniscus or crescent sign). After the cyst has ruptured into an airway, its membrane may float on residual fluid within the cyst and give rise to the classic water lily sign.

Differential Diagnosis

- Bronchogenic cyst
- Fluid-filled bullae

Discussion

The main differential diagnosis includes other conditions that may result in fluid-filled lung lesions, particularly bronchogenic cysts and fluid-filled bullae. Diagnosis of hydatid disease is based on clinical history, presence of blood eosinophilia (usually mild and seen in 25% to 50% of cases), and positive laboratory test results for hydatid disease.

Diagnosis

Hydatid disease

Suggested Readings

Kilic D, Tercan F, Sahin E, et al: Unusual radiologic manifestations of the echinococcus infection in the thorax. J Thorac Imaging 21: 32-36, 2006.

Martinez S, Restrepo CS, Carrillo JA, et al: Thoracic manifestations of tropical parasitic infections: A pictorial review. Radiographics 25:135-155, 2005.

von Sinner WN: New diagnostic signs in hydatid disease: Radiography, ultrasound, CT and MRI correlated to pathology. Eur J Radiol 12:150-159, 1991.

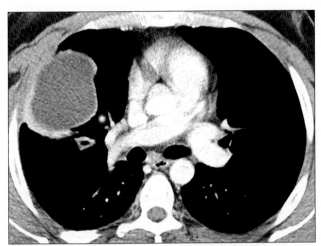

Figure 1. Contrast-enhanced CT at the level of the bronchus intermedius shows a cystic mass with homogeneous fluid density and adjacent compressive atelectasis in the right middle lobe. The patient was a 27-year-old man with hydatid disease.

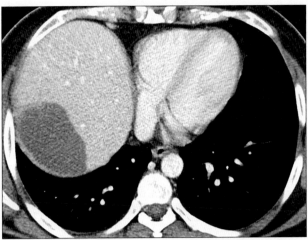

Figure 2. In the same patient, CT at the level of the upper abdomen shows a cystic mass with homogeneous fluid density in the right lobe of the liver.

Case 83

DEMOGRAPHICS/CLINICAL HISTORY

A 59-year-old man with progressive shortness of breath over 2 years, undergoing radiography and computed tomography (CT)

FINDINGS

Chest radiography (Fig. 1) shows low lung volumes and a reticular pattern involving mainly the lower lung zones. High-resolution CT images at the level of the aortic arch (Fig. 2), right upper lobe bronchus (Fig. 3), and basal segmental bronchi (Fig. 4) show a reticular pattern and honeycombing, predominantly in the peripheral lung regions and lower lung zones. Notice the increasing extent of reticulation and honeycombing from the uppermost (Fig. 2) to the lowest section (Fig. 4).

DISCUSSION

Definition/Background

Idiopathic pulmonary fibrosis (IPF) is a form of chronic, fibrosing interstitial pneumonia limited to the lungs and characterized by a histologic pattern of usual interstitial pneumonia (UIP). By definition, IPF is idiopathic UIP. IPF is the most common idiopathic interstitial lung disease. Patients are typically older than 50 years, and approximately 80% are 65 years old or older. IPF has a poor prognosis; the mean survival time after diagnosis is approximately 3 to 5 years.

Characteristic Clinical Features

Patients may have progressive dyspnea, nonproductive cough, and fatigue. The clinical course of IPF is one of relentless progressive increase in the extent of fibrosis and the severity of clinical manifestations.

Characteristic Radiologic Findings

The radiographic findings consist of symmetric, bilateral, predominantly basal reticular opacities. High-resolution CT shows irregular intralobular lines resulting in a reticular pattern involving mainly the subpleural regions and lower lung zones. Other findings of fibrosis include architectural distortion; dilation of bronchi and bronchioles (e.g., traction bronchiectasis, bronchiolectasis); irregular pleural, vascular, and bronchial interfaces; and honeycombing. Ground-glass opacities are common but limited in extent and usually associated with findings of fibrosis.

Less Common Radiologic Manifestations

Most patients with IPF are smokers, and they may have associated findings of emphysema. Occasionally, ground-glass opacities may be more extensive than reticular opacities.

Differential Diagnosis

- Nonspecific interstitial pneumonia (NSIP)
- Chronic hypersensitivity pneumonitis (HP)
- Asbestosis
- Collagen vascular disease

Discussion

In the proper clinical context, a confident diagnosis can be made using high-resolution CT in 50% to 70% of cases. A confident high-resolution CT diagnosis of IPF requires clinical exclusion of known causes of UIP and the presence of all three of the following high-resolution CT criteria: a reticular pattern in a predominantly peripheral and basal distribution, honeycombing in a predominantly peripheral and basal distribution, and absence of atypical features (e.g., centrilobular nodules, peribronchovascular nodules, extensive consolidation, extensive ground-glass opacities). In the remaining cases, a confident diagnosis requires surgical biopsy.

The interstitial lung disease that most commonly mimics IPF is NSIP, whether idiopathic or associated with connective tissue disease. Findings that favor NSIP include a predominance of ground-glass opacities, relative subpleural sparing, and absence of honeycombing.

A reticular pattern and honeycombing are commonly seen in chronic HP. Differentiation from IPF often can be based on high-resolution CT findings of centrilobular nodules, lobular areas of decreased attenuation and vascularity, and the relative sparing of the lung bases in patients with HP.

Asbestosis usually can be differentiated from IPF by the presence of pleural plaques or diffuse pleural thickening.

Diagnosis

Idiopathic pulmonary fibrosis

Suggested Readings

Hunninghake GW, Zimmerman MB, Schwartz DA, et al: Utility of a lung biopsy for the diagnosis of idiopathic pulmonary fibrosis. Am J Respir Crit Care Med 164:193-196, 2001.

Lynch DA, Travis WD, Müller NL, et al: Idiopathic interstitial pneumonias: CT features. Radiology 236:10-21, 2005.

Silva CI, Müller NL, Lynch DA, et al: Chronic hypersensitivity pneumonitis: Differentiation from idiopathic pulmonary fibrosis and nonspecific interstitial pneumonia by using thin-section CT. Radiology 246:288-297, 2008.

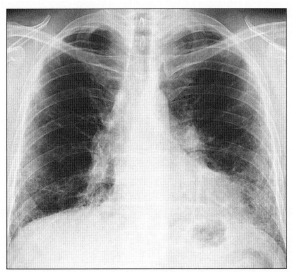

Figure 1. Chest radiograph shows a bilateral reticular pattern involving mainly the lower lung zones and decreased lung volumes. The patient was a 59-year-old man with idiopathic pulmonary fibrosis.

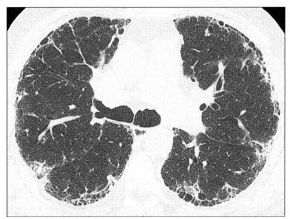

Figure 3. In the same patient, high-resolution CT at the level of the right upper lobe bronchus shows bilateral, subpleural reticulation and honeycombing.

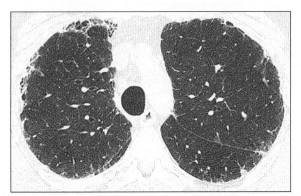

Figure 2. In the same patient, high-resolution CT at the level of the aortic arch shows mild reticulation in a patchy distribution in the subpleural regions of both lungs and honeycombing mainly in the right upper lobe.

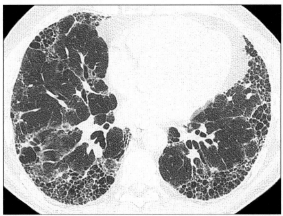

Figure 4. In the same patient, high-resolution CT at the level of the lower lung zones shows extensive, bilateral honeycombing in the peripheral lung regions.

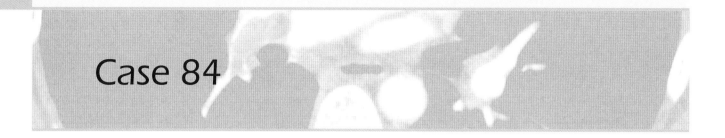

Case 84

DEMOGRAPHICS/CLINICAL HISTORY

A 60-year-old man with chronic interstitial fibrosis and acute, rapidly progressing shortness of breath, undergoing computed tomography (CT).

FINDINGS

High-resolution CT images at the level of the upper (Fig. 1) and lower (Fig. 2) lung zones show extensive, bilateral ground-glass opacities and mild, peripheral honeycombing.

DISCUSSION

Definition/Background

Idiopathic pulmonary fibrosis (IPF) is a form of chronic, fibrosing interstitial pneumonia limited to the lungs and characterized by a histologic pattern of usual interstitial pneumonia (UIP). The clinical course of IPF is one of relentlessly progressive increase in the severity of clinical manifestations and fibrosis. Acute deterioration with an abrupt and unexpected worsening of symptoms may occur because of infection, pulmonary embolism, pneumothorax, or heart failure. Often, however, no identifiable cause for the acute decline is identified, and these episodes are called *acute exacerbations*. Diagnostic criteria for acute exacerbation of IPF include the following:

1. Subjective worsening of dyspnea or cough within the past 30 days
2. New ground-glass opacities or consolidation seen on the chest radiograph or high-resolution CT
3. Decline of 10% or more in the absolute forced vital capacity (FVC) or decline of 10 mm Hg or more in the PaO_2
4. Negative respiratory culture results for respiratory pathogens (positive culture defined as moderate or heavy growth of sputum or endotracheal aspirate or bronchoalveolar lavage)
5. No evidence of pulmonary embolism, congestive heart failure, or pneumothorax as the cause of acute worsening

Characteristic Clinical Features

Patients may have rapidly progressing dyspnea, hypoxemia, and a history of clinical and radiologic findings consistent with IPF.

Characteristic Radiologic Findings

The high-resolution CT manifestations of acute exacerbation of IPF consist of extensive ground-glass opacities superimposed on a predominantly peripheral and basal reticular pattern and honeycombing. The ground-glass opacities may be diffuse, multifocal, or peripheral.

Less Common Radiologic Manifestations

Imaging may show consolidation superimposed on the ground-glass opacities and usually involving mainly the dependent lung regions.

Differential Diagnosis

- *Pneumocystis* pneumonia
- Acute interstitial pneumonia
- Acute respiratory distress syndrome (ARDS)
- Drug reaction

Discussion

The main differential diagnosis for patients with acute clinical deterioration and acute exacerbation of IPF observed on high-resolution CT is opportunistic infection, particularly *Pneumocystis jiroveci* pneumonia (PCP). Exclusion of PCP in these patients usually requires bronchoalveolar lavage or biopsy.

In patients with no known history of IPF, the findings resemble those of ARDS and acute interstitial pneumonia. Definitive diagnosis requires surgical biopsy.

Diagnosis

Acute exacerbation of idiopathic pulmonary fibrosis

Suggested Readings

Collard HR, Moore BB, Flaherty KR, et al: Acute exacerbations of idiopathic pulmonary fibrosis. Am J Respir Crit Care Med1;176:636-643, 2007.

Kim DS, Park JH, Park BK, et al: Acute exacerbation of idiopathic pulmonary fibrosis: Frequency and clinical features. Eur Respir J 27:143-150, 2006.

Lynch DA, Travis WD, Müller NL, et al: Idiopathic interstitial pneumonias: CT features. Radiology 236:10-21, 2005.

Silva CI, Müller NL, Fujimoto K, et al: Acute exacerbation of chronic interstitial pneumonia: High-resolution computed tomography and pathologic findings. J Thorac Imaging 22:221-9, 2007.

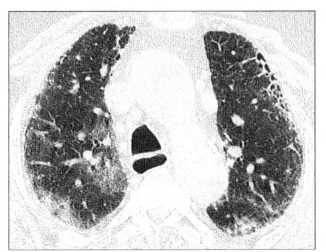

Figure 1. High-resolution CT at the level of the upper lung zones shows patchy, bilateral ground-glass opacities and mild, peripheral honeycombing. The patient was a 60-year-old man with acute exacerbation of IPF.

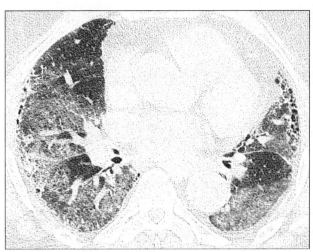

Figure 2. In the same patient, high-resolution CT at the level of the lower lung zones shows extensive, bilateral ground-glass opacities and mild, peripheral honeycombing.

Case 85

DEMOGRAPHICS/CLINICAL HISTORY

A 77-year-old man with a dry cough and progressive shortness of breath over 1 year, undergoing computed tomography (CT).

FINDINGS

Axial high-resolution CT images at the level of the aortopulmonary window (Fig. 1), right inferior pulmonary vein (Fig. 2), and lung bases (Fig. 3) and coronal, reformatted CT (Fig. 4) show extensive, bilateral ground-glass opacities; mild reticulation; and traction bronchiectasis mainly in the lower lung zones. Notice the relative sparing of the lung immediately adjacent to the pleura in the dorsal regions of the lower lung zones (Figs. 2 and 3).

DISCUSSION

Definition/Background
Nonspecific interstitial pneumonia (NSIP) is a chronic interstitial lung disease characterized by relatively homogeneous expansion of the alveolar walls by inflammation or fibrosis. NSIP is the second most common chronic interstitial pneumonia (after usual interstitial pneumonia [UIP]), accounting for 14% to 35% of cases. NSIP may be idiopathic but more commonly is a manifestation of connective tissue disease, hypersensitivity pneumonitis, drug-induced lung disease, or chronic interstitial lung disease complicating diffuse alveolar damage (DAD).

Characteristic Clinical Features
Patient may have progressive dyspnea and dry cough, with a duration ranging from 6 months to 3 years before the diagnosis. The median age at onset of symptoms in NSIP is 40 to 50 years, but the disease may occur at any age and has been reported in patients between 9 and 78 years old. Idiopathic NSIP occurs mostly in middle-aged women who have never been smokers.

Characteristic Radiologic Findings
The most common radiographic and high-resolution CT abnormalities consist of bilateral, patchy or confluent, hazy areas of increased opacity (i.e., ground-glass opacities) involving mainly the middle and lower lung zones. Most patients have a fine reticular pattern and traction bronchiectasis superimposed on the ground-glass opacities. Relative sparing of the lung immediately adjacent to the pleura in the dorsal regions of the lower lung zones is common.

Less Common Radiologic Manifestations
Honeycombing is seen in 10% to 30% of patients, and it tends to be mild, involving less than 10% of the parenchyma.

Differential Diagnosis
- Idiopathic pulmonary fibrosis (IPF)
- Hypersensitivity pneumonitis (HP)
- Cryptogenic organizing pneumonia (COP)

Discussion
The high-resolution CT manifestations of NSIP can mimic those of IPF, HP, and COP. The most important and often the most difficult differential diagnosis is between fibrotic NSIP and IPF. The most helpful findings in distinguishing these two conditions are the greater extent of ground-glass opacities and the lack or limited extent of honeycombing in NSIP.

HP typically manifests with bilateral ground-glass opacities, poorly defined centrilobular nodules, and lobular areas of air trapping. Occasionally, NSIP may be the predominant or only histologic pattern of HP, and the high-resolution CT findings may sometimes be identical.

COP (i.e., idiopathic bronchiolitis obliterans organizing pneumonia [BOOP]) usually can be distinguished by the predominance of consolidation, which typically involves mainly the peribronchial and subpleural lung regions.

Although certain CT findings may suggest NSIP, definitive diagnosis requires surgical biopsy. Even a histologic diagnosis of NSIP does not establish a final diagnosis. NSIP is a common reaction pattern to various drugs; is commonly associated with connective tissue diseases, particularly scleroderma; and can be a histologic manifestation of HP. These conditions must be excluded by careful clinical assessment before making a diagnosis of idiopathic NSIP.

Diagnosis
Nonspecific interstitial pneumonia

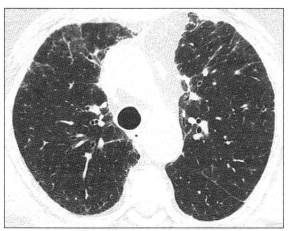

Figure 1. High-resolution CT at the level of the aortopulmonary window shows patchy, bilateral ground-glass opacities and mild, subpleural reticulation in the anterior lung regions. The patient was a 77-year-old man with NSIP.

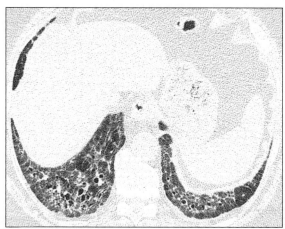

Figure 3. In the same patient, high-resolution CT at the level of the lung bases shows extensive, bilateral ground-glass opacities; mild reticulation; and traction bronchiectasis. Notice the relative sparing of the lung immediately adjacent to the pleura in the dorsal regions of the lower lobes.

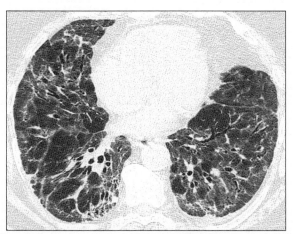

Figure 2. In the same patient, high-resolution CT at the level of the right inferior pulmonary vein shows extensive, bilateral ground-glass opacities; mild reticulation; and traction bronchiectasis. Notice the relative sparing of the lung immediately adjacent to the pleura in the dorsal regions of the lower lobes.

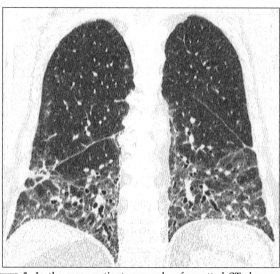

Figure 4. In the same patient, coronal, reformatted CT shows extensive, bilateral ground-glass opacities; mild reticulation; and traction bronchiectasis mainly in the lower lung zones.

Suggested Readings

American Thoracic Society, European Respiratory Society: American Thoracic Society/European Respiratory Society International Multidisciplinary Consensus classification of the idiopathic interstitial pneumonias. Am J Respir Crit Care Med 165:277-304, 2002.

Lynch DA, Travis WD, Müller NL, et al: Idiopathic interstitial pneumonias: CT features. Radiology 236:10-21, 2005.

Silva CI, Müller NL, Hansell DM, et al: Nonspecific interstitial pneumonia and idiopathic pulmonary fibrosis: Changes in pattern and distribution of disease over time. Radiology 247:251-259, 2008.

Travis WD, Hunninghake G, King TE Jr, et al: Idiopathic nonspecific interstitial pneumonia: Report of an American Thoracic Society project. Am J Respir Crit Care Med 177:1338-1347, 2008.

Case 86

DEMOGRAPHICS/CLINICAL HISTORY

A 43-year-old woman with dry cough, low-grade fever, and progressive shortness of breath over several weeks, undergoing radiography and computed tomography (CT)

FINDINGS

Chest radiography (Fig. 1) reveals bilateral, asymmetric, confluent areas of consolidation mainly in the upper and middle lung zones. High-resolution CT images at the level of the upper (Fig. 2), middle (Fig. 3), and lower (Fig. 4) lung zones show bilateral areas of consolidation in a peribronchial and peripheral distribution. CT images also show mild, patchy, bilateral ground-glass opacities.

DISCUSSION

Definition/Background

Organizing pneumonia has a histologic pattern characterized by intraluminal granulation tissue polyps within alveolar ducts and surrounding alveoli associated with chronic inflammation of the surrounding lung parenchyma. Because the granulation tissue polyps usually involve the bronchioles, the pattern is also commonly known as *bronchiolitis obliterans organizing pneumonia* (BOOP). Organizing pneumonia may be associated with several underlying causes, including infections, connective tissue diseases, inflammatory bowel disease, inhalational injury, hypersensitivity pneumonitis, drug reaction, radiation therapy, and aspiration. In some patients, however, no underlying cause is found, and the condition is called cryptogenic organizing pneumonia (COP) (the preferred term) or BOOP. COP accounts for 4% to 12% of cases of idiopathic interstitial pneumonias.

Characteristic Clinical Features

Patients may have cough and progressive dyspnea of relatively short duration (median, less than 3 months). The cough may be dry or produce clear sputum. Other common manifestations include weight loss, chills, and intermittent, low-grade fever.

Characteristic Radiologic Findings

The most common radiographic manifestation of COP consists of bilateral, symmetric or asymmetric areas of consolidation. On high-resolution CT, the consolidation has a predominantly peribronchial or subpleural distribution in 60% to 80% of cases. Another characteristic feature of COP is a perilobular pattern, seen in approximately 60% of patients and defined as linear opacities that are of greater thickness and are less sharply defined than those encountered in thickened interlobular septa and that have an arcade-like or polygonal appearance.

Less Common Radiologic Manifestations

In approximately 20% of patients, organizing pneumonia may result in crescentic or ring-shaped opacities surrounding areas of ground-glass opacification (i.e., reversed halo sign). Ground-glass opacities are commonly observed but are seldom the predominant finding. Centrilobular nodules are seen in 30% to 50% of patients and usually are associated with areas of consolidation.

Differential Diagnosis

- Bronchopneumonia
- Chronic eosinophilic pneumonia
- Nonspecific interstitial pneumonia

Discussion

The differential diagnosis for COP includes organizing pneumonia related to infection, connective tissue disease (particularly rheumatoid arthritis and polymyositis), inflammatory bowel disease, inhalational injury, hypersensitivity pneumonitis, drug reaction, radiation therapy, and aspiration. In the appropriate clinical context, peribronchial or subpleural consolidations that increase over several weeks despite antibiotics strongly suggest COP. The radiologic differential diagnosis in patients presenting with patchy, bilateral consolidations includes bacterial, fungal, and viral pneumonia; bronchioloalveolar cell carcinoma; lymphoma; vasculitis; sarcoidosis; and chronic eosinophilic pneumonia. Most of these entities can be excluded by a combination of clinical findings, bronchoalveolar lavage, and transbronchial biopsy.

Diagnosis

Cryptogenic organizing pneumonia

Suggested Readings

American Thoracic Society: European Respiratory Society: American Thoracic Society/European Respiratory Society International Multidisciplinary Consensus classification of the idiopathic interstitial pneumonias. Am J Respir Crit Care Med 165:277-304, 2002.

Cordier JF: Cryptogenic organising pneumonia. Eur Respir J 28:422-446, 2006.

Lynch DA, Travis WD, Müller NL, et al: Idiopathic interstitial pneumonias: CT features. Radiology 236:10-21, 2005.

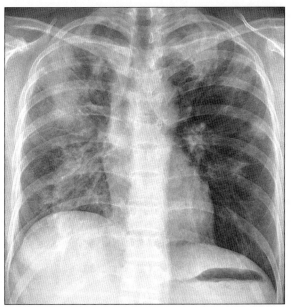

Figure 1. The chest radiograph reveals bilateral, asymmetric, confluent areas of consolidation mainly in the upper and middle lung zones. The patient was a 43-year-old woman with COP.

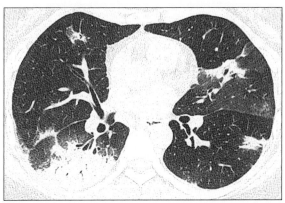

Figure 3. In the same patient, high-resolution CT at the level of the middle lobe bronchus shows bilateral areas of consolidation in a peribronchial and peripheral distribution. Mild, patchy, bilateral ground-glass opacities also can be seen.

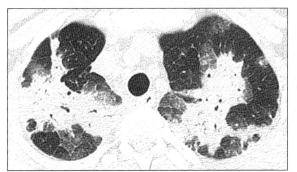

Figure 2. In the same patient, high-resolution CT at the level of the lung apices shows confluent, bilateral areas of consolidation in a peribronchial distribution. Notice the mild, bilateral ground-glass opacities.

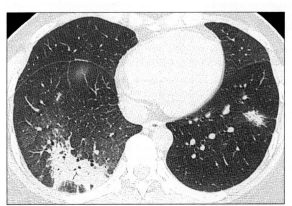

Figure 4. In the same patient, high-resolution CT at the level of the lower lung zones shows asymmetric, bilateral areas of consolidation in a peribronchial distribution. Notice the mild, patchy, bilateral ground-glass opacities.

Case 87

DEMOGRAPHICS/CLINICAL HISTORY

A 70-year-old man who was previously well but now has acute, severe shortness of breath and hypoxemia, undergoing computed tomography (CT).

FINDINGS

High-resolution CT images (Figs. 1 and 2) show extensive, bilateral ground-glass opacities with superimposed smooth, linear opacities (i.e., crazy-paving pattern) and dependent areas of consolidation. Traction bronchiectasis also can be seen.

DISCUSSION

Definition/Background

Acute interstitial pneumonia (AIP) is a severe, acute disease of unknown origin that usually occurs in a previously healthy person and produces histologic findings of diffuse alveolar damage (DAD). The clinical, radiologic, and pathologic manifestations are identical to those of acute respiratory distress syndrome (ARDS); the only distinction is that no cause is found. AIP is quite uncommon, has no sex predominance, and has no association with cigarette smoking. The typical age at presentation is 50 to 60 years (range, 7 to 83 years).

Characteristic Clinical Features

Patients commonly have a prodromal illness associated with symptoms suggesting a viral upper respiratory tract infection, with fever, chills, myalgias, and arthralgias. This is followed by a dry cough and rapidly progressing and severe dyspnea.

Characteristic Radiologic Findings

The radiographic manifestations are similar to those of ARDS and consist of bilateral air space consolidation with air bronchograms. The earliest manifestations of AIP on high-resolution CT consist mainly of patchy or diffuse, bilateral ground-glass opacities. Most patients have smooth septal thickening and intralobular lines superimposed on the ground-glass pattern, resulting in a crazy-paving pattern. The consolidation seen in most patients may be patchy or confluent, and it tends to involve mainly the dependent lung portions.

Less Common Radiologic Manifestations

Small pleural effusions are seen in about 30% of patients, and mild mediastinal lymphadenopathy is seen in 5% to 10%.

Differential Diagnosis

- Acute respiratory distress syndrome (ARDS)
- Pneumonia
- Aspiration
- Diffuse pulmonary hemorrhage

Discussion

Because AIP is essentially idiopathic ARDS, the numerous possible causes of ARDS need to be excluded before making a diagnosis of AIP. They include infection, aspiration, drug-induced lung disease, and ARDS superimposed on previous interstitial lung disease (i.e., acute exacerbation of idiopathic pulmonary fibrosis or nonspecific interstitial pneumonia).

Diagnosis

Acute interstitial pneumonia

Suggested Readings

American Thoracic Society, European Respiratory Society: American Thoracic Society/European Respiratory Society International Multidisciplinary Consensus classification of the idiopathic interstitial pneumonias. Am J Respir Crit Care Med 165:277-304, 2002.

Lynch DA, Travis WD, Müller NL, et al: Idiopathic interstitial pneumonias: CT features. Radiology 236:10-21, 2005.

Tomiyama N, Müller NL, Johkoh T, et al: Acute respiratory distress syndrome and acute interstitial pneumonia: Comparison of thin-section CT findings. J Comput Assist Tomogr 25:28-33, 2001.

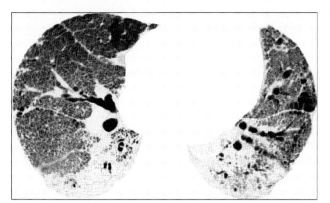

Figure 1. High-resolution CT at the level of the right middle lobe bronchus shows extensive, bilateral ground-glass opacities with superimposed smooth linear opacities (i.e., crazy-paving pattern) and dependent areas of consolidation. Traction bronchiectasis also can be seen. The patient was a 70-year-old man with AIP.

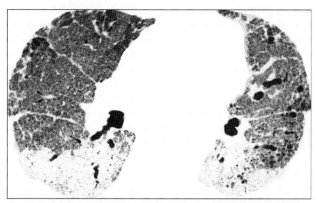

Figure 2. In the same patient, high-resolution CT at the level of the lower lobe bronchi shows extensive, bilateral ground-glass opacities with superimposed smooth linear opacities (i.e., crazy-paving pattern) and dependent areas of consolidation. CT also shows traction bronchiectasis.

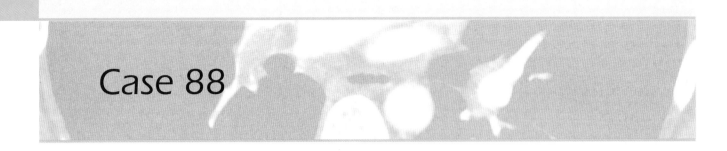

Case 88

DEMOGRAPHICS/CLINICAL HISTORY

A 45-year-old, 40-pack-year smoker with progressive shortness of breath for 6 months, undergoing computed tomography (CT).

FINDINGS

High-resolution CT shows extensive, bilateral ground-glass opacities; bronchial wall thickening; and mild emphysema (Fig.1).

DISCUSSION

Definition/Background

Respiratory bronchiolitis–interstitial lung disease (RBILD) is an interstitial lung disease seen almost exclusively in cigarette smokers. It is characterized histologically by the presence of numerous macrophages filling respiratory bronchioles and adjacent alveolar ducts and alveoli with or without associated interstitial fibrosis. RBILD typically has a bronchiolocentric distribution and involves the lung parenchyma in a patchy fashion. This pattern is distinct from desquamative interstitial pneumonia (DIP), for which the findings are diffuse.

Characteristic Clinical Features

Patients may have a chronic cough and progressive shortness of breath over 1 or 2 years. Patients with RBILD are typically young, usually in their 30s and 40s, and most are current smokers, with an average of more than 30 pack-years of cigarette smoking.

Characteristic Radiologic Findings

Chest radiographs can show normal anatomy or show airway wall thickening, diffuse ground-glass opacities, or poorly defined, fine reticulonodular opacities that can be diffuse or have a lower zonal predominance. The characteristic high-resolution CT findings consist of poorly defined centrilobular nodules and ground-glass opacities, which may be diffuse or involve mainly the upper or lower lung zones. Upper lobe emphysema is common, usually mild, and caused by smoking.

Less Common Radiologic Manifestations

A small percentage of patients with RBILD have a reticular pattern due to fibrosis. The fibrosis is mild and tends to involve mainly the peripheral regions of the lower lung zones.

Differential Diagnosis

- Respiratory bronchiolitis
- Desquamative interstitial pneumonia (DIP)
- Hypersensitivity pneumonitis (HP)
- Nonspecific interstitial pneumonia (NSIP)

Discussion

Respiratory bronchiolitis is a common histopathologic finding in smokers that may result in poorly defined centrilobular nodules and ground-glass opacities mainly in the upper lobes, but it is by definition not associated with clinical symptoms.

DIP is an uncommon condition that is characterized histologically by the presence of numerous macrophages filling the alveolar air spaces, mild inflammation of the alveolar walls, and minimal fibrosis. Approximately 90% of patients who have DIP are cigarette smokers. There is considerable overlap between the clinical, radiologic, and histologic findings of RBILD and DIP, and they usually are considered part of the spectrum of the same disease process.

The high-resolution CT manifestations of RBILD can be identical to those of HP. The differential diagnosis is based on clinical history of exposure to precipitating antigens in HP and a history of cigarette smoking in virtually all patients with RBILD but in only 6% of patients with HP.

The diffuse ground-glass opacities in RBILD, with or without mild reticulation, often resemble the CT findings of NSIP. However, RBILD most commonly has upper lobe predominance, whereas NSIP usually involves mainly the lower lung zones. Although high-resolution CT can suggest RBILD in the appropriate clinical setting, definitive diagnosis requires surgical biopsy.

Diagnosis

Respiratory bronchiolitis–interstitial lung disease

Suggested Readings

Heyneman LE, Ward S, Lynch DA, et al: Respiratory bronchiolitis, respiratory bronchiolitis-associated interstitial lung disease, and desquamative interstitial pneumonia: Different entities or part of the spectrum of the same disease process? AJR Am J Roentgenol 173:1617-1622, 1999.

Lynch DA, Travis WD, Müller NL, et al: Idiopathic interstitial pneumonias: CT features. Radiology 236:10-21, 2005.

Park JS, Brown KK, Tuder RM, et al: Respiratory bronchiolitis-associated interstitial lung disease: Radiologic features with clinical and pathologic correlation. J Comput Assist Tomogr 26:13-20, 2002.

Wells AU, Nicholson AG, Hansell DM: Challenges in pulmonary fibrosis. 4. Smoking-induced diffuse interstitial lung diseases. Thorax 62:904-910, 2007.

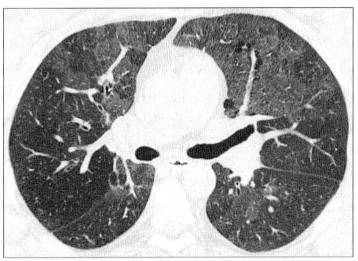

Figure 1. High-resolution CT shows extensive, bilateral ground-glass opacities and mild emphysema. The patient was 45-year-old, male, 40-pack-year smoker, with RBILD.

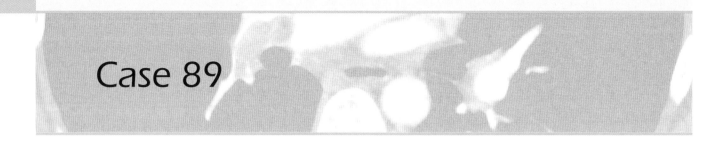

Case 89

DEMOGRAPHICS/CLINICAL HISTORY

A 57-year-old, female smoker with a 1-year history of progressive shortness of breath and dry cough, undergoing computed tomography (CT).

FINDINGS

High-resolution CT images at the level of the inferior pulmonary veins (Fig. 1) and dome of the left hemidiaphragm (Fig. 2) show bilateral ground-glass opacities involving mainly the peripheral lung regions (Fig. 1) and lung bases (Fig. 2). Mild reticulation and mild right lower lobe emphysema also can be seen.

DISCUSSION

Definition/Background
Desquamative interstitial pneumonia (DIP) is an uncommon interstitial lung disease, characterized histologically by the presence of numerous macrophages filling the alveolar airspaces, mild inflammation of the alveolar walls, and mild fibrosis. Approximately 90% of patients who have DIP are cigarette smokers. Occasionally, it may be associated with dust exposure (e.g., asbestos, aluminum, toxic agents), drug reaction, or leukemia.

Characteristic Clinical Features
Patients may have a chronic cough and progressive shortness of breath over 1 or 2 years. The patients are usually between 30 and 50 years old.

Characteristic Radiologic Findings
Chest radiographs can show normal anatomy or show increased hazy opacities (i.e., ground-glass opacities) mainly in the lower lobes. The characteristic high-resolution CT findings consist of extensive, symmetric, bilateral ground-glass opacities involving predominantly the lower lobes. The ground-glass opacities may be diffuse or involve mainly the peripheral lung regions.

Less Common Radiologic Manifestations
A fine reticular pattern involving mainly the subpleural regions and lower lobes is observed in approximately 60% of patients with DIP. Honeycombing may be seen, but it is uncommon and, when present, usually involves less than 10% of the lung bases.

Differential Diagnosis
- Respiratory bronchiolitis–interstitial lung disease (RBILD)
- Hypersensitivity pneumonitis (HP)
- Nonspecific interstitial pneumonia (NSIP)

Discussion
The differential diagnosis for patients with chronic symptoms who present with bilateral ground-glass opacities as the predominant or only finding is broad. The main considerations are HP, NSIP, RBILD, and DIP.

The high-resolution CT manifestations of DIP can resemble to those of HP. The differential diagnosis is based on a clinical history of exposure to precipitating antigens in HP and a history of cigarette smoking for 90% patients with DIP but only 6% of patients with HP.

Bilateral, predominantly basal ground-glass opacities in DIP, with or without mild reticulation, resemble the CT findings for NSIP. There is considerable overlap between the clinical, radiologic, and histologic findings of RBILD and those of DIP, and they usually are considered part of the spectrum of the same disease process. Because DIP is uncommon and has nonspecific radiologic findings of bilateral ground-glass opacities, the diagnosis is usually made histologically after surgical lung biopsy.

Diagnosis
Desquamative interstitial pneumonia

Suggested Readings
Hartman TE, Primack SL, Swensen SJ, et al: Desquamative interstitial pneumonia: Thin-section CT findings in 22 patients. Radiology 187:787-790, 1993.

Heyneman LE, Ward S, Lynch DA, et al: Respiratory bronchiolitis, respiratory bronchiolitis-associated interstitial lung disease, and desquamative interstitial pneumonia: Different entities or part of the spectrum of the same disease process? AJR Am J Roentgenol 173:1617-1622, 1999.

Lynch DA, Travis WD, Müller NL, et al: Idiopathic interstitial pneumonias: CT features. Radiology 236:10-21, 2005.

Wells AU, Nicholson AG, Hansell DM: Challenges in pulmonary fibrosis. 4. Smoking-induced diffuse interstitial lung diseases. Thorax 62:904-910, 2007.

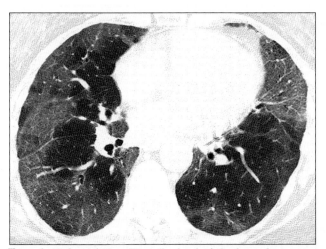

Figure 1. High-resolution CT at the level of the lower lung zones shows extensive, bilateral ground-glass opacities mainly in the peripheral lung regions. The patient was a 57-year-old woman with DIP.

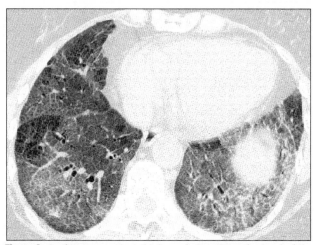

Figure 2. In the same patient, high-resolution CT at the level of the left hemidiaphragm shows diffuse ground-glass opacities, mild reticulation, and a few, small, localized areas of decreased attenuation in the right lung, consistent with emphysema.

Case 90

DEMOGRAPHICS/CLINICAL HISTORY

A 54-year-old woman with chronic cough and progressive shortness of breath, undergoing radiography and computed tomography (CT).

FINDINGS

Chest radiograph (Fig. 1) shows an extensive, bilateral reticulonodular pattern involving mainly the upper lobes and with associated elevation of the hila. High-resolution CT at the level of the upper lobes (Fig. 2) shows extensive reticulation with associated distortion of architecture, traction bronchiectasis, and subpleural honeycombing. Coronal, reformatted CT (Fig. 3) shows an upper lobe distribution of the reticulation, traction bronchiectasis, and subpleural honeycombing. Notice the superior retraction of the hila and compensatory overinflation of the lower lobes. In another patient with sarcoidosis, high-resolution CT (Fig. 4) at the level of the upper lobes shows architectural distortion, posterior displacement of the upper lobe bronchi, extensive traction bronchiectasis and bronchiolectasis, and a few subpleural cysts, consistent with honeycombing.

DISCUSSION

Definition/Background

Sarcoidosis is a systemic inflammatory disorder of unknown origin that affects multiple organs and is characterized by the formation of noncaseating granulomas. Fibrosis is seen at presentation in approximately 5% of cases and eventually develops in 20% to 25% of patients.

Characteristic Clinical Features

The most common clinical manifestations are dyspnea, cough, and chest pain.

Characteristic Radiologic Findings

The fibrosis in sarcoidosis typically involves mainly the perihilar regions of the middle and upper lung zones. It is usually associated with superior retraction of the hila, distortion of the bronchovascular bundles, bulla formation, traction bronchiectasis, and compensatory overinflation of the lower lobes. High-resolution CT frequently shows an abnormal central conglomeration of dilated and distorted perihilar bronchi (i.e., traction bronchiectasis) that is associated with masses of fibrous tissue and typically is most evident in the upper lobes. Subpleural honeycombing occurs in a small percentage of patients. The patients usually have enlarged bilateral hilar and mediastinal lymph nodes or extensively calcified nodes.

Less Common Radiologic Manifestations

Fibrosis may result in large cystic spaces due to traction bronchiectasis or bullae and in the development of intracavitary mycetomas.

Differential Diagnosis

- Silicosis
- Hypersensitivity pneumonitis
- Tuberculosis
- Pulmonary Langerhans histiocytosis
- Talcosia

Discussion

In most patients, the radiographic and CT findings of predominantly upper and middle lung zone fibrosis with a perihilar predominance and associated with enlarged or calcified, symmetric, bilateral hilar and mediastinal lymph nodes are characteristic enough to allow a diagnosis of sarcoidosis based on the imaging evidence. Silicosis may result in calcified nodes and conglomerate upper lobe fibrosis, but it tends to result in dense large opacities without perihilar traction bronchiectasis. Tuberculosis typically results in unilateral or bilateral, asymmetric upper lobe scarring. Pulmonary Langerhans histiocytosis also results in a predominantly middle and upper lung zone reticulonodular pattern with relative sparing of the lung bases seen on the radiograph. However, it is not associated with lymphadenopathy. High-resolution CT typically shows cystic spaces and nodules in a random distribution in the upper lobes and allows confident distinction of pulmonary Langerhans histiocytosis from sarcoidosis.

Diagnosis

Sarcoidosis with pulmonary fibrosis.

Suggested Readings

Abehsera M, Valeyre D, Grenier P, et al: Sarcoidosis with pulmonary fibrosis: CT patterns and correlation with pulmonary function. AJR Am J Roentgenol 174:1751-1757, 2000.

Nunes H, Brillet PY, Valeyre D, et al: Imaging in sarcoidosis. Semin Respir Crit Care Med 28:102-120, 2007.

Primack SL, Hartman TE, Hansell DM, Müller NL: End-stage lung disease: CT findings in 61 patients. Radiology 189:681-686, 1993.

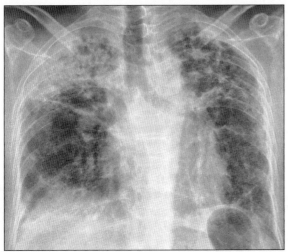

Figure 1. Chest radiograph shows an extensive, bilateral reticulonodular pattern involving mainly the upper lobes and associated elevation of the hila. The patient was a 54-year-old woman with pulmonary fibrosis due to sarcoidosis.

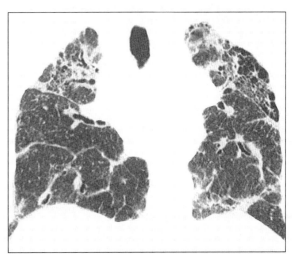

Figure 3. In the same patient, coronal, reformatted CT shows an upper lobe distribution of the reticulation, traction bronchiectasis, and subpleural honeycombing. Notice the superior retraction of the hila and compensatory overinflation of the lower lobes.

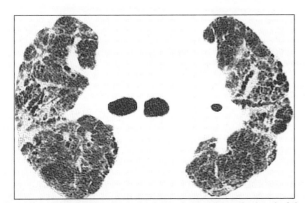

Figure 2. In the same patient, high-resolution CT at the level of the upper lobes shows extensive reticulation with associated distortion of architecture, traction bronchiectasis, and subpleural honeycombing.

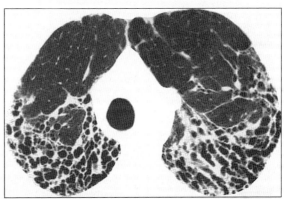

Figure 4. High-resolution CT at the level of the upper lobes shows architectural distortion, posterior displacement of the upper lobe bronchi, extensive traction bronchiectasis and bronchiolectasis, and a few subpleural cysts, consistent with honeycombing. The patient was a 46-year-old man with chronic sarcoidosis.

Case 91

DEMOGRAPHICS/CLINICAL HISTORY

A 41-year-old man who was a bird fancier and had progressive shortness of breath over several weeks, undergoing computed tomography (CT)

FINDINGS

High-resolution CT images at the level of the left upper lobe bronchus (Fig. 1) and basal segmental bronchi (Fig. 2) show diffuse, bilateral parenchymal abnormalities consisting of poorly defined, centrilobular, nodular ground-glass opacities. In another patient with hypersensitivity pneumonitis, expiratory high-resolution CT (Fig. 3) shows bilateral ground-glass opacities and lobular areas of air trapping.

DISCUSSION

Definition/Background

Hypersensitivity pneumonitis (HP), also known as extrinsic allergic alveolitis, is an immune-mediated inflammatory form of diffuse interstitial pulmonary disease caused by inhalation of various antigens that affect susceptible patients. A wide spectrum of antigens may cause HP, including thermophilic bacteria, fungi, mycobacteria, animal proteins, and certain small-molecular-weight chemical compounds such as isocyanates. The two most common forms are bird fancier's lung due to exposure to avian proteins and farmer's lung due to exposure to *Thermoactinomyces* in moldy hay. HP may be acute, subacute (the most common form), or chronic. Subacute HP is caused by intermittent or continuous exposure to low doses of antigen.

Characteristic Clinical Features

Patients with subacute HP typically present with exertional dyspnea and cough developing over several weeks or months.

Characteristic Radiologic Findings

The chest radiograph is of limited value in the diagnosis. The characteristic high-resolution CT findings of subacute HP consist of symmetric, patchy or diffuse, bilateral ground-glass opacities and lobular areas of decreased attenuation and vascularity on inspiratory images and air trapping on expiratory images. Numerous bilateral, symmetric, poorly defined, centrilobular ground-glass nodules are seen in 40% to 80% of patients.

Less Common Radiologic Manifestations

Thin-walled cysts in a random distribution are found in 13% of patients with subacute HP. The cysts typically are few (1 to 15), are 3 to 25 mm in the maximal diameter, and are associated with ground-glass opacities.

Differential Diagnosis

- Nonspecific interstitial pneumonia (NSIP)
- Respiratory bronchiolitis–interstitial lung disease (RBILD)
- Desquamative interstitial pneumonia (DIP)
- Lymphoid interstitial pneumonia (LIP)

Discussion

Ground-glass opacity is a relatively nonspecific finding seen in a variety of interstitial and air space lung diseases. The differential diagnosis for patients with chronic respiratory symptoms and exclusively ground-glass opacities includes NSIP, RBILD, DIP, and LIP. Although HP is probably the most common cause of diffuse ground-glass opacities in normal hosts, a confident diagnosis can be made only for patients with a clinical history of inhalation of antigens known to cause HP, particularly when the ground-glass opacities are associated with lobular areas of air trapping or centrilobular nodules. For the remaining patients, biopsy is required for a definitive diagnosis.

Diagnosis

Hypersensitivity pneumonitis: acute and subacute disease

Suggested Readings

Mohr LC: Hypersensitivity pneumonitis. Curr Opin Pulm Med 10:401-411, 2004.

Silva CIS, Müller NL, Churg A: Hypersensitivity pneumonitis: Spectrum of high-resolution CT and pathologic findings. AJR Am J Roentgenol 188:334-344, 2007.

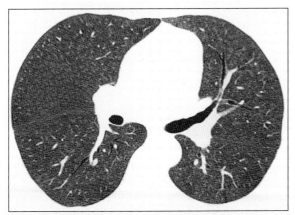

Figure 1. High-resolution CT at the level of the left upper lobe bronchus shows diffuse, bilateral parenchymal abnormalities consisting of poorly defined, centrilobular, nodular ground-glass opacities. The patient was a 41-year-old man with subacute HP.

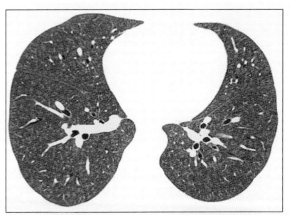

Figure 2. In the same patient, high-resolution CT at the level of the basal segmental bronchi shows diffuse, bilateral parenchymal abnormalities consisting of poorly defined, centrilobular, nodular ground-glass opacities.

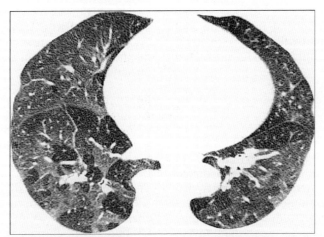

Figure 3. Expiratory, high-resolution CT shows bilateral ground-glass opacities and lobular areas of air trapping. The patient was an 85-year-old woman with subacute HP.

Case 92

DEMOGRAPHICS/CLINICAL HISTORY

A 76-year-old man with progressive shortness of breath over 2 years, undergoing computed tomography (CT).

FINDINGS

Axial, high-resolution CT at the level of the upper lung zones (Fig. 1), lower lung zones (Fig. 2), and lung bases (Fig. 3) and coronal, reformatted CT (Fig. 4) images show patchy and predominantly peripheral reticulation and architectural distortion consistent with fibrosis, bilateral ground-glass opacities, and lobular areas of decreased attenuation and vascularity.

DISCUSSION

Definition/Background

Hypersensitivity pneumonitis (HP), also known as extrinsic allergic alveolitis, is an immune-mediated inflammatory form of diffuse interstitial pulmonary disease caused by inhalation of various antigens that affect susceptible patients. A wide spectrum of antigens may cause HP, including thermophilic bacteria, fungi, mycobacteria, animal proteins, and certain small-molecular-weight chemical compounds such as isocyanates. The two most common forms are bird fancier's lung due to exposure to avian proteins and farmer's lung due to exposure to *Thermoactinomyces* in moldy hay. HP may be acute, subacute (the most common form), or chronic. Chronic HP results from very low-level, persistent or recurrent exposure to antigen and is distinguished from subacute HP by the presence of fibrosis.

Characteristic Clinical Features

Patients with chronic HP typically present with exertional dyspnea and cough developing over several months or years.

Characteristic Radiologic Findings

The chest radiograph is of limited value in the diagnosis. The characteristic high-resolution CT findings of chronic HP consist of fibrosis (i.e., reticulation, architectural distortion, traction bronchiectasis and bronchiolectasis, and honeycombing) and superimposed findings of acute or subacute disease (i.e., centrilobular nodules, ground-glass opacities, and lobular areas of air trapping) (Fig. 1,

Fig. 2, Fig. 3, Fig. 4). The reticulation in chronic HP can be patchy, random, or peribronchovascular or can have a predominantly subpleural distribution, mimicking idiopathic pulmonary fibrosis. The distribution of chronic HP in the cephalocaudal plane varies greatly. CT may show middle lung zone predominance of fibrosis with sparing of the lung apices and bases, upper lung zone, lower lobe predominance, or no zonal predominance.

Less Common Radiologic Manifestations

Thin-walled cysts in a random distribution are found in approximately 40% of the patients with chronic HP. The cysts are typically few (1 to 15), are 3 to 25 mm in the maximal diameter, and are associated with ground-glass opacities.

Differential Diagnosis

- Nonspecific interstitial pneumonia (NSIP)
- Idiopathic pulmonary fibrosis (IPF)
- Respiratory bronchiolitis—interstitial lung disease

Discussion

The main differential diagnosis of chronic HP is with NSIP and IPF. In approximately 50% of patients, the characteristic pattern and distribution of high-resolution CT findings of chronic HP, IPF, and NSIP allow confident distinction between these entities. The CT features that best differentiate chronic HP from IPF and NSIP are lobular areas of decreased attenuation and vascularity, centrilobular nodules, and absence of lower zonal predominance of abnormalities in chronic HP. The CT findings combined with the clinical history may preclude the need for surgical biopsy in selected patients, but biopsy is often required for a definitive diagnosis.

Diagnosis

Hypersensitivity pneumonitis: chronic disease

Suggested Readings

Mohr LC: Hypersensitivity pneumonitis. Curr Opin Pulm Med 10:401-411, 2004.

Silva CIS, Müller NL, Churg A: Hypersensitivity pneumonitis: Spectrum of high-resolution CT and pathologic findings. AJR Am J Roentgenol 188:334-344, 2007.

Silva CI, Müller NL, Lynch DA, et al: Chronic hypersensitivity pneumonitis: Differentiation from idiopathic pulmonary fibrosis and nonspecific interstitial pneumonia by using thin-section CT. Radiology 246:288-297, 2008.

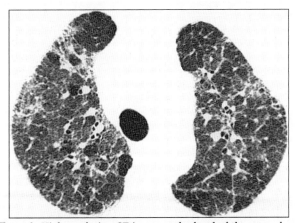

Figure 1. High-resolution CT image at the level of the upper lung zones shows patchy reticulation and architectural distortion consistent with fibrosis and mainly in the peripheral lung regions. Bilateral ground-glass opacities and lobular areas of decreased attenuation and vascularity also can be seen. The patient was a 76-year-old man with chronic HP.

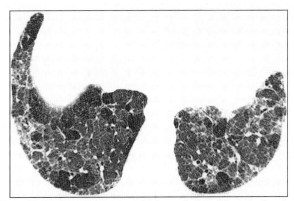

Figure 3. In the same patient, high-resolution CT at the level of the lung bases shows mild, patchy, peripheral reticulation and bilateral ground-glass opacities and lobular areas of decreased attenuation and vascularity.

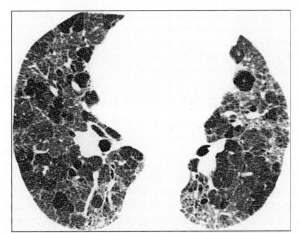

Figure 2. In the same patient, high-resolution CT at the level of the lower lobe bronchi shows patchy, peripheral reticulation and architectural distortion consistent with fibrosis. Bilateral ground-glass opacities and lobular areas of decreased attenuation and vascularity also can be seen.

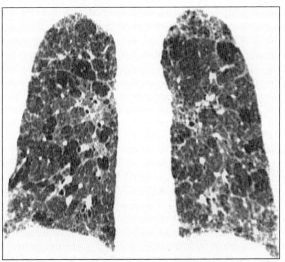

Figure 4. In the same patient, coronal, reformatted CT shows patchy, predominantly peripheral reticulation; extensive, bilateral ground-glass opacities; and lobular areas of decreased attenuation and vascularity.

Case 93

DEMOGRAPHICS/CLINICAL HISTORY

A 52-year-old man with cough and progressive shortness of breath over 1 year, undergoing radiography and computed tomography (CT).

FINDINGS

A chest radiograph (Fig. 1) shows a diffuse, reticular pattern in the upper and middle lung zones, with sparing of the lower lung zones. High-resolution CT at the level of the lung apices (Fig. 2) shows numerous bilateral, thin-walled cysts. Conglomeration of cysts in the left upper lobe has led to the formation of large cysts with bizarre shapes. High-resolution CT slightly above the level of the aortic arch (Fig. 3) shows numerous, bilateral cysts; a few, small nodules; and ground-glass opacities. High-resolution CT at the level of the lung bases (Fig. 4) shows minimal abnormalities.

DISCUSSION

Definition/Background

Pulmonary Langerhans cell histiocytosis (LCH) is an uncommon interstitial lung disease seen mainly in young adults. It is characterized by peribronchiolar proliferation of Langerhans cells. LCH is subdivided into two types: single-organ or multiorgan involvement. Pulmonary LCH usually occurs in isolation, but it is also found in most adult cases with multiorgan involvement. Most patients with pulmonary LCH are current or former smokers.

Characteristic Clinical Features

Most patients present with cough and progressive dyspnea. Approximately 10% to 15% of patients present with pneumothorax. Approximately 25% of patients are asymptomatic.

Characteristic Radiologic Findings

The chest radiograph most commonly shows a nodular or reticulonodular pattern involving the upper and middle lung zones and sparing the costophrenic angles. The characteristic high-resolution CT findings consist of cysts and nodules predominantly in the upper and middle lung regions and relative sparing of the lung bases. The nodules are well defined, are usually small, and tend to have a centrilobular distribution. The cysts can be small or large and often exhibit bizarre configurations.

Patients with pulmonary LCH are usually smokers and frequently have centrilobular emphysema.

Less Common Radiologic Manifestations

Imaging may show poorly defined centrilobular nodules or ground-glass opacities due to respiratory bronchiolitis and may reveal pneumothorax.

Differential Diagnosis

- Emphysema
- Lymphangioleiomyomatosis
- Idiopathic pulmonary fibrosis
- *Pneumocystis* pneumonia
- Sarcoidosis

Discussion

The characteristic findings of cysts and nodules throughout the middle and upper lung zones with relative sparing of the lung bases in an adult smoker allow confident diagnosis of pulmonary LCH in most cases. However, there is some overlap of appearances with other cystic lung diseases, and biopsy confirmation may be required in atypical cases. Centrilobular emphysema can usually be readily distinguished by the lack of visible walls and the presence of vessels within the focal areas of lung destruction. The cysts in lymphangioleiomyomatosis are typically seen throughout the lungs, without any zonal predominance, and they are not associated with nodules. The cysts of honeycombing in idiopathic pulmonary fibrosis typically involve mainly the subpleural and basilar lung regions and are associated with reticulation and decreased lung volumes. Upper lobe cystic lesions identical to those in pulmonary LCH may be seen in *Pneumocystis* pneumonia. The two can be distinguished by the clinical history and presence of extensive ground-glass opacities in patients with *Pneumocystis* pneumonia.

Diagnosis

Pulmonary Langerhans cell histiocytosis

Suggested Readings

Abbott GF, Rosado-de-Christenson ML, Franks TJ, et al: From the archives of the AFIP: Pulmonary Langerhans cell histiocytosis. Radiographics 24:821-841, 2004.

Bonelli FS, Hartman TE, Swensen SJ, Sherrick A: Accuracy of high-resolution CT in diagnosing lung diseases. AJR Am J Roentgenol 170:1507-1512, 1998.

Koyama M, Johkoh T, Honda O, et al: Chronic cystic lung disease: Diagnostic accuracy of high-resolution CT in 92 patients. AJR Am J Roentgenol 180:827-835, 2003.

Tazi A: Adult pulmonary Langerhans' cell histiocytosis. Eur Respir J 27:1272-1285, 2006.

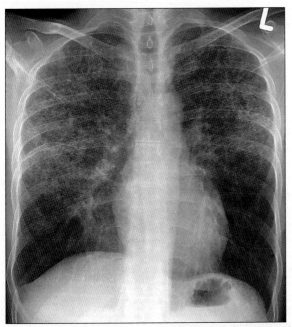

Figure 1. Chest radiograph shows a diffuse, reticular pattern in the upper and middle lung zones and sparing of the lower lung zones. The patient was a 52-year-old male smoker with pulmonary LCH.

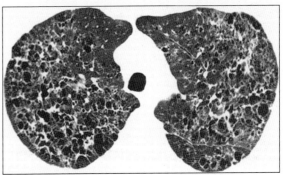

Figure 3. In the same patient, high-resolution CT slightly above the level of the aortic arch shows numerous, bilateral cysts; a few, small nodules; and ground-glass opacities. The ground-glass opacities reflect the presence of respiratory bronchiolitis (i.e., smoker's bronchiolitis).

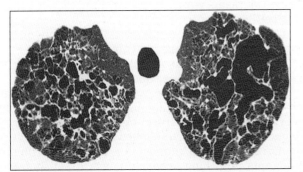

Figure 2. In the same patient, high-resolution CT at the level of the lung apices shows numerous bilateral, thin-walled cysts. Conglomeration of cysts in the left upper lobe has led to the formation of large cysts with bizarre shapes.

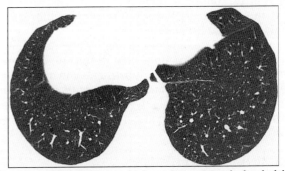

Figure 4. In the same patient, high-resolution CT at the level of the lung bases shows minimal abnormalities.

Case 94

DEMOGRAPHICS/CLINICAL HISTORY

A 48-year-old woman with progressive shortness of breath over several years, undergoing computed tomography (CT).

FINDINGS

Numerous, bilateral, thin-walled cysts are distributed diffusely throughout the lung parenchyma (Figs. 1 to 3).

DISCUSSION

Definition/Background

Lymphangioleiomyomatosis (LAM) is an uncommon disease of unknown origin. It is characterized by proliferation of abnormal smooth muscle cells (i.e., LAM cells) throughout the bronchioles, perivascular spaces, and lymphatics. Bronchiolar obstruction results in pulmonary cyst formation and, commonly, in pneumothorax; vessel obstruction may result in pulmonary hemorrhage and lymphatic obstruction in chylothorax and lymph node enlargement. LAM occurs in a sporadic form, which affects only women (typically of childbearing age) and in a small percentage of patients with tuberous sclerosis.

Characteristic Clinical Features

The most common symptoms are progressive dyspnea and recurrent pneumothorax. Approximately 40% to 50% of patients present with pneumothorax and 15% with chylothorax. The patients are women, who usually are of childbearing age.

Characteristic Radiologic Findings

The chest radiograph may show normal anatomy or show diffuse, bilateral reticulation; normal or increased lung volumes; and commonly, recurrent pneumothorax and pleural effusion. The characteristic high-resolution CT findings consist of thin-walled cysts, usually measuring a few millimeters to 2 cm in diameter and distributed diffusely throughout the lungs without any upper or lower lung zone predominance.

Less Common Radiologic Manifestations

Ground-glass opacities may be seen because of pulmonary edema and hemorrhage resulting from involvement of the venules and leading to vascular occlusion. Small, centrilobular nodules may be seen and reflect the presence of peribronchiolar accumulation of smooth muscle cells. Pleural effusion can result from chylothorax. Mediastinal lymphadenopathy and renal angiomyolipomas may also occur.

Differential Diagnosis

- Pulmonary Langerhans cell histiocytosis
- Emphysema

Discussion

Many small, thin-walled cysts scattered through both lungs in a young woman strongly suggests LAM. The cystic changes in LAM may be identical to those of Langerhans cell histiocytosis. However, the cysts in Langerhans cell histiocytosis tend to show relative sparing of the lung bases, whereas the cysts in LAM involve all lung zones to a similar extent. Other helpful findings are the frequent presence of nodules and bizarrely shaped cysts in Langerhans cell histiocytosis.

The cysts in LAM have well-defined, smooth walls and therefore can be readily distinguished from emphysema, which is characterized by localized areas of low attenuation without identifiable walls. Emphysema usually has upper lobe predominance. Uniform distribution throughout both lungs strongly favors the diagnosis of LAM.

Diagnosis

Lymphangioleiomyomatosis

Suggested Readings

Abbott GF, Rosado-de-Christenson ML, Frazier AA, et al: From the archives of the AFIP: Lymphangioleiomyomatosis: Radiologic-pathologic correlation. Radiographics 25:803-828, 2005.

Johnson SR: Lymphangioleiomyomatosis. Eur Respir J 27:1056-1065, 2006.

Pallisa E, Sanz P, Roman A, et al: Lymphangioleiomyomatosis: Pulmonary and abdominal findings with pathologic correlation. Radiographics 22:S185-S198, 2002.

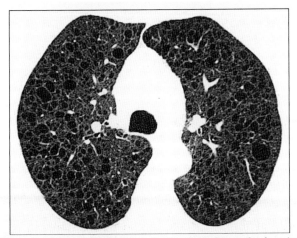

Figure 1. High-resolution CT at the level of the tracheal carina shows numerous, thin-walled cysts throughout both lungs. The patient was a 48-year-old woman with lymphangioleiomyomatosis.

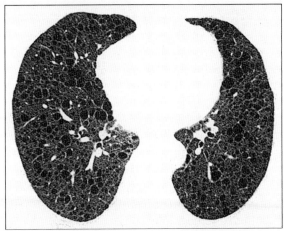

Figure 2. In the same patient, high-resolution CT at the level of basal segmental bronchi shows numerous, thin-walled cysts throughout both lungs.

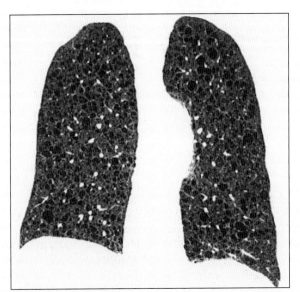

Figure 3. In the same patient, coronal, reformatted CT shows numerous, thin-walled cysts throughout both lungs.

Case 95

DEMOGRAPHICS/CLINICAL HISTORY

A 56-year-old woman with rheumatoid arthritis and a 1-year history of progressive shortness of breath, undergoing computed tomography (CT).

FINDINGS

High-resolution CT images at the level of the basal segmental bronchi (Fig. 1) and at the level of the diaphragm (Fig. 2) show minimal bilateral ground-glass opacities; a reticular pattern; and honeycombing, occurring mainly in the posterior peripheral lung regions and consistent with the usual interstitial pneumonia pattern. Notice the associated volume loss with posterior displacement of the major fissures (Fig. 1).

DISCUSSION

Definition/Background

Rheumatoid arthritis is an autoimmune disorder of unknown origin with various clinical manifestations. Interstitial lung disease occurs in 5% to 20% of patients and most commonly has a pattern of usual interstitial pneumonia (UIP) and, less commonly, of nonspecific interstitial pneumonia (NSIP).

Characteristic Clinical Features

The most common symptoms related to parenchymal disease are dry cough and progressive shortness of breath.

Characteristic Radiologic Findings

The characteristic radiologic pattern of pulmonary fibrosis in rheumatoid arthritis is a reticular or reticulonodular pattern involving mainly the lung bases. High-resolution CT shows reticulation, traction bronchiectasis, traction bronchiolectasis, and honeycombing mainly in the peripheral lung regions and lung bases. These findings are typical of UIP. In patients with rheumatoid arthritis and NSIP, high-resolution CT shows a predominant ground-glass pattern with or without superimposed fine reticulation and traction bronchiectasis but little or no honeycombing.

Less Common Radiologic Manifestations

Occasionally, rheumatoid arthritis may be associated with organizing pneumonia, which typically manifests as bilateral areas of consolidation in a predominantly peribronchial and peripheral distribution, or as lymphoid interstitial pneumonia (LIP), which typically manifests with bilateral ground-glass opacities, poorly defined centrilobular nodules, and several thin-walled cysts involving mainly the lower lung zones. Necrobiotic nodules are rare.

Differential Diagnosis

- Idiopathic pulmonary fibrosis
- Nonspecific interstitial pneumonia (NSIP)
- Drug-induced lung disease

Discussion

The radiologic findings of UIP related to rheumatoid arthritis are identical to those of idiopathic pulmonary fibrosis, and the findings of NSIP are identical to those seen in idiopathic NSIP, NSIP related to other connective tissue diseases, drug reaction, or hypersensitivity pneumonitis. The differential diagnosis is based on the clinical history of rheumatoid arthritis.

Diagnosis

Pulmonary parenchymal manifestations of rheumatoid arthritis.

Suggested Readings

Anaya JM, Diethelm L, Ortiz LA, et al: Pulmonary involvement in rheumatoid arthritis. Semin Arthritis Rheum 24:242-254, 1995.

Gabbay E, Tarala R, Will R, et al: Interstitial lung disease in recent onset rheumatoid arthritis. Am J Respir Crit Care Med 156(Pt 1): 528-535, 1997.

Remy-Jardin M, Remy J, Cortet B, et al: Lung changes in rheumatoid arthritis. CT findings 193:375-382, 1994.

Tanaka N, Kim JS, Newell JD, et al: Rheumatoid arthritis-related lung diseases: CT findings. Radiology 232:81-91, 2004.

Tansey D, Wells AU, Colby TV, et al: Variations in histological patterns of interstitial pneumonia between connective tissue disorders and their relationship to prognosis. Histopathology 44:585-596, 2004.

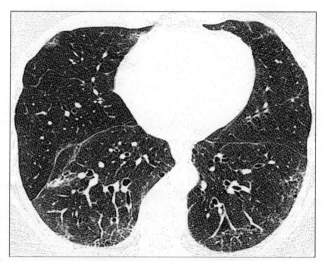

Figure 1. High-resolution CT at the level of the basal segmental bronchi shows minimal, bilateral ground-glass opacities; a reticular pattern; and honeycombing, mainly in the posterior peripheral lung regions. Notice the associated volume loss with posterior displacement of the major fissures. The patient was a 56-year-old woman with a long-standing history of rheumatoid arthritis and parenchymal findings consistent with UIP.

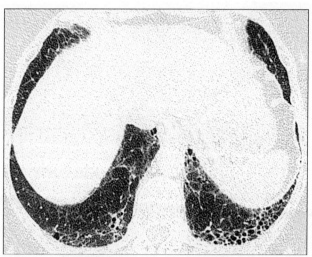

Figure 2. In the same patient, high-resolution CT at the level of the diaphragm shows extensive, subpleural honeycombing.

Case 96

DEMOGRAPHICS/CLINICAL HISTORY

A 41-year-old woman with scleroderma and progressive shortness of breath over several months, undergoing computed tomography (CT)

FINDINGS

High-resolution CT shows bilateral reticulation, mild ground-glass opacities, traction bronchiectasis, and traction bronchiolectasis mainly in the peripheral lung regions (Fig. 1). Notice the relative sparing of the subpleural regions of the right lower lobe and a fluid level in the dilated esophagus. In another patient, high-resolution CT at the level of the upper lobes (Fig. 2) shows bilateral areas of ground-glass opacities involving predominantly the peripheral lung regions, and CT at the level of the lung bases (Fig. 3) shows diffuse bilateral areas of ground-glass opacities and mild reticulation.

DISCUSSION

Definition/Background

Scleroderma is an autoimmune disorder of unknown cause that is characterized by excessive deposits of collagen, resulting in thickening of the skin. It may be localized or systemic (i.e., progressive systemic sclerosis). Systemic sclerosis is uncommon, with an estimated prevalence of 1 case per 2000 members of the population. It most frequently affects women in their childbearing years. Pulmonary fibrosis ultimately develops in 80% of patients with systemic sclerosis. In a small percentage of patients, pulmonary fibrosis may precede other clinical manifestations of systemic sclerosis. The most frequent histologic subtype of pulmonary fibrosis is nonspecific interstitial pneumonia (NSIP). Usual interstitial pneumonia (UIP) and diffuse alveolar damage (DAD) are much less common.

Characteristic Clinical Features

The most common pulmonary symptom of systemic sclerosis is dyspnea, which eventually occurs in approximately 60% of patients.

Characteristic Radiologic Findings

The most frequent abnormality on chest radiography consists of a widespread, symmetric basal reticulonodular pattern or hazy increase in opacity (ground-glass opacity). High-resolution CT typically shows findings of NSIP consisting mainly of ground-glass opacities involving mainly the lower lung zones with or without associated fine reticulation, traction bronchiectasis, traction bronchiolectasis, and volume loss. Honeycombing is characteristically absent in the early stages, although it may develop as the fibrosis progresses. The fibrosis in NSIP tends to spare the immediate subpleural lung in the dorsal regions of the lower lobes. Most patients with progressive systemic sclerosis have a dilated esophagus evident on CT.

Less Common Radiologic Manifestations

Less common findings are a predominant reticulation pattern due to UIP or extensive ground-glass opacities and dependent consolidation due to DAD. Patients may have enlarged central pulmonary arteries due to pulmonary artery hypertension. Pleural effusions occur in 5% to 10% of patients

Differential Diagnosis

- Nonspecific interstitial pneumonia from other causes
- Usual interstitial pneumonia

Discussion

The radiologic findings of NSIP in progressive systemic sclerosis are identical to those seen in idiopathic NSIP, NSIP related to other connective tissue diseases, drug reactions, or hypersensitivity pneumonitis. The differential diagnosis is based on the clinical history of systemic sclerosis.

Diagnosis

Nonspecific interstitial pneumonia in scleroderma

Suggested Readings

Desai SR, Veeraraghavan S, Hansell DM, et al: CT features of lung disease in patients with systemic sclerosis: Comparison with idiopathic pulmonary fibrosis and nonspecific interstitial pneumonia. Radiology 232:560-567, 2004.

Devaraj A, Wells AU, Hansell DM: Computed tomographic imaging in connective tissue diseases. Semin Respir Crit Care Med 28:389-397, 2007.

Highland KB, Garin MC, Brown KK: The spectrum of scleroderma lung disease. Semin Respir Crit Care Med 28:418-429, 2007.

Orlandi I, Camiciottoli G, Diciotti S, et al: Thin-section and low-dose volumetric computed tomographic densitometry of the lung in systemic sclerosis. J Comput Assist Tomogr 30:823-827, 2006.

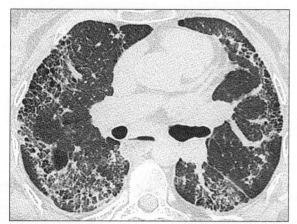

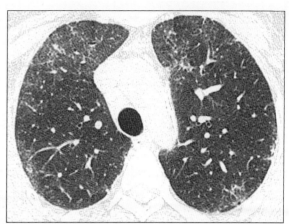

Figure 1. High-resolution CT at the level of the bronchus intermedius shows bilateral reticulation, mild ground-glass opacities, and findings of fibrosis (i.e., honeycombing, traction bronchiectasis, and traction bronchiolectasis) occurring mainly in the peripheral lung regions. Notice the relative sparing of the subpleural regions of the right lower lobe and a fluid level in the dilated esophagus. The patient was a 41-year-old woman with a fibrotic NSIP pattern associated with scleroderma.

Figure 2. High-resolution CT at the level of the upper lobes shows bilateral areas of ground-glass opacities involving predominantly the peripheral lung regions, mild reticulation, and traction bronchiectasis. The patient was a 39-year-old woman with an NSIP pattern associated with scleroderma.

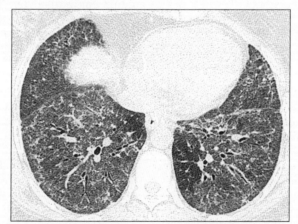

Figure 3. In a 39-year-old woman with an NSIP pattern associated with scleroderma, high-resolution CT at the level of the lung bases shows diffuse bilateral areas of ground-glass opacities and mild reticulation.

Case 97

DEMOGRAPHICS/CLINICAL HISTORY

A 73-year-old woman with cough and hemoptysis, undergoing radiography and computed tomography (CT)

FINDINGS

Posteroanterior (Fig. 1) and lateral (Fig. 2) chest radiographs show bilateral, large, thick-walled cavitating masses. CT at the level of the pulmonary ligaments shows bilateral cavitating masses with thick walls (Fig. 3). In another patient, high-resolution CT shows bilateral ground-glass opacities in a patchy distribution (Fig. 4).

DISCUSSION

Definition/Background

Wegener granulomatosis (WG) is a multisystem disease characterized by necrotizing granulomatous inflammation of the upper and lower respiratory tracts, glomerulonephritis, and necrotizing vasculitis of the lungs and of a variety of other organs and tissues. The diagnosis often can be made by the combination of clinical and radiologic findings and serum positive for antineutrophil classic pattern cytoplasmic antibodies (c-ANCAs).

Characteristic Clinical Features

Most patients present with upper and lower respiratory symptoms, which include epistaxis, sinusitis, cough, hemoptysis, dyspnea, and pleuritic chest pain.

Characteristic Radiologic Findings

The most common radiographic abnormality consists of lung nodules or masses, which are seen in up to 90% of patients with WG. The nodules or masses range from a few millimeters to 10 cm in diameter. Cavitation occurs eventually in approximately 50% of cases. The second most common radiographic manifestation consists of areas of air-space consolidation or ground-glass opacities, seen in approximately 50% of patients.

Less Common Radiologic Manifestations

Imaging may reveal subglottic stenosis, focal tracheal stenosis, or bronchial stenosis. Pleural effusion is seen in 15% to 20% of cases and pleural thickening in 10%.

Differential Diagnosis
- Septic embolism
- Metastases
- Lymphoma

Discussion

The main differential diagnosis is with conditions that may result in multiple pulmonary nodules or masses, with or without cavitation. They include mainly infections (e.g., septic embolism, multiple lung abscesses) and neoplasms (e.g., hematogenous metastases, lymphoma). Multiple lung abscesses associated with bacteremia and septic emboli usually are associated with fever, tend to involve mainly the lower lobes, and seldom are more than 3 cm in diameter. The nodules and masses in WG can be up to 10 cm in diameter and show no predilection for the upper or lower lung zones. Hematogenous metastases may be multiple and range from a few millimeters to more than 10 cm in diameter; approximately 5% cavitate. Typically, metastatic nodules and masses have a wide range in size in any patient and tend to involve mainly the lower lobes. Multiple nodules and masses may be seen in patients with lymphoma. Cavitation, which occurs in about 50% of cases of WG, is uncommon in lymphoma. Differentiation of WG from these other conditions usually can be made clinically by the presence of upper respiratory symptoms (including sinusitis and epistaxis), laboratory findings indicative of glomerulonephritis, and serum positive for c-ANCAs.

Diagnosis

Wegener granulomatosis

Suggested Readings

Lee KS, Kim TS, Fujimoto K, et al: Thoracic manifestations of Wegener's granulomatosis: CT findings in 30 patients. Eur Radiol 13:43-51, 2003.

Lohrmann C, Uhl M, Kotter E, et al: Pulmonary manifestations of Wegener granulomatosis: CT findings in 57 patients and a review of the literature. Eur J Radiol 53:471-477, 2005.

Lohrmann C, Uhl M, Schaefer O, et al: Serial high-resolution computed tomography imaging in patients with Wegener granulomatosis: Differentiation between active inflammatory and chronic fibrotic lesions. Acta Radiol 46:484-491, 2005.

Sheehan RE, Flint JD, Müller NL: Computed tomography features of the thoracic manifestations of Wegener granulomatosis. J Thorac Imaging 18:34-41, 2003.

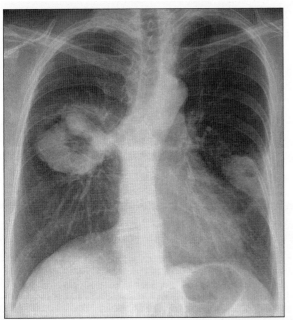

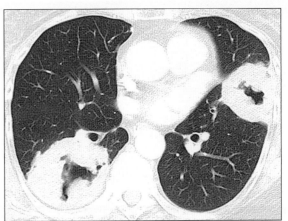

Figure 3. CT at the level of the pulmonary ligaments shows bilateral cavitating masses with thick walls in a 73-year-old woman with WG.

Figure 1. Posteroanterior chest radiograph shows bilateral cavitating masses with thick walls. The patient was a 73-year-old woman with WG.

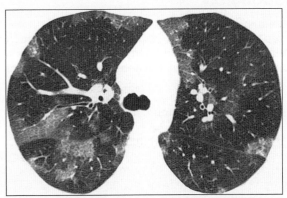

Figure 4. High-resolution CT shows bilateral ground-glass opacities in a patchy distribution. The patient was a 35 year-old-man with diffuse pulmonary hemorrhage caused by WG.

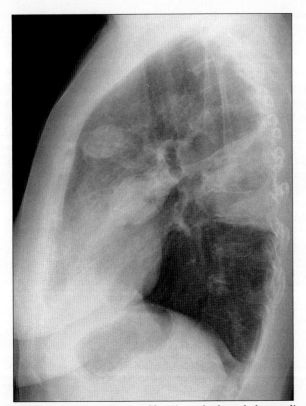

Figure 2. In the same 73-year-old patient, the lateral chest radiograph shows pulmonary masses, two of which are cavitating.

Case 98

DEMOGRAPHICS/CLINICAL HISTORY

A 78-year-old woman with hemoptysis and gromerulonephritis, undergoing computed tomography (CT).

FINDINGS

CT images at the level of the great vessels (Fig. 1) and the aortic arch (Fig. 2) show extensive, bilateral ground-glass opacities and areas of consolidation involving mainly the right upper lobe, which is consistent with diffuse pulmonary hemorrhage.

DISCUSSION

Definition/Background

Goodpasture syndrome, also known as anti-glomerular basement membrane antibody disease, is an autoimmune disorder characterized by repeated episodes of pulmonary hemorrhage that is usually associated with glomerulonephritis and the presence of anti-glomerular basement membrane (anti-GBM) antibodies.

Characteristic Clinical Features

The most common presenting symptom is hemoptysis, which occurs in about 80% to 95% of patients. The hemoptysis may range from mild to copious and can be a life-threatening condition. In more than 50% of patients, it precedes glomerulonephritis.

Characteristic Radiologic Findings

The most common radiologic manifestations consist of patchy hazy areas of increased opacity (i.e., ground-glass opacities) that are scattered fairly evenly throughout the lungs. With more severe hemorrhage, the pattern may progress to focal or confluent areas of consolidation, which often are associated with air bronchograms. The opacities usually are widespread but may be more prominent in the perihilar areas and in the middle and lower lung zones. The apices and costophrenic angles are almost invariably spared. Parenchymal involvement usually is bilateral.

Less Common Radiologic Manifestations

Imaging may show unilateral or bilateral, asymmetric ground-glass opacities or consolidation.

Differential Diagnosis

- Microscopic polyangiitis
- Wegener granulomatosis
- Systemic lupus erythematosus
- Mixed connective tissue disease

Discussion

The diagnosis of Goodpasture syndrome should be suspected when an adult patient has hemoptysis and bilateral air-space consolidation on the chest radiograph, particularly when manifestations of renal disease are also present. Confirmation can be obtained by demonstration of circulating or tissue-bound anti-GBM antibodies. If the diagnosis remains uncertain, it can be confirmed by demonstrating autoantibodies on kidney biopsy. Most other conditions characterized by hemoptysis and renal dysfunction can be recognized by associated clinical and laboratory manifestations of vasculitis or by the observation of immunoglobulin and complement deposition in a granular pattern on immunofluorescent examination of a kidney biopsy specimen. Because renal involvement in Goodpasture syndrome may not be apparent initially, the diagnosis must considered in any patient who has radiologic and clinical findings consistent with diffuse alveolar hemorrhage and no evidence of kidney disease. The differential diagnosis in this situation is large and includes various connective tissue diseases (especially systemic lupus erythematosus), systemic vasculitis (e.g., Wegener granulomatosis), aspirated blood after vascular disruption, and some metastatic neoplasms, such as choriocarcinoma.

Diagnosis

Goodpasture syndrome (antibasement membrane antibody disease)

Suggested Readings

Erlich JH, Sevastos J, Pussell BA: Goodpasture's disease: Antiglomerular basement membrane disease. Nephrology (Carlton) 9:49-51, 2004.

Frankel SK, Cosgrove GP, Fischer A, et al: Update in the diagnosis and management of pulmonary vasculitis. Chest 129:452-465, 2006.

Hansell DM: Small-vessel diseases of the lung: CT-pathologic correlates. Radiology 225:639-653, 2002.

Mayberry JP, Primack SL, Müller NL: Thoracic manifestations of systemic autoimmune diseases: Radiographic and high-resolution CT findings. Radiographics 20:1623-1635, 2000.

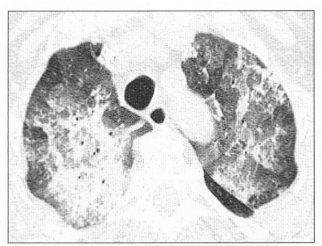

Figure 1. CT at the level of the great vessels shows extensive bilateral ground-glass opacities and areas of consolidation involving mainly the right upper lobe consistent with diffuse pulmonary hemorrhage. The patient was a 78-year-old woman with Goodpasture syndrome.

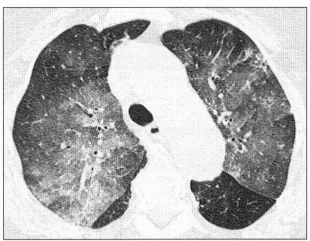

Figure 2. CT at the level of the aortic arch shows extensive bilateral ground-glass opacities consistent with diffuse pulmonary hemorrhage in a 78-year-old woman with Goodpasture syndrome.

Case 99

DEMOGRAPHICS/CLINICAL HISTORY

A 34-year-old woman with rapidly progressive glomerulonephritis, hemoptysis, and positive results for perinuclear-staining antineutrophil cytoplasmic antibodies (p-ANCAs), undergoing computed tomography (CT)

FINDINGS

CT images at the level of the aortic arch (Fig. 1) and the lung bases (Fig. 2) show patchy, bilateral ground-glass opacities and small areas of consolidation consistent with diffuse pulmonary hemorrhage. Also noted are a few septal lines.

DISCUSSION

Definition/Background
Microscopic polyangiitis is a necrotizing vasculitis that involves small vessels (i.e., arterioles, venules, and capillaries) and has few or no immune deposits. It is the most common cause of the pulmonary-renal syndrome, which is characterized by the coexistence of pulmonary hemorrhage and glomerulonephritis.

Characteristic Clinical Features
The clinical manifestations are usually renal and, less commonly, pulmonary. Rapidly progressive glomerulonephritis occurs in more than 90% of patients, and diffuse pulmonary hemorrhage with associated hemoptysis occurs in 10% to 30%.

Characteristic Radiologic Findings
The most common radiologic manifestations consist of patchy, hazy areas of increased opacity (i.e., ground-glass opacities) scattered fairly evenly throughout the lungs. With more severe hemorrhage, the pattern may progress to focal or confluent areas of consolidation that often are associated with air bronchograms. The opacities usually are widespread but may be more prominent in the perihilar areas and in the middle and lower lung zones. The apices and costophrenic angles are almost invariably spared. Parenchymal involvement usually is bilateral. Septal lines and ground-glass centrilobular nodules may be seen.

Less Common Radiologic Manifestations
Imaging may reveal unilateral or bilateral, asymmetric ground-glass opacities or consolidation.

Differential Diagnosis
- Goodpasture syndrome
- Wegener granulomatosis
- Systemic lupus erythematosus
- Mixed connective tissue disease

Discussion
The diagnosis of microscopic polyangiitis should be suspected in patients with rapidly progressive glomerulonephritis and serum positive for p-ANCA who present with clinical and radiologic findings consistent with diffuse pulmonary hemorrhage. A positive p-ANCA result lacks specificity because it is found in a wide variety of settings, including microscopic polyangiitis, Churg-Strauss syndrome, rheumatoid arthritis, and Goodpasture syndrome.

Microscopic polyangiitis is the most common cause of the pulmonary-renal syndrome. The main differential diagnosis clinically is with other conditions that may cause pulmonary and renal manifestations, particularly Goodpasture syndrome, Wegener granulomatosis, and systemic lupus erythematosus. Goodpasture syndrome is usually diagnosed by demonstration of circulating or tissue-bound anti-glomerular basement membrane (anti-GBM) antibodies. Microscopic polyangiitis is distinguished from Wegener granulomatosis by the lack of granulomatous inflammation and from systemic lupus erythematosus and other small-vessel vasculitides by the lack of immune deposits on surgical lung biopsy.

Diagnosis
Microscopic polyangiitis

Suggested Readings
Collins CE, Quismorio FP Jr: Pulmonary involvement in microscopic polyangiitis. Curr Opin Pulm Med 11:447-451, 2005.
Brown KK: Pulmonary vasculitis. Proc Am Thorac Soc 3:48-57, 2006.
Heeringa P, Schreiber A, Falk RJ, Jennette JC: Pathogenesis of pulmonary vasculitis. Semin Respir Crit Care Med 25:465-474, 2004.
Lauque D, Cadranel J, Lazor R, et al: Microscopic polyangiitis with alveolar hemorrhage. A study of 29 cases and review of the literature. Groupe d'Etudes et de Recherche sur les Maladies "Orphelines" Pulmonaires (GERM"O"P). Medicine (Baltimore) 79: 222-233, 2000.

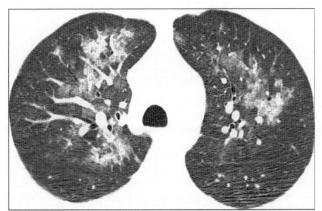

Figure 1. Diffuse pulmonary hemorrhage in microscopic polyangiitis is seen in a 34-year-old woman with rapidly progressive glomerulonephritis, hemoptysis, and a positive p-ANCA result. CT at the level of the aortic arch shows patchy, bilateral ground-glass opacities and small areas of consolidation.

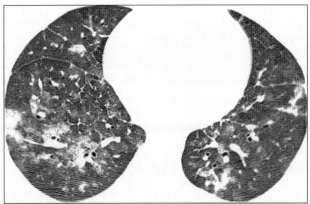

Figure 2. In the same patient, CT at the level of the lung bases shows patchy, bilateral ground-glass opacities, small areas of consolidation, ground-glass centrilobular nodules, and a few septal lines.

Case 100

DEMOGRAPHICS/CLINICAL HISTORY

A 50-year-old man with recurrent genital ulcerations, relapsing uveitis, and hemoptysis, undergoing radiography and computed tomography (CT).

FINDINGS

Chest radiograph reveals increased size and opacity of the right interlobar and lower lobe pulmonary arteries (Fig. 1). Contrast-enhanced CT shows a partially thrombosed aneurysm of the right interlobar pulmonary artery (Fig. 2). CT at a slightly lower level shows thrombosis of the right lower lobe pulmonary artery (Fig. 3). CT using lung windows shows the increased diameter of the right interlobar and lower lobe pulmonary arteries and asymmetric, bilateral ground-glass opacities, which are consistent with pulmonary hemorrhage (Fig. 4).

DISCUSSION

Definition/Background

Behçet disease is an uncommon systemic disorder characterized by vasculitis and the triad of recurrent ulcers of the oral and genital mucosa with relapsing uveitis. Vascular complications develop in 20% to 40% of patients with Behçet disease and include subcutaneous thrombophlebitis, deep venous thrombosis, and pulmonary and systemic arterial aneurysms and occlusions. Although it has a worldwide distribution, it occurs most commonly in Turkey and in Eastern Asia.

Characteristic Clinical Features

Pulmonary manifestations may be the initial features of the disease, but they more commonly develop several years after the diagnosis. Most patients with pulmonary artery aneurysms have hemoptysis. Other symptoms include chest pain, dyspnea, and cough.

Characteristic Radiologic Findings

The radiologic manifestations are usually those of pulmonary artery aneurysms and thrombosis of the pulmonary arteries and systemic veins. Radiographically, pulmonary artery aneurysms manifest as round, perihilar opacities or as a rapidly developing, unilateral hilar enlargement. The presence, size, and location of the pulmonary aneurysms are best assessed on contrast-enhanced CT. Aneurysms are seen as saccular or fusiform dilatations, which

show homogeneous contrast filling simultaneously with the pulmonary artery. The aneurysms are often multiple and range from 1 to 7 cm in diameter. The wall of the involved pulmonary artery is often thickened and enhances after intravenous administration of contrast.

Less Common Radiologic Manifestations

Partial or complete thrombosis of the aneurysm may occur and result in localized areas of consolidation as a result of infarction, areas of decreased attenuation and vascularity, and atelectasis. Pulmonary hemorrhage as a result of vasculitis or pulmonary artery rupture can cause focal, multifocal, or diffuse ground-glass opacities or consolidations. Thrombosis of major veins, including the superior vena cava, is a common finding in patients with or without pulmonary artery aneurysms.

Differential Diagnosis

- Mycotic pulmonary artery pseudoaneurysm
- Traumatic pulmonary artery aneurysm
- Hughes-Stovin syndrome

Discussion

Pulmonary artery aneurysms and pseudoaneurysms are uncommon. The differential diagnosis includes Behçet disease, Hughes-Stovin syndrome, infection (e.g., mycotic pseudoaneurysm), and previous trauma, often iatrogenic (e.g., malpositioned Swan-Ganz catheter). Hughes-Stovin syndrome is characterized by recurrent thrombophlebitis, pulmonary artery aneurysm formation, and rupture. The diagnosis of Behçet disease as the cause of pulmonary artery aneurysm is usually straightforward and based on the characteristic history of associated recurrent oral and genital ulcerations and uveitis.

Diagnosis

Behçet disease

Suggested Readings

Alpagut U, Ugurlucan M, Dayioglu E: Major arterial involvement and review of Behcet's disease. Ann Vasc Surg 21:232-239, 2007.

Erkan F, Gul A, Tasali E: Pulmonary manifestations of Behçet disease. Thorax 56:572-578, 2001.

Hiller N, Lieberman S, Chajek-Shaul T, et al: Thoracic manifestations of Behçet disease at CT. Radiographics 24:801-808, 2004.

Nguyen ET, Silva CI, Seely JM, et al: Pulmonary artery aneurysms and pseudoaneurysms in adults: Findings at CT and radiography. AJR Am J Roentgenol 188:W126-W134, 2007.

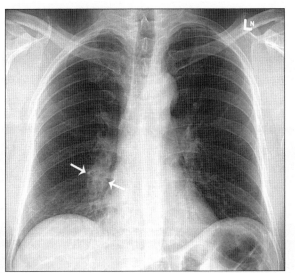

Figure 1. Chest radiograph reveals an increase in the size and opacity of the right interlobar and lower lobe pulmonary arteries *(arrows)*. The patient was a 50-year-old man with Behçet disease and pulmonary artery aneurysm.

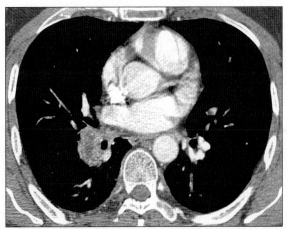

Figure 3. Contrast-enhanced CT at a slightly lower level in the same patient shows thrombosis of the aneurysmal right lower lobe pulmonary artery.

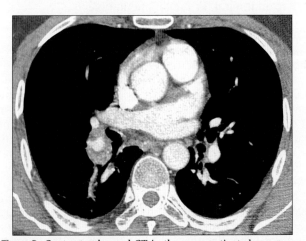

Figure 2. Contrast-enhanced CT in the same patient shows a partially thrombosed aneurysm of the right interlobar pulmonary artery.

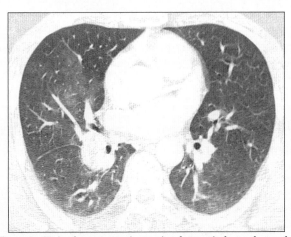

Figure 4. CT in the same patient using lung windows shows the increased diameter of the right interlobar and lower lobe pulmonary arteries and asymmetric, bilateral ground-glass opacities, which are consistent with pulmonary hemorrhage.

Case 101

DEMOGRAPHICS/CLINICAL HISTORY

A 57-year-old man with a history of asthma, peripheral eosinophilia, and serum perinuclear-staining antineutrophil cytoplasmic antibodies (p-ANCAs) undergoing radiography and computed tomography (CT).

FINDINGS

Posteroanterior chest radiograph shows patchy, bilateral areas of hazy, increased opacity and consolidation (Fig. 1). Axial (Fig. 2) and coronal (Fig. 3) CT images show patchy, bilateral, focal ground-glass opacities and consolidation.

DISCUSSION

Definition/Background

Churg-Strauss syndrome (CSS) is a p-ANCA–associated, small-vessel vasculitis characterized clinically by asthma, allergic rhinitis, and peripheral eosinophilia and pathologically by necrotizing vasculitis and extravascular granulomatous inflammation.

Characteristic Clinical Features

Pulmonary involvement results in cough and shortness of breath and, occasionally, in hemoptysis.

Characteristic Radiologic Findings

The most common radiologic finding consists of transient, patchy, nonsegmental ground-glass opacities or areas of consolidation without predilection for any lung zone. The ground-glass opacities and areas of consolidation often have a peripheral distribution and may be indistinguishable from those of simple pulmonary eosinophilia (i.e., Löffler syndrome) and chronic eosinophilic pneumonia.

Less Common Radiologic Manifestations

Interlobular septal thickening is seen on high-resolution CT in approximately 50% of patients. Thickening may reflect the presence of interstitial pulmonary edema resulting from cardiac involvement or eosinophilic infiltration of the septa. Less common findings include small centrilobular nodules and multiple nodules or masses measuring 0.5 to 3.5 cm in diameter, with or without a halo of ground-glass attenuation.

Differential Diagnosis

- Simple pulmonary eosinophilia
- Chronic eosinophilic pneumonia
- *Pneumocystis* pneumonia
- Allergic bronchopulmonary aspergillosis
- Bacterial, viral, or fungal pneumonia

Discussion

The radiologic manifestations of CSS can be similar to those of simple pulmonary eosinophilia and chronic eosinophilic pneumonia. Simple pulmonary eosinophilia is characterized by patchy, nonsegmental ground-glass opacities or consolidation that usually is transient and migratory and associated with eosinophilia. Most patients have a history of asthma or atopy. The cause is unknown. Chronic eosinophilic pneumonia is characterized radiologically by the presence of bilateral areas of consolidation that involve predominananntly or exclusively the outer thirds of the lungs. This peripheral distribution is evident on the radiograph in only 50% to 60% of patients but can be seen on CT in virtually all cases. The diagnosis of CSS, as distinct from simple pulmonary eosinophilia or chronic eosinophilic lung disease in patients with asthma, is based on the presence of systemic manifestations of CSS, including rash, peripheral neuropathy, and presence of serum p-ANCAs. The association of CSS with p-ANCAs has greatly facilitated the diagnosis of this disease. Bacterial, fungal, and viral pneumonias as the cause of bilateral opacities in patients with asthma, similar to other patients, need to be excluded based on clinical findings and appropriate cultures or serologic tests. The main considerations are infections that may result in symmetric, bilateral ground-glass opacities or consolidation. These infections include mainly bacterial bronchopneumonia and opportunistic infections such as *Pneumocystis jiroveci* and cytomegalovirus; the latter two organisms should be suspected in asthmatic patients being treated with corticosteroids.

Diagnosis

Chung-Strauss syndrome

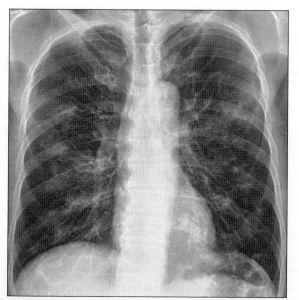

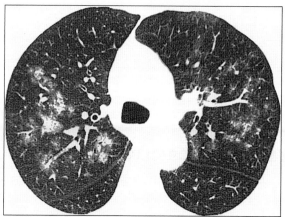

Figure 2. Axial CT in the same patient shows patchy, bilateral, focal ground-glass opacities and consolidation.

Figure 1. Posteroanterior chest radiograph shows patchy, bilateral areas of hazy, increased opacities and consolidation. The patient was a 57-year-old man with the diagnosis of Churg-Strauss syndrome based on a history of asthma, peripheral eosinophilia, and serum positive for p-ANCAs.

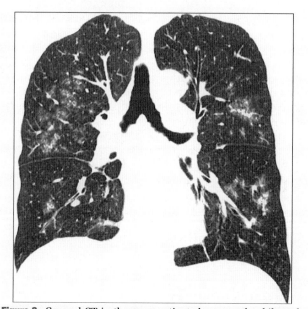

Figure 3. Coronal CT in the same patient shows patchy, bilateral, focal ground-glass opacities and consolidation.

Suggested Readings

Keogh KA, Specks U: Churg-Strauss syndrome. Semin Respir Crit Care Med 27:148-157, 2006.

Kim YK, Lee KS, Chung MP, et al: Pulmonary involvement in Churg-Strauss syndrome: An analysis of CT, clinical, and pathologic findings. Eur Radiol 17:3157-3165, 2007.

Silva CI, Müller NL, Fujimoto K, et al: Churg-Strauss syndrome: High resolution CT and pathologic findings. J Thorac Imaging 20:74-80, 2005.

Case 102

DEMOGRAPHICS/CLINICAL HISTORY

A 60-year-old woman with a dry cough and low-grade fever, undergoing radiography.

FINDINGS

Posteroanterior chest radiograph (Fig. 1) shows focal consolidation in the left middle lung zone and poorly defined ground-glass opacity in the right upper lung zone. Chest radiograph a few weeks later (Fig. 2) shows resolution of the previous findings and new focal areas of consolidation in the right middle lung zone and left upper and lower lung zones.

DISCUSSION

Definition/Background
Simple pulmonary eosinophilia, also known as Loeffler syndrome, is characterized by blood eosinophilia and migratory areas of consolidation, usually transient, visible on chest radiographs. The term *simple pulmonary eosinophilia* should be reserved for cases with no known cause, which occurs in approximately one third of cases.

Characteristic Clinical Features
Patients are frequently asymptomatic or have only mild symptoms, most commonly fever and cough.

Characteristic Radiologic Findings
Characteristic radiographic manifestations consist of transient and migratory areas of consolidation that typically clear spontaneously within 1 month. The foci of consolidation may be single or multiple, and they usually have ill-defined margins. The distribution is typically patchy, although a peripheral predominance may be seen.

Less Common Radiologic Manifestations
Mediastinal lymphadenopathy is seen on CT in approximately 15% of patients.

Differential Diagnosis
- Pneumonia
- Parasitic infection
- Drug-induced lung diseases
- Chronic eosinophilic pneumonia

Discussion
On a single chest radiograph, the findings of patchy consolidation are nonspecific and most commonly result from pneumonia, edema, or hemorrhage. However, the presence of transient migratory areas of consolidation on sequential radiographs and peripheral eosinophilia strongly suggest simple pulmonary eosinophilia. The main differential diagnosis clinically includes known causes of pulmonary eosinophilia, particularly parasitic infestation and drug-induced lung disease. Simple pulmonary eosinophilia can be differentiated from the more serious chronic eosinophilic pneumonia (CEP) by the clinical course, which is typically mild and less than 4 weeks in simple pulmonary eosinophilia and more severe and chronic in CEP.

Diagnosis
Simple pulmonary eosinophilia (Loeffler syndrome)

Suggested Readings
Alberts WM: Eosinophilic interstitial lung disease. Curr Opin Pulm Med 10:419-424, 2004.

Bain GA, Flower CD: Pulmonary eosinophilia. Eur J Radiol 23:3-8, 1996.

Cottin V, Cordier JF: Eosinophilic pneumonias. Allergy 60:841-857, 2005.

Kim Y, Lee KS, Choi DC, et al: The spectrum of eosinophilic lung disease: Radiologic findings. J Comput Assist Tomogr 21:920-930, 1997.

Johkoh T, Müller NL, Akira M, et al: Eosinophilic lung diseases: Diagnostic accuracy of thin-section CT in 111 patients. Radiology 216:773-780, 2000.

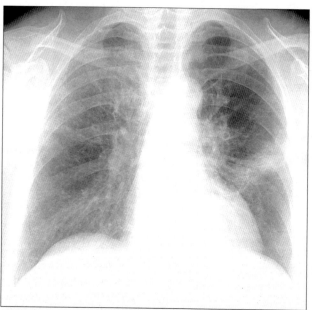

Figure 1. Posteroanterior chest radiograph shows focal consolidation in the left middle lung zone and poorly defined, increased ground-glass opacity in the right upper lung zone. The patient was a 60-year-old woman with simple pulmonary eosinophilia.

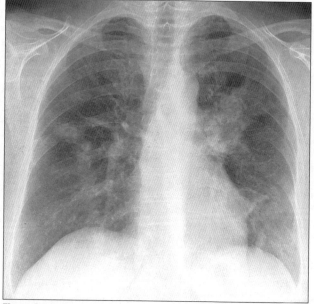

Figure 2. In the same patient, the chest radiograph a few weeks later shows resolution of the previous findings and new focal areas of consolidation in the right middle lung zone and the left upper and lower lung zones.

Case 103

DEMOGRAPHICS/CLINICAL HISTORY

A 41-year-old woman with peripheral eosinophilia and a chronic cough, undergoing computed tomography (CT).

FINDINGS

CT images at the level of the upper lobes (Fig. 1) and the lung bases (Fig. 2) show bilateral, peripheral, nonsegmental areas of consolidation and ground-glass opacities.

DISCUSSION

Definition/Background

Chronic eosinophilic pneumonia (CEP) is an idiopathic condition characterized by extensive filling of alveoli by a mixed inflammatory infiltrate consisting primarily of eosinophils. CEP is almost always associated with an increased number of eosinophils in the bronchoalveolar lavage (BAL) fluid and in peripheral blood. Approximately 50% of patients have a history of asthma or atopy.

Characteristic Clinical Features

Patients may have a dry cough, shortness of breath, fever, weight loss, and malaise. Symptoms are usually present for a least 1 month before diagnosis.

Characteristic Radiologic Findings

The characteristic radiographic pattern consists of bilateral, nonsegmental consolidation involving predominately or exclusively the outer two thirds of the lungs. This peripheral distribution, typically involving mainly the upper lobes, is apparent on the chest radiograph in approximately 60% of patients. The characteristic CT manifestations consist of bilateral, peripheral, nonsegmental areas of consolidation and ground-glass opacities involving the upper lobes. A peripheral distribution of consolidation is seen on CT in 85% to 100% of cases.

Less Common Radiologic Manifestations

Imaging may show unilateral or asymmetric consolidation. Consolidation can occur in a random distribution or mainly involve the lower lung zones.

Differential Diagnosis

- Simple pulmonary eosinophilia
- Churg-Strauss syndrome
- Drug-induced lung disease
- Cryptogenic organizing pneumonia (bronchiolitis obliterans organizing pneumonia [BOOP])

Discussion

An appearance identical to that of CEP can be seen in patients who have simple pulmonary eosinophilia (i.e., Loeffler syndrome) or Churg-Strauss syndrome. Simple pulmonary eosinophilia, however, is usually self-limited and associated with pulmonary infiltrates that are transient or fleeting; patients with Churg-Strauss syndrome frequently have systemic manifestations such as skin lesions and peripheral neuropathy. With simple pulmonary eosinophilia, areas of consolidation can appear and disappear within days; chronic eosinophilic pneumonia has a more protracted course, and areas of consolidation remain unchanged over weeks or months. Patients with chronic eosinophilic pneumonia are more likely to have peripheral consolidation than patients with simple pulmonary eosinophilia or Churg-Strauss syndrome.

The presence of peripheral airspace consolidation can be considered suggestive of chronic eosinophilic pneumonia only in the appropriate clinical setting; that is, in patients who have eosinophilia. An identical appearance of peripheral air-space consolidation can be seen in cryptogenic organizing pneumonia. Occasionally, a peripheral distribution of consolidation mimicking chronic eosinophilic pneumonia may be seen in patients who have sarcoidosis or pulmonary lymphoma.

For most patients, a diagnosis of CEP can be made based on the presence of chronic symptoms, peripheral consolidation on the radiograph or CT scan, and peripheral eosinophilia. BAL fluid analysis may be helpful in the diagnosis by showing increased levels of eosinophils.

Diagnosis

Chronic eosinophilic pneumonia

Suggested Readings

Alberts WM: Eosinophilic interstitial lung disease. Curr Opin Pulm Med 10:419-424, 2004.

Bain GA, Flower CD: Pulmonary eosinophilia. Eur J Radiol 23:3-8, 1996.

Cottin V, Cordier JF: Eosinophilic pneumonias. Allergy 60:841-857, 2005.

Kim Y, Lee KS, Choi DC, et al: The spectrum of eosinophilic lung disease: Radiologic findings. J Comput Assist Tomogr 21:920-930, 21.

Johkoh T, Müller NL, Akira M, et al: Eosinophilic lung diseases: Diagnostic accuracy of thin-section CT in 111 patients. Radiology 216:773-780, 2000.

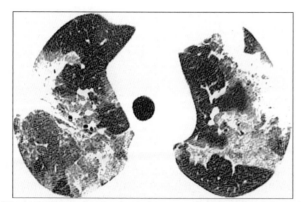

Figure 1. CT at the level of the upper lobes shows bilateral, peripheral, nonsegmental areas of consolidation and ground-glass opacities.

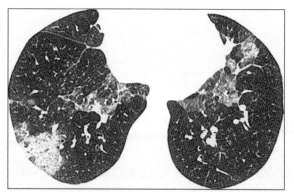

Figure 2. CT at the level of the lung bases shows bilateral, peripheral, nonsegmental areas of consolidation and ground-glass opacities. The patient was a 41-year-old woman with chronic eosinophilic pneumonia who presented with chronic cough and peripheral eosinophilia.

Case 104

DEMOGRAPHICS/CLINICAL HISTORY

A 60-year-old man with chronic renal failure and an incidental finding on imaging, undergoing computed tomography (CT).

FINDINGS

High-resolution CT at the level of the upper lobes (Fig. 1) shows poorly defined, centrilobular nodular opacities. CT using a soft tissue window (Fig. 2) shows that a couple of the nodular opacities contain foci of calcification and calcification in the chest wall vessels. In another patient, CT at the level of lung bases shows numerous, well-defined, small nodules mainly in the peripheral lung regions and bilateral consolidation (Fig. 3), and CT using a soft tissue window shows calcification within the consolidation and in some of the small nodules (Fig. 4).

DISCUSSION

Definition/Background

Metastatic calcification is characterized by calcium salt deposition in normal lung parenchyma. It typically occurs in patients who have hypercalcemia, which usually is associated with chronic renal failure and less often with an intraosseous malignancy such as multiple myeloma.

Characteristic Clinical Features

Most patients are asymptomatic. Rarely, patients may develop progressive shortness of breath.

Characteristic Radiologic Findings

For most patients with metastatic calcification, the chest radiograph shows normal anatomy. When present, the findings consist of numerous 3- to 10-mm-diameter, fluffy, poorly defined nodular opacities mimicking air space nodules or patchy areas of parenchymal opacification. The high-resolution CT manifestations of metastatic calcification typically consist of fluffy, poorly defined nodular opacities that are 3 to 10 mm in diameter. The nodules have a centrilobular distribution and tend to be most numerous in the upper lung zones. In approximately 50% of cases, calcification is evident on thin-section CT.

The calcific nature of the opacities can be confirmed by scanning with bone-imaging agents such as technetium 99m methylene diphosphonate (^{99m}Tc-MDP).

Less Common Radiologic Manifestations

Imaging may show diffuse calcification of the nodules, air space consolidation, or extensive ground-glass opacities.

Differential Diagnosis

- Pneumonia
- Sarcoidosis
- Silicosis
- Amyloidosis
- Idiopathic pulmonary ossification

Discussion

The differential diagnosis for metastatic pulmonary calcification includes pneumonia, sarcoidosis, silicosis, talcosis, amyloidosis, and idiopathic pulmonary ossification. The diagnosis of metastatic calcification can usually be made based on a clinical history of chronic renal failure; lack of significant respiratory symptoms; and characteristic appearance of fluffy, poorly defined, 3- to 10-mm-diameter, upper lobe nodules on high-resolution CT and by demonstration of calcification on CT or ^{99m}Tc-MDP scintigraphy. When looking for metastatic calcification, it is important to use thin-section CT (≤ 1 mm) to minimize volume averaging and to reformat the images using a standard algorithm to minimize artifacts due to the reconstruction algorithm.

Diagnosis

Metastatic pulmonary calcification

Suggested Readings

Hartman TE, Müller NL, Primack SL, et al: Metastatic pulmonary calcification in patients with hypercalcemia: Findings on chest radiographs and CT scans. AJR Am J Roentgenol 162:799-802, 1994.

Marchiori E, Müller NL, Souza AS Jr, et al: Unusual manifestations of metastatic pulmonary calcification: High-resolution CT and pathological findings. J Thorac Imaging 20:66-70, 2005.

Marchiori E, Souza AS Jr, Franquet T, Müller NL: Diffuse high-attenuation pulmonary abnormalities: A pattern-oriented diagnostic approach on high-resolution CT. AJR Am J Roentgenol 184:273-282, 2005.

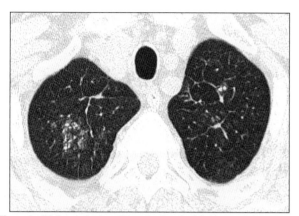

Figure 1. High-resolution CT at the level of the upper lobes shows poorly defined, centrilobular, nodular opacities. The patient was a 60-year-old man with chronic renal failure and metastatic pulmonary calcification.

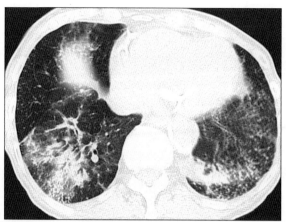

Figure 3. CT at the level of lung bases shows numerous, well-defined, small nodules mainly in the peripheral lung regions and reveals bilateral consolidation. The patient was a 74-year-old man with chronic renal failure and metastatic pulmonary calcification.

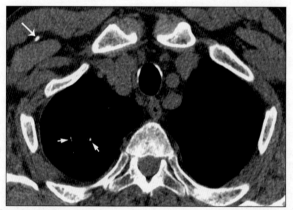

Figure 2. In the same patient, CT photographed using a soft tissue window shows that a couple of the nodular opacities contain foci of calcification *(short arrows)*. Notice the calcification in the chest wall vessels *(long arrow)*.

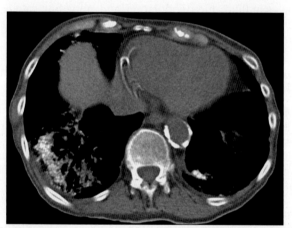

Figure 4. CT using a soft tissue window shows calcification within the consolidation and in some of the small nodules in a 74-year-old man with chronic renal failure and metastatic pulmonary calcification.

Case 105

DEMOGRAPHICS/CLINICAL HISTORY

A middle-aged man with mild, chronic shortness of breath, undergoing computed tomography (CT).

FINDINGS

High-resolution CT images at the level of the lung bases using lung (Fig. 1) and soft tissue (Fig. 2) windows show fine, sandlike micronodulation and apparent calcification of the interlobular septa. Notice the small, subpleural cysts or paraseptal emphysema (Fig. 1).

DISCUSSION

Definition/Background

Pulmonary alveolar microlithiasis is a rare, idiopathic disease characterized by innumerable tiny calculi (i.e., microliths) within alveolar air spaces. Although it can occur at any age, most reported cases have described patients between the ages of 20 and 50 years.

Characteristic Clinical Features

There is typically dissociation between the radiologic findings, which can be striking and extensive, and the clinical manifestations, which are usually mild. More than 50% of patients are asymptomatic when the disease is discovered.

Characteristic Radiologic Findings

The characteristic radiographic pattern is one of a fine, sandlike micronodulation (i.e., sandstorm lung) that may be diffuse but tends to be most severe in the middle and lower lung zones. High-resolution CT manifestations consist of calcific nodules that are 1 mm or less in diameter, sometimes confluent, and distributed predominantly along the cardiac borders and dorsal portions of the lower lung zones. Other common findings on high-resolution CT include ground-glass opacities and interlobular septal thickening (often with apparent extensive calcification).

Less Common Radiologic Manifestations

Imaging may show subpleural interstitial thickening and paraseptal emphysema.

Differential Diagnosis

- Miliary tuberculosis
- Talcosis
- Amyloidosis
- Idiopathic pulmonary ossification

Discussion

The differential diagnosis for microlithiasis includes miliary tuberculosis, talcosis due to intravenous drug use, amyloidosis, and idiopathic pulmonary ossification. The diagnosis usually can be made with confidence based on the classic radiographic pattern of sandlike nodules in a predominantly middle and lower lung zone distribution and the striking radiologic-clinical disparity in the severity of disease. Microliths can be identified in sputum, bronchoalveolar lavage fluid, and transbronchial biopsy specimens.

Diagnosis

Pulmonary alveolar microlithiasis

Suggested Readings

Castellana G, Lamorgese V: Pulmonary alveolar microlithiasis. World cases and review of the literature. Respiration 70:549-555, 2003.
Lauta VM: Pulmonary alveolar microlithiasis: An overview of clinical and pathological features together with possible therapies. Respir Med 97:1081-1085, 2003.
Marchiori E, Souza AS Jr, Franquet T, Müller NL: Diffuse high-attenuation pulmonary abnormalities: A pattern-oriented diagnostic approach on high-resolution CT. AJR Am J Roentgenol 184: 273-282, 2005.

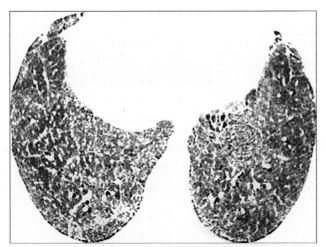

Figure 1. High-resolution CT at the level of the lung bases and using lung windows shows fine, sandlike micronodulation and small, subpleural cysts or paraseptal emphysema. The patient was a middle-aged man with alveolar microlithiasis. (Case courtesy of Dr. Marcos Manzini, Sao Paulo, Brazil.)

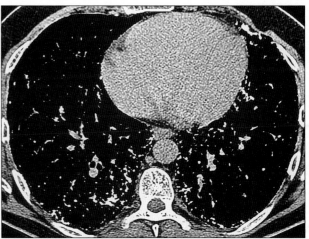

Figure 2. In the same patient, high-resolution CT at the level of the lung bases and using soft tissue windows shows fine, sandlike micronodulation and apparent calcification of the interlobular septa. (Case courtesy of Dr. Marcos Manzini, Sao Paulo, Brazil.)

Case 106

DEMOGRAPHICS/CLINICAL HISTORY

A 55-year-old man with slowly progressing shortness of breath, undergoing radiography and computed tomography (CT).

FINDINGS

Posteroanterior chest radiograph shows extensive hazy areas of increased opacities and faint reticulonodular pattern (Fig. 1). High-resolution CT images at the level of upper lobes (Fig. 2) and left inferior pulmonary vein (Fig. 3) show extensive ground-glass opacities and superimposed thickening of the interlobular and intralobular septa (i.e., crazy-paving pattern), which is clearly demarcated from adjacent normal lung.

DISCUSSION

Definition/Background
Pulmonary alveolar proteinosis (PAP), also called alveolar lipoproteinosis, is a rare disease characterized by the accumulation of protein- and lipid-rich material resembling surfactant within the parenchymal air spaces. More than 90% of cases occur as an acquired disease of unknown origin.

Characteristic Clinical Features
Patients have a dry cough and slowly progressing shortness of breath.

Characteristic Radiologic Findings
The chest radiograph usually shows bilateral, patchy areas of consolidation that have a vaguely nodular appearance. The characteristic high-resolution CT findings consist of extensive bilateral, ground-glass opacities with a superimposed fine linear pattern (i.e., interlobular and intralobular septal thickening) forming polygonal shapes measuring 3 to 10 mm in diameter (i.e., crazy-paving pattern). There is typically sharp demarcation between normal and abnormal parenchyma.

Less Common Radiologic Manifestations
Occasionally, patients may develop interstitial fibrosis.

Differential Diagnosis
- Pneumonia
- Pulmonary hemorrhage
- Pulmonary edema
- Lipoid pneumonia

Discussion
The findings on the chest radiograph mimic those of pneumonia, pulmonary edema, and hemorrhage. The diagnosis of PAP can be based on the characteristic manifestations on high-resolution CT. However, although characteristic of PAP, the crazy-paving pattern also can be seen in a variety of other conditions, including bronchioloalveolar cell carcinoma, lipoid pneumonia, pulmonary hemorrhage or edema, Kaposi sarcoma, and bacterial pneumonia. The diagnosis of PAP usually can be confirmed by examination of bronchoalveolar lavage (BAL) fluid, which is typically milky and contains periodic acid–Schiff (PAS) staining of the proteinaceous material.

Diagnosis
Alveolar proteinosis

Suggested Readings
Chung MJ, Lee KS, Franquet T, et al: Metabolic lung disease: Imaging and histopathologic findings. Eur J Radiol 54:233-245, 2005.
Inoue Y, Trapnell BC, Tazawa R, et al: Characteristics of a large cohort of patients with autoimmune pulmonary alveolar proteinosis in Japan. Am J Respir Crit Care Med 177:752-762, 2008.
Seymour JF, Presneill JJ: Pulmonary alveolar proteinosis: Progress in the first 44 years. Am J Respir Crit Care Med 166:215-235, 2002.

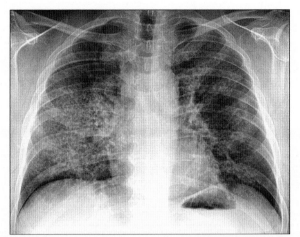

Figure 1. Posteroanterior chest radiograph shows extensive hazy areas of increased opacities and a faint reticulonodular pattern. The patient was a 55-year-old man with pulmonary alveolar proteinosis.

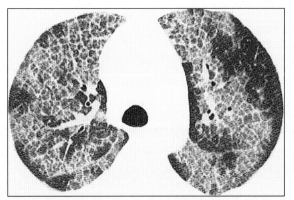

Figure 2. High-resolution CT at the level of upper lobes in the same patient shows extensive ground-glass opacities and superimposed thickening of the interlobular and intralobular septa (i.e., crazy-paving pattern), which is clearly demarcated from adjacent normal lung.

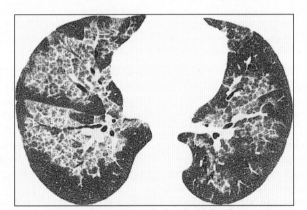

Figure 3. High-resolution CT at the level of left inferior pulmonary vein in the same patient shows extensive ground-glass opacities and superimposed thickening of the interlobular and intralobular septa (i.e., crazy-paving pattern), which is clearly demarcated from adjacent normal lung.

Case 107

DEMOGRAPHICS/CLINICAL HISTORY

A 54-year-old woman with mild, chronic shortness of breath and splenomegaly, undergoing computed tomography (CT).

FINDINGS

High-resolution CT images at the level of the aortic arch (Fig. 1) and at the level of the inferior pulmonary veins (Fig.2) show extensive, bilateral, interlobular septal thickening. Ground-glass opacities and poorly defined, small, centrilobular nodules can be seen.

DISCUSSION

Definition/Background

Niemann-Pick disease is caused by an inherited defect in the production of sphingomyelinase, a deficiency that results in the deposition of sphingomyelin in the liver, spleen, lung, bone marrow, and brain. Many patients die in infancy or childhood; however, some survive into adulthood, occasionally exhibiting the first manifestations of their disease at that time.

Characteristic Clinical Features

Patients may be asymptomatic or present with progressive shortness of breath.

Characteristic Radiologic Findings

The radiographic manifestations consist of a reticular or reticulonodular pattern involving mainly the lower lung zones. High-resolution CT shows patchy, bilateral ground-glass opacities; smooth or nodular thickening of the interlobular septa; and commonly smooth, intralobular lines. The various patterns may occur separate from each other or be admixed, resulting in a crazy-paving pattern. The abnormalities may be diffuse but tend to involve mainly the lower lung zones. Hepatomegaly and splenomegaly are common.

Less Common Radiologic Manifestations
- Lymphadenopathy

Differential Diagnosis
- Interstitial pulmonary edema
- Lymphangitic carcinomatosis
- Lymphoma

Discussion

Bilateral ground-glass opacities associated with diffuse, smooth thickening of the interlobular septa in a young adult with no symptoms or only mild symptoms suggest the possibility of Niemann-Pick disease. When associated with hepatomegaly and splenomegaly, these findings strongly suggest the diagnosis. Although lymphoma may result in similar findings, patients with lymphoma usually have systemic symptoms and extensive mediastinal lymphadenopathy rather than septal lines without lymphadenopathy. Patients with interstitial pulmonary edema usually present with acute shortness of breath.

Diagnosis

Niemann-Pick disease

Suggested Readings

Duchateau F, Dechambre S, Coche E: Imaging of pulmonary manifestations in subtype B of Niemann-Pick disease. Br J Radiol 74:1059-1061, 2001.

Mendelson DS, Wasserstein MP, Desnick RJ, et al: Type B Niemann-Pick disease: Findings at chest radiography, thin-section CT, and pulmonary function testing. Radiology 238:339-345, 2006.

Nicholson AG, Florio R, Hansell DM, et al: Pulmonary involvement by Niemann-Pick disease. A report of six cases. Histopathology 48:596-603, 2006.

Rodrigues R, Marchiori E, Müller NL: Niemann-Pick disease: High-resolution CT findings in two siblings. J Comput Assist Tomogr 28:52-54, 2004.

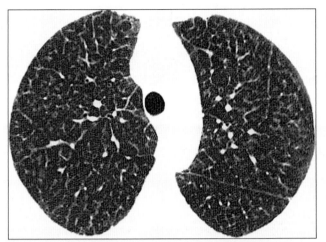

Figure 1. High-resolution CT at the level of the aortic arch shows extensive, bilateral, interlobular septal thickening. Ground-glass opacities and poorly defined, small, centrilobular nodules can be seen. The patient was a 54-year-old woman with Niemann-Pick disease.

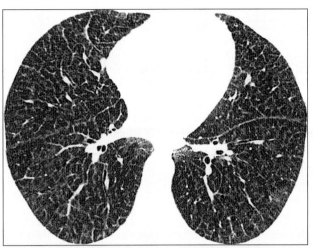

Figure 2. In the same patient, high-resolution CT at the level of the inferior pulmonary veins shows extensive, bilateral, interlobular septal thickening. Ground-glass opacities and poorly defined, small centrilobular nodules can be seen.

Case 108

DEMOGRAPHICS/CLINICAL HISTORY

A 43-year-old woman with acute shortness of breath, undergoing computed tomography (CT).

FINDINGS

Contrast-enhanced CT images show filling defects in the right lower lobe artery (Fig. 1) and anterior and lateral basal segmental arteries of the right lower lobe (Fig. 2). In another patient, contrast-enhanced CT at the level of the lower lobe arteries shows a complete filling defect in the right lower lobe artery (Fig. 3).

DISCUSSION

Definition/Background
Acute pulmonary thromboembolism (PE) is a common cause of morbidity and mortality; it is associated with an estimated 300,000 to 600,000 hospitalizations and approximately 50,000 deaths each year in the United States. Pulmonary emboli usually result from the migration of clots initially developed in deep veins of the legs (i.e., deep vein thrombosis), accounting for the term thromboembolism.

Characteristic Clinical Features
Patients may have acute onset of dyspnea, tachypnea, and pleuritic chest pain

Characteristic Radiologic Findings
The chest radiograph has very low sensitivity and specificity in the diagnosis of acute PE. The diagnostic findings consist of partial or complete filling defects seen within one or more pulmonary arteries on contrast-enhanced CT.

Less Common Radiologic Manifestations
Imaging may show pleura-based, commonly wedge-shaped areas of consolidation or ground-glass opacities due to pulmonary hemorrhage or infarction; small, unilateral or bilateral pleural effusions; and distal oligemia (i.e., Westermark sign).

Differential Diagnosis
- Chronic pulmonary thromboembolism (PE)
- Air embolism
- Fat embolism
- Pulmonary artery sarcoma

Discussion
Partial filling defects seen within one or more pulmonary arteries on contrast-enhanced CT is diagnostic of acute PE. A complete filling defect, defined as an intraluminal area of low attenuation that occupies the entire lumen, is a common finding in acute PE, but it may also be seen in chronic PE. The completely occluded artery typically has an increased diameter at the site of occlusion in acute PE and decreased diameter in chronic PE. Other findings of chronic PE include emboli that are eccentric and contiguous with the vessel wall, arterial stenosis or web, and reduction of more than 50% of the overall arterial diameter.

Rarely, intraluminal filling defects within the pulmonary arteries may result from air embolism, large fat emboli after major trauma, and intravascular tumors, particularly pulmonary artery sarcoma. Air and fat emboli can be readily recognized on CT by their characteristic attenuation values. Large pulmonary artery sarcomas are easily recognized because they extend beyond the vessel lumen. However, smaller tumors may mimic acute or chronic PE. Delayed enhancement of the filling defect on contrast-enhanced CT or enhancement with gadolinium on magnetic resonance imaging can help in differentiating a tumor mass from a thrombus. The tumor has positive radiotracer uptake on ^{18}F-fluorodeoxyglucose positron emission tomography (FDG-PET).

Diagnosis
Acute pulmonary thromboembolism

Suggested Readings
Bhalla S, Lopez-Costa I: MDCT of acute thrombotic and nonthrombotic pulmonary emboli. Eur J Radiol 64:54-64, 2007.

Han D, Lee KS, Franquet T, et al: Thrombotic and nonthrombotic pulmonary arterial embolism: Spectrum of imaging findings. Radiographics 23:1521-1539, 2003.

Tapson VF: Acute pulmonary embolism. N Engl J Med 358:1037-1052, 2008.

Wittram C, Maher MM, Yoo AJ, et al: CT angiography of pulmonary embolism: 4. Diagnostic criteria and causes of misdiagnosis. Radiographics 24:1219-1238, 2004.

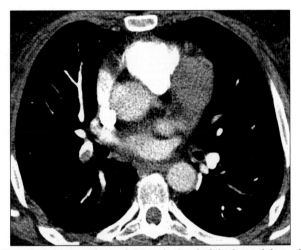

Figure 1. Contrast-enhanced CT at the level of the lower lobe and right middle lobe arteries shows a filling defect in the right lower lobe artery. The patient was a 43-year-old woman with acute PE.

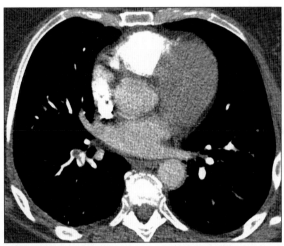

Figure 2. In the same patient, contrast-enhanced CT at the level of the basal segmental arteries shows filling defects in the anterior and lateral basal segmental arteries of the right lower lobe.

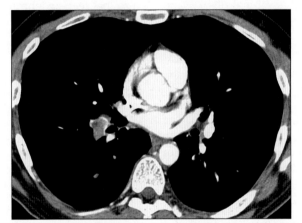

Figure 3. Contrast-enhanced CT at the level of the lower lobe arteries shows a complete filling defect in the right lower lobe artery. Notice that the diameter of the occluded vessel is larger than the corresponding left lower lobe vessel. The patient was a 39-year-old man with acute PE.

Case 109

DEMOGRAPHICS/CLINICAL HISTORY

An 88-year-old woman with acute shortness of breath and pleuritic chest pain, undergoing computed tomography (CT).

FINDINGS

Contrast-enhanced CT (Fig. 1) shows a complete filling defect in the lingular artery. Cross-sectional (Fig. 2) and coronal, reformatted (Fig. 3) CT images show a pleural-based, focal consolidation with central lucency that is characteristic of pulmonary infarction.

DISCUSSION

Definition/Background
Acute pulmonary embolism (PE) is a common cause of morbidity and mortality. Potential complications of acute PE include pulmonary hemorrhage or, less commonly, infarction; acute pulmonary hypertension; right ventricular dysfunction; and right and left ventricular failure.

Characteristic Clinical Features
Patients may have acute onset of dyspnea, tachypnea, and pleuritic chest pain.

Characteristic Radiologic Findings
The diagnostic findings of acute PE consist of partial or complete filling defects within one or more pulmonary arteries on contrast-enhanced CT. Pulmonary hemorrhage typically results in pleural-based, wedge-shaped areas of consolidation or ground-glass opacities. Infarction is characterized by pleural-based consolidation with no contrast-enhancement that may contain a central lucency.

Less Common Radiologic Manifestations
Cavitation of pulmonary infarction can occur but is rare.

Differential Diagnosis
- Chronic pulmonary embolism
- Pneumonia

Discussion
The presence of partial filling defects within one or more pulmonary arteries on contrast-enhanced CT is diagnostic of acute PE. A complete filling defect, defined as an intraluminal area of low attenuation that occupies the entire lumen, is a common finding in acute PE but may also be seen in chronic PE. The completely occluded artery typically has an increased diameter at the site of occlusion in acute PE and decreased diameter in chronic PE. Other findings of chronic PE typically include emboli eccentric and contiguous with the vessel wall, arterial stenosis or web, and reduction of more than 50% of the overall arterial diameter.

Focal areas of hemorrhage or atelectasis are relatively common in patients with acute PE, but infarction is uncommon. Areas of hemorrhage typically resolve over several days, whereas areas of infarction become better defined over several days and resolve slowly over several months. Areas of hemorrhage or infarction typically are seen distal to occlusive emboli and are pleural based and wedge shaped and therefore usually readily distinguished from pneumonia.

Diagnosis
Hemorrhage and infarction in acute pulmonary embolism

Suggested Readings

He H, Stein MW, Zalta B, Haramati LB: Pulmonary infarction: Spectrum of findings on multidetector helical CT. J Thorac Imaging 21:1-7, 2006.

Revel MP, Triki R, Chatellier G, et al: Is it possible to recognize pulmonary infarction on multisection CT images? Radiology 244:875-882, 2007.

Tapson VF: Acute pulmonary embolism. N Engl J Med 358:1037-1052, 2008.

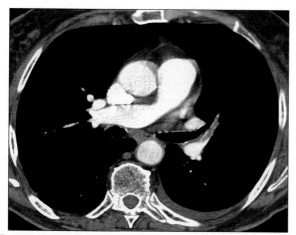

Figure 1. Contrast-enhanced CT shows a complete filling defect in the lingular artery. The patient was an 88-year-old woman with acute PE and infarction.

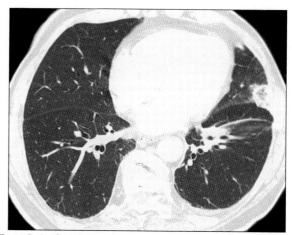

Figure 2. In the same patient, cross-sectional CT shows a pleural-based, focal consolidation with a central lucency that is characteristic of pulmonary infarction.

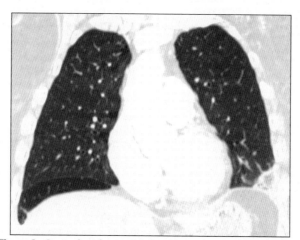

Figure 3. Coronal, reformatted CT shows a pleural-based, focal consolidation with an appearance resembling a truncated cone and with central lucency characteristic of pulmonary infarction in the same patient.

Case 110

DEMOGRAPHICS/CLINICAL HISTORY

A 52-year-old woman with progressive shortness of breath, undergoing computed tomography (CT).

FINDINGS

CT pulmonary angiogram (Fig. 1) shows a complete filling defect and markedly narrowed, right lower lobe pulmonary artery.

DISCUSSION

Definition/Background

Chronic pulmonary embolism (PE) is an uncommon entity resulting from an incomplete resolution of pulmonary emboli. Although it was previously believed that only 0.1% to 0.5% of patients with acute PE develop chronic thromboembolic hypertension (CTPH), studies suggest that up to 4% of patients with symptomatic acute PE may develop CTPH.

Characteristic Clinical Features

Slowly progressive dyspnea and exercise intolerance

Characteristic Radiologic Findings

The characteristic findings of chronic PE on contrast-enhanced CT consist of eccentric filling defects that are contiguous with the vessel wall, evidence of recanalization within an area of arterial hypoattenuation, arterial stenosis or web, reduction of more than 50% of the overall arterial diameter, and a complete filling defect at the level of stenosed pulmonary arteries. Findings of pulmonary hypertension include a diameter of the main pulmonary artery that is more than 2.9 cm or larger than the adjacent ascending aorta.

Less Common Radiologic Manifestations

Calcifications within chronic thrombi or in the wall of the enlarged central pulmonary arteries are seen in a small percentage of cases.

Differential Diagnosis

- Acute pulmonary embolism
- Pulmonary artery sarcoma

Discussion

The partial filling defects seen in chronic PE are typically eccentric and attached to the vessel wall, whereas those in acute PE are typically in the center of the vessel. Complete filling defects, defined as intraluminal areas of low attenuation that occupy the entire lumen, are common in acute and chronic PE. The completely occluded artery typically has a decreased diameter in chronic PE due to organization and fibrosis, whereas a normal or increased diameter is seen in acute PE. Large pulmonary artery sarcomas can be readily recognized because they extend beyond the vessel lumen. However, smaller tumors may mimic acute or chronic PE. Delayed enhancement of the filling defect on contrast-enhanced CT or enhancement with gadolinium on magnetic resonance imaging (MRI) can be helpful in differentiating a tumor mass from a thrombus. The tumor also has positive uptake on ^{18}F-fluorodeoxyglucose positron emission tomography (FDG-PET).

Diagnosis

Chronic pulmonary embolism

Suggested Readings

Auger WR, Kim NH, Kerr KM, et al: Chronic thromboembolic pulmonary hypertension. Clin Chest Med 28:255-269, 2007.
Coulden R: State-of-the-art imaging techniques in chronic thromboembolic pulmonary hypertension. Proc Am Thorac Soc 3:577-583, 2006.
Reddy GP, Gotway MB, Araoz PA: Imaging of chronic thromboembolic pulmonary hypertension. Semin Roentgenol 40:41-47, 2005.
Tapson VF, Humbert M: Incidence and prevalence of chronic thromboembolic pulmonary hypertension: From acute to chronic pulmonary embolism. Proc Am Thorac Soc 3:564-567, 2006.

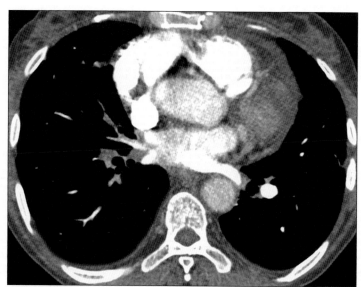

Figure 1. CT pulmonary angiogram shows a complete filling defect and markedly narrowed, right lower lobe pulmonary artery. The patient was a 52-year-old woman with chronic PE.

Case 111

DEMOGRAPHICS/CLINICAL HISTORY

A 17-year-old boy with acute shortness of breath 2 days after hip arthroplasty, undergoing computed tomography (CT).

FINDINGS

Cross-sectional CT (Fig. 1) and coronal, reformatted, high-resolution CT (Fig. 2) show extensive bilateral ground-glass opacities; areas of consolidation mainly in the dependent lung regions and lower lobes; and a few centrilobular nodules.

DISCUSSION

Definition/Background
The term *fat embolism* refers to the presence of globules of free fat within the pulmonary vasculature. Fat embolism is very common among trauma patients, especially those with long bone or pelvic fractures. Fat embolism must be differentiated from fat embolism syndrome, which is defined by the presence of clinical signs and symptoms resulting from fat emboli.

Characteristic Clinical Features
The symptoms of fat embolism syndrome usually appear gradually, with dyspnea, neurologic symptoms, fever, and petechial rash typically developing 12 to 36 hours after injury.

Characteristic Radiologic Findings
The radiologic findings are nonspecific. The chest radiograph may be normal or show bilateral, hazy areas of increased opacity (i.e., ground-glass opacities) or patchy or confluent consolidation. The CT findings include bilateral, patchy or diffuse ground-glass opacities; patchy or confluent areas of consolidation; and poorly defined centrilobular nodules less than 10 mm in diameter.

Less Common Radiologic Manifestations
Imaging may show interlobular septal thickening.

Differential Diagnosis
- Lug contusion
- Pneumonia
- Aspiration

Discussion
The time lapse between trauma and radiographic signs of fat embolism is usually 12 to 36 hours. This delay differentiates fat embolism from traumatic lung contusion, in which the radiographic opacity invariably appears immediately after injury. Although the latter opacity usually clears rapidly (in about 24 hours), resolution of fat embolism typically takes 7 to 10 days and occasionally as long as 4 weeks. Further differentiation lies in the extent of lung involvement, with contusion seldom affecting both lungs diffusely and symmetrically.

Diagnosis
Pulmonary fat embolism

Suggested Readings
Han D, Lee KS, Franquet T, et al: Thrombotic and nonthrombotic pulmonary arterial embolism: Spectrum of imaging findings. Radiographics 23:1521-1539, 2003.

Malagari K, Economopoulos N, Stoupis C, et al: High-resolution CT findings in mild pulmonary fat embolism. Chest 123:1196-11201, 2003.

Talbot M, Schemitsch EH: Fat embolism syndrome: History, definition, epidemiology. Injury 37:S3-S7, 2006.

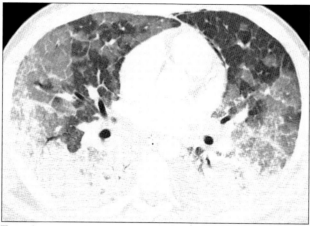

Figure 1. Cross-sectional, high-resolution CT shows extensive, bilateral ground-glass opacities; areas of consolidation mainly in the dependent lung regions; and a few centrilobular nodules. The patient was a 17-year-old boy with severe fat embolism syndrome after hip arthroplasty.

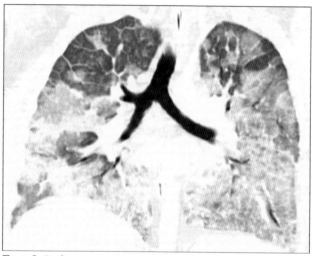

Figure 2. In the same patient, coronal, reformatted, high-resolution CT shows extensive, bilateral ground-glass opacities; areas of consolidation mainly in the dependent lower lobes; and a few centrilobular nodules.

Case 112

DEMOGRAPHICS/CLINICAL HISTORY

A 55-year-old man with progressive shortness of breath, undergoing radiography.

FINDINGS

Posteroanterior (Fig. 1) and lateral (Fig. 2) chest radiographs show marked enlargement of the central pulmonary arteries, with rapid pruning leading to decreased vascularity in the peripheral lung regions. Notice the focal convexity inferior to the aortic arch and lateral to the left main bronchus (Fig. 1), which is consistent with enlargement of the main pulmonary artery.

DISCUSSION

Definition/Background

Pulmonary arterial hypertension is defined as a mean pulmonary arterial pressure of more than 25 mm Hg at rest or 30 mm Hg with exercise. Chest radiography is usually the initial imaging study in patients with suspected pulmonary hypertension because it is useful in assessing heart size, the pattern of cardiac chamber dilatation, enlargement of proximal pulmonary arteries, and the presence of underlying pulmonary parenchymal abnormalities.

Characteristic Clinical Features

Patients may have exertional breathlessness progressing to exertional syncope or chest pain.

Characteristic Radiologic Findings

The characteristic radiographic manifestations of pulmonary hypertension consist of enlarged central pulmonary arteries down to the segmental level with decreased size of the peripheral pulmonary vessels (i.e., peripheral pruning). The upper limit for the transverse diameter of the right interlobar artery measured from its lateral aspect to the intermediate bronchus is 15 mm in women

and 16 mm in men. The transverse diameter of the left interlobar artery is difficult to appreciate on the frontal view. On the lateral radiograph, the upper limit measured from the circular lucency of the left upper lobe bronchus to the posterior margin of the vessel is 18 mm.

Less Common Radiologic Manifestations

Calcification within the pulmonary arteries may be seen in cases of prolonged and severe pulmonary hypertension.

Differential Diagnosis

- Left-to-right shunts
- Idiopathic dilatation of the pulmonary artery
- Hilar lymphadenopathy

Discussion

Left-to-right shunts, such as atrial septal defect (ASD), may result in enlargement of the pulmonary arteries because of increased blood flow in the absence of pulmonary artery hypertension. Occasionally, the central pulmonary arteries may be dilated without an apparent cause (i.e., idiopathic dilatation). Bilateral enlargement of the hila may result from the increased size of the pulmonary arteries (typically with a smooth contour) or from lymphadenopathy (typically with a lobulated contour).

Diagnosis

Pulmonary arterial hypertension: radiographic findings

Suggested Readings

Frazier AA, Galvin JR, Franks TJ, Rosado-De-Christenson ML: From the archives of the AFIP: Pulmonary vasculature: Hypertension and infarction. Radiographics 20:491-524; quiz 530-531, 532, 2000.

McGoon MD: The assessment of pulmonary hypertension. Clin Chest Med 22:493-508, ix, 2001.

Trow TK, McArdle JR: Diagnosis of pulmonary arterial hypertension. Clin Chest Med 28:59-73, viii, 2007.

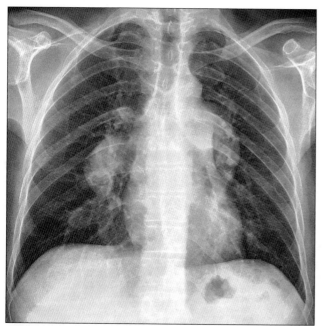

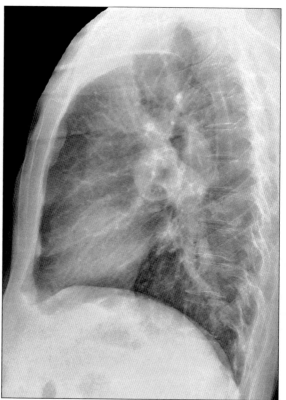

Figure 1. Posteroanterior chest radiograph shows marked enlargement of the central pulmonary arteries, with rapid pruning leading to decreased vascularity in the peripheral lung regions. Notice the focal convexity inferior to the aortic arch and lateral to the left main bronchus consistent with enlargement of the main pulmonary artery. The patient was a 55-year-old man with pulmonary arterial hypertension.

Figure 2. In the same patient, the lateral chest radiograph shows marked enlargement of the right and left pulmonary arteries.

Case 113

DEMOGRAPHICS/CLINICAL HISTORY

A 69-year-old woman with dyspnea on exertion, undergoing computed tomography (CT).

FINDINGS

Contrast-enhanced CT shows enlargement of the main pulmonary artery. Notice that the diameter of the pulmonary artery is larger than that of the adjacent ascending aorta.

DISCUSSION

Definition/Background

Pulmonary arterial hypertension is defined as a mean pulmonary arterial pressure of more than 25 mm Hg at rest or 30 mm Hg with exercise. Manifestations of pulmonary arterial hypertension on CT include dilation of central pulmonary arteries, dilatation of the right heart chambers, and hypertrophy of the right ventricle.

Characteristic Clinical Features

Patients may have exertional breathlessness progressing to exertional syncope or chest pain.

Characteristic Radiologic Findings

The characteristic radiographic manifestations of pulmonary hypertension consist of enlarged central pulmonary arteries down to the segmental level with decreased size of peripheral pulmonary vessels (i.e., peripheral pruning). A diameter of the main pulmonary artery (measured at the level of its bifurcation at a right angle to its long axis and just lateral to the ascending aorta) of 29 mm or larger suggests pulmonary hypertension, with a sensitivity of 69% to 87% and a specificity of 89% to 100%.

When the pulmonary artery diameter at the level of its bifurcation exceeds that of the adjacent ascending aorta, pulmonary hypertension is likely, with a specificity of 92% and a positive predictive value 93%. However, because the aorta dilates in the elderly, the pulmonary artery to aorta ratio has a relatively low negative predictive value of 44% and sensitivity of 70%.

Less Common Radiologic Manifestations

Calcification within the pulmonary arteries may be seen in cases of prolonged and severe pulmonary hypertension. Severe pulmonary arterial hypertension is commonly associated with small pericardial effusion.

Differential Diagnosis
- Left-to-right shunts
- Idiopathic dilatation of the pulmonary artery

Discussion

Left-to-right shunts, such as atrial septal defect (ASD), may result in enlargement of the pulmonary arteries because of increased blood flow in the absence of pulmonary arterial hypertension. Occasionally, the central pulmonary arteries may be dilated without apparent cause (i.e., idiopathic dilatation).

Diagnosis

Pulmonary arterial hypertension: computed tomography findings

Suggested Readings

Frazier AA, Galvin JR, Franks TJ, Rosado-de-Christenson ML: From the archives of the AFIP: Pulmonary vasculature: Hypertension and infarction. Radiographics 20:491-524; quiz 530-531, 532, 2000.

McGoon MD: The assessment of pulmonary hypertension. Clin Chest Med 22:493-508, ix, 2001.

Trow TK, McArdle JR: Diagnosis of pulmonary arterial hypertension. Clin Chest Med 28:59-73, viii, 2007.

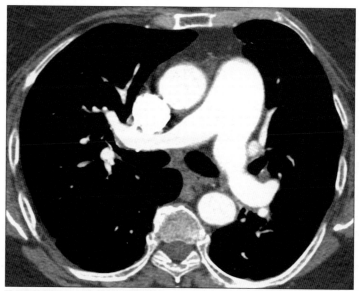

Figure 1. Contrast-enhanced CT shows enlargement of the main pulmonary artery. Notice that the diameter of the pulmonary artery is larger than that of the adjacent ascending aorta. The patient was a 69-year-old woman with pulmonary arterial hypertension.

Case 114

DEMOGRAPHICS/CLINICAL HISTORY

A 39-year-old man with dyspnea on exertion, undergoing computed tomography (CT).

FINDINGS

Contrast-enhanced CT (Fig. 1) shows enlargement of the main and left pulmonary arteries. CT at the level of the ventricles (Fig. 2) shows enlargement of the right ventricle and atrium, slight leftward bowing of the interventricular septum, and a small pericardial effusion. CT using lung windows (Fig. 3) shows bilateral, poorly defined, centrilobular nodules and a halo of ground-glass signal attenuation surrounding small pulmonary vessels.

DISCUSSION

Definition/Background

Pulmonary arterial hypertension is defined as a mean pulmonary arterial pressure of more than 25 mm Hg at rest or 30 mm Hg with exercise. Idiopathic pulmonary arterial hypertension (previously known as primary pulmonary hypertension) is precapillary pulmonary hypertension without an identifiable cause.

Characteristic Clinical Features

Patients may have exertional breathlessness progressing to exertional syncope or chest pain.

Characteristic Radiologic Findings

The characteristic radiographic manifestations of pulmonary hypertension consist of enlarged central pulmonary arteries down to the segmental level with decreased size of peripheral pulmonary vessels (i.e., peripheral pruning). The diameter of the main pulmonary artery (measured at the level of its bifurcation at a right angle to its long axis and just lateral to the ascending aorta) is usually 29 mm or larger. Other common findings include enlargement of the right ventricle and right atrium, thickening of the right ventricular wall, straightening or leftward bowing of the interventricular septum, and pericardial effusion.

Less Common Radiologic Manifestations

The lungs are usually normal, but severe pulmonary hypertension may be associated with small, poorly defined, centrilobular nodules because of capillary congestion or accumulation of cholesterol granulomas.

Differential Diagnosis

- Left-to-right shunts
- Chronic thromboembolic pulmonary arterial hypertension
- Pulmonary hypertension secondary to collagen vascular disease
- Capillary hemangiomatosis

Discussion

Left-to-right shunts, such as atrial septal defect (ASD), may result in enlargement of the pulmonary arteries due to increased blood flow in the absence of pulmonary arterial hypertension. The characteristic findings of chronic thromboembolic pulmonary arterial hypertension on contrast-enhanced CT consist of eccentric filling defects that are contiguous with the vessel wall, evidence of recanalization within an area of arterial hypoattenuation, arterial stenosis or web, reduction of more than 50% of the overall arterial diameter, and a complete filling defect at the level of stenosed pulmonary arteries. Pulmonary arterial hypertension is a relatively common complication of collagen vascular disease and may occur in the absence of parenchymal disease. The differential diagnosis is based on the clinical history and laboratory findings.

The lung parenchyma in idiopathic pulmonary arterial hypertension is usually normal, but severe pulmonary hypertension may be associated with small, poorly defined, centrilobular nodules because of capillary congestion or accumulation of cholesterol granulomas. These findings may resemble those of pulmonary capillary hemangiomatosis. Definitive diagnosis requires surgical lung biopsy.

Diagnosis

Idiopathic pulmonary arterial hypertension

Suggested Readings

Frazier AA, Galvin JR, Franks TJ, Rosado-de-Christenson ML: From the archives of the AFIP: Pulmonary vasculature: Hypertension and infarction. Radiographics 20:491-524, 2000.

McGoon MD: The assessment of pulmonary hypertension. Clin Chest Med 22:493-508, ix, 2001.

Trow TK, McArdle JR: Diagnosis of pulmonary arterial hypertension. Clin Chest Med 28:59-73, viii, 2007.

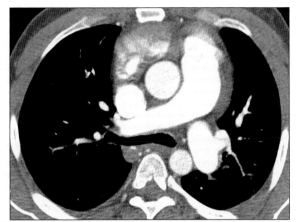

Figure 1. Contrast-enhanced CT shows enlargement of the main and left pulmonary arteries. The patient was a 39-year-old man with idiopathic pulmonary arterial hypertension.

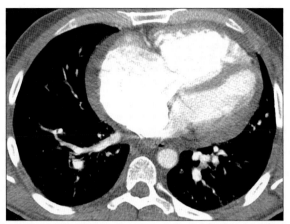

Figure 2. In the same patient, CT at the level of the ventricles shows enlargement of the right ventricle and atrium, a slight leftward bulge of the interventricular septum, and a small pericardial effusion.

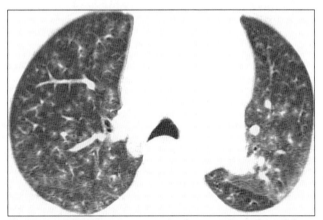

Figure 3. In the same patient, CT using lung windows shows bilateral, poorly defined, centrilobular nodules and a halo of ground-glass signal attenuation surrounding small pulmonary vessels.

Case 115

DEMOGRAPHICS/CLINICAL HISTORY

A 55-year-old man with progressive shortness of breath, undergoing computed tomography (CT).

FINDINGS

Contrast-enhanced CT (Fig. 1) shows dilatation of the central pulmonary arteries and large, eccentric filling defects in the right main, right interlobar, and left lower lobe pulmonary arteries. In another patient, CT using lung windows (Fig. 2) shows bilateral areas of decreased attenuation and vascularity and adjacent areas of increased attenuation and vascularity, resulting in a mosaic attenuation and perfusion pattern.

DISCUSSION

Definition/Background

Chronic thromboembolic pulmonary hypertension (CTEPH) results from thrombi from untreated or recurrent acute emboli that organize and become incorporated into the wall of the pulmonary arteries. CTEPH may complicate up to 3.8% of cases of acute pulmonary embolism and carries a poor prognosis if left untreated.

Characteristic Clinical Features

Patients may have exertional breathlessness progressing to exertional syncope or chest pain. Most patients have a history of previous acute pulmonary thromboembolism.

Characteristic Radiologic Findings

The characteristic findings of CTEPH on contrast-enhanced CT consist of eccentric filling defects that are contiguous with the vessel wall, evidence of recanalization within an area of arterial hypoattenuation, arterial stenosis or web, reduction of more than 50% of the overall arterial diameter, and a complete filling defect at the level of stenosed pulmonary arteries. A mosaic attenuation and perfusion pattern with areas of decreased attenuation and vascularity and areas of increased attenuation and vascularity is evident on CT in 77% to 100% of patients.

Less Common Radiologic Manifestations

Calcifications within chronic thrombi or in the wall of the enlarged central pulmonary arteries are seen in a small percentage of cases.

Differential Diagnosis

- Acute pulmonary embolism
- Pulmonary artery sarcoma

Discussion

The partial filling defects seen in chronic pulmonary embolism (PE) are typically eccentric and attached to the vessel wall, whereas those in acute PE are typically in the center of the vessel. Complete filling defects, defined as intraluminal areas of low attenuation that occupy the entire lumen, are common in acute and chronic PE. The completely occluded artery typically has a decreased diameter in chronic PE caused by organization and fibrosis, as compared with the normal or increased diameter seen in acute PE.

Large pulmonary artery sarcomas can be readily recognized because they extend beyond the vessel lumen. However, smaller tumors may mimic acute or chronic PE. Delayed enhancement of the filling defect on contrast-enhanced CT or enhancement with gadolinium on magnetic resonance imaging (MRI) can be helpful in differentiating a tumor mass from a thrombus. The tumor also has positive uptake on ^{18}F-fluorodeoxyglucose positron emission tomography (FDG-PET).

Diagnosis

Chronic thromboembolic pulmonary arterial hypertension

Suggested Readings

Frazier AA, Galvin JR, Franks TJ, Rosado-de-Christenson ML: From the archives of the AFIP: Pulmonary vasculature: Hypertension and infarction. Radiographics 20:491-524, 2000.

McGoon MD: The assessment of pulmonary hypertension. Clin Chest Med 22:493-508, ix, 2001.

Trow TK, McArdle JR: Diagnosis of pulmonary arterial hypertension. Clin Chest Med 28:59-73, viii, 2007.

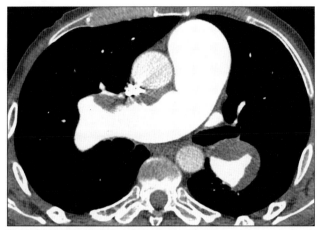

Figure 1. Contrast-enhanced CT shows dilatation of the central pulmonary arteries and large, eccentric filling defects in the right main, right interlobar, and left lower lobe pulmonary arteries. The patient was a 55-year-old man with chronic thromboembolic pulmonary arterial hypertension.

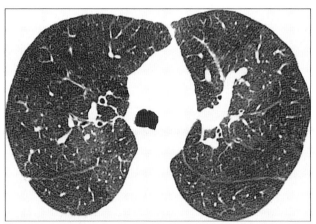

Figure 2. CT using lung windows shows bilateral areas of decreased attenuation and vascularity and adjacent areas of increased attenuation and vascularity resulting in a mosaic attenuation and perfusion pattern. Notice the enlarged left upper lobe segmental and subsegmental pulmonary arteries. The patient was a 43-year-old woman with chronic thromboembolic pulmonary arterial hypertension.

Case 116

DEMOGRAPHICS/CLINICAL HISTORY

A 54-year-old woman with progressive shortness of breath and previous trauma, undergoing radiography and computed tomography (CT).

FINDINGS

Posteroanterior chest radiograph (Fig. 1) shows cardiomegaly and enlargement of the central pulmonary vessels. Contrast-enhanced CT image (Fig. 2) shows dilatation of the main and right pulmonary arteries. Contrast-enhanced CT at the level of the pubic bones (Fig. 3) shows a complex tangle of enlarged enhancing vessels in the left inguinal region.

DISCUSSION

Definition/Background
Pulmonary arterial hypertension is a common complication of congenital left-to-right shunts. It may occur in high-pressure shunts, such as ventricular septal defects and patent ductus arteriosus, and in low-pressure, high-flow shunts, such as atrial septal defects and partial anomalous pulmonary venous drainage.

Characteristic Clinical Features
Patients may have progressive dyspnea.

Characteristic Radiologic Findings
Increased flow from a left-to-right shunt initially results in enlargement of peripheral pulmonary vessels in proportion to the proximal vessels, with pulmonary vessels visible within 2 cm of the pleural surface. Pulmonary hypertension results in gradual reversal of the shunt (i.e., Eisenmenger syndrome) and rapid tapering of the peripheral vessels and increased diameter of the proximal arteries.

Less Common Radiologic Manifestations
Calcification within the pulmonary arteries may be seen in cases of prolonged and severe pulmonary hypertension.

Differential Diagnosis
- Idiopathic pulmonary hypertension
- Chronic thromboembolic pulmonary hypertension

Discussion
The diagnosis of the left-to-right shunt usually can be made on echocardiography and magnetic resonance imaging (MRI). Peripheral arteriovenous fistulas can be diagnosed with ultrasound, CT, MRI, and angiography.

Diagnosis
Pulmonary hypertension in left-to-right shunt

Suggested Readings
Ferguson EC, Krishnamurthy R, Oldham SA: Classic imaging signs of congenital cardiovascular abnormalities. Radiographics 27:1323-1334, 2007.

Sommer RJ, Hijazi ZM, Rhodes JF Jr: Pathophysiology of congenital heart disease in the adult. Part I. Shunt lesions. Circulation 117:1090-1099, 2008.

Wang ZJ, Reddy GP, Gotway MB, et al: Cardiovascular shunts: MR imaging evaluation. Radiographics 23:S181-S194, 2003.

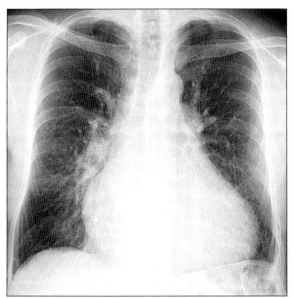

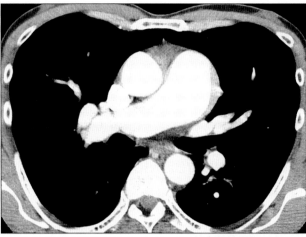

Figure 2. In the same patient, contrast-enhanced CT shows dilatation of the main and right pulmonary arteries.

Figure 1. Posteroanterior chest radiograph shows cardiomegaly and enlargement of the central pulmonary vessels. The patient was a 54-year-old woman with pulmonary arterial hypertension resulting from post-traumatic, left femoral arteriovenous fistula.

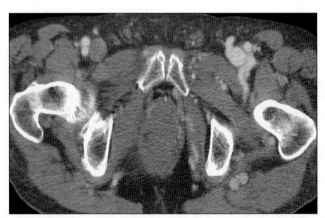

Figure 3. In the same patient, contrast-enhanced CT at the level of the pubic bones shows a complex tangle of enlarged enhancing vessels in the left inguinal region.

Case 117

DEMOGRAPHICS/CLINICAL HISTORY

A 21-year-old man with chronic shortness of breath and severe pulmonary arterial hypertension, undergoing computed tomography (CT).

FINDINGS

CT images at the level of the bronchus intermedius (Fig. 1) and inferior pulmonary veins (Fig. 2) show bilateral, smooth thickening of the interlobular septa and patchy ground-glass opacities.

DISCUSSION

Definition/Background

Pulmonary veno-occlusive disease (PVOD) is a rare, idiopathic condition characterized by gradual obliteration of the pulmonary veins and venules. Increased venous pressure results in postcapillary pulmonary hypertension, interstitial pulmonary edema, and focal areas of hemorrhage.

Characteristic Clinical Features

Patients may have insidious onset of dyspnea and intermittent hemoptysis, with reduced gas transfer and arterial desaturation on exercise.

Characteristic Radiologic Findings

The specific diagnosis of PVOD is suggested radiologically when features of pulmonary arterial hypertension are accompanied by evidence of diffuse interstitial pulmonary edema, particularly extensive interlobular septal thickening and a normal-sized left atrium. Small pleural effusions and slightly enlarged mediastinal lymph nodes are common.

Less Common Radiologic Manifestations

Imaging may show poorly defined centrilobular nodules.

Differential Diagnosis

- Idiopathic pulmonary arterial hypertension
- Pulmonary capillary hemangiomatosis
- Valvular (mitral) stenosis

Discussion

Although the clinical manifestations are often similar, PVOD usually can be distinguished radiologically from idiopathic pulmonary hypertension by the presence of extensive interlobular septal thickening.

Pulmonary capillary hemangiomatosis (PCH) typically results in pulmonary arterial hypertension associated with poorly defined centrilobular nodules due to abnormal capillary proliferation. However, there is considerable overlap between the radiologic manifestations of PCH and PVOD. Both are characterized by elevated pulmonary arterial pressures and normal or low pulmonary capillary wedge pressures. Definitive diagnosis of PVOD and PCH requires surgical lung biopsy.

In PVOD, the central pulmonary veins and the left atrium are not enlarged, in contrast to patients with mitral stenosis, cor triatriatum, or left atrial myxoma.

Diagnosis

Pulmonary veno-occlusive disease

Suggested Readings

Frazier AA, Franks TJ, Mohammed TL, et al: From the archives of the AFIP: Pulmonary veno-occlusive disease and pulmonary capillary hemangiomatosis. Radiographics 27:867-882, 2007.

Resten A, Maitre S, Humbert M, et al: Pulmonary hypertension: CT of the chest in pulmonary venoocclusive disease. AJR Am J Roentgenol 183:65-70, 2004.

Trow TK, McArdle JR: Diagnosis of pulmonary arterial hypertension. Clin Chest Med 28:59-73, viii, 2007.

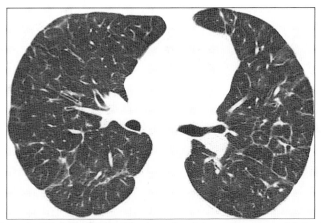

Figure 1. CT at the level of the bronchus intermedius shows bilateral, smooth thickening of the interlobular septa and patchy ground-glass opacities. The patient was a 21-year-old man with severe pulmonary arterial hypertension and histologically proven pulmonary veno-occlusive disease.

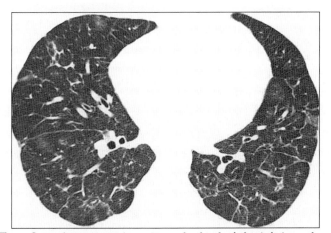

Figure 2. In the same patient, CT at the level of the inferior pulmonary veins shows bilateral septal thickening and patchy ground-glass opacities.

Case 118

DEMOGRAPHICS/CLINICAL HISTORY

Young man with known pulmonary arterial hypertension, undergoing computed tomography (CT).

FINDINGS

High-resolution CT shows extensive bilateral ground-glass opacities (Fig. 1).

DISCUSSION

Definition/Background

Pulmonary capillary hemangiomatosis (PCH) is a rare condition characterized by diffuse interstitial proliferation of thin-walled capillaries in and around pulmonary vessels and airways. It results in progressive pulmonary arterial hypertension; venous occlusion results in increased hydrostatic pressure with consequent focal areas of edema and hemorrhage.

Characteristic Clinical Features

Patients may have slowly progressive dyspnea and intermittent hemoptysis.

Characteristic Radiologic Findings

The high-resolution CT manifestations of pulmonary capillary hemangiomatosis consist of enlargement of the central pulmonary arteries due to pulmonary arterial hypertension, patchy or confluent ground-glass opacities, and poorly defined, centrilobular ground-glass nodules caused by capillary proliferation. Pericardial effusion results from severe pulmonary arterial hypertension.

Less Common Radiologic Manifestations

Imaging may show smooth interlobular septal thickening.

Differential Diagnosis

- Idiopathic pulmonary arterial hypertension
- Pulmonary veno-occlusive disease

Discussion

Although the clinical manifestations are often similar to those of idiopathic pulmonary hypertension, the diagnosis of PCH should be suspected in patients with diffuse, poorly defined, centrilobular nodules. However, similar nodular opacities may be seen in some patients with idiopathic pulmonary hypertension due to capillary congestion or the presence of cholesterol granulomas.

Pulmonary veno-occlusive disease (PVOD) typically results in pulmonary arterial hypertension associated with extensive interlobular septal thickening. However, poorly defined, centrilobular nodules may be seen in PVOD and interlobular septal thickening in some patients with PCH. There is considerable overlap between the radiologic manifestations of PCH and PVOD. Both are characterized by elevated pulmonary arterial pressures and normal or low pulmonary capillary wedge pressures. Definitive diagnosis of PVOD and PCH requires surgical lung biopsy.

Diagnosis

Pulmonary capillary hemangiomatosis

Suggested Readings

Frazier AA, Franks TJ, Mohammed TL, et al: From the archives of the AFIP: Pulmonary veno-occlusive disease and pulmonary capillary hemangiomatosis. Radiographics 27:867-882, 2007.

Lawler LP, Askin FB: Pulmonary capillary hemangiomatosis: Multidetector row CT findings and clinico-pathologic correlation. J Thorac Imaging 20:61-63, 2005.

Trow TK, McArdle JR: Diagnosis of pulmonary arterial hypertension. Clin Chest Med 28:59-73, viii, 2007.

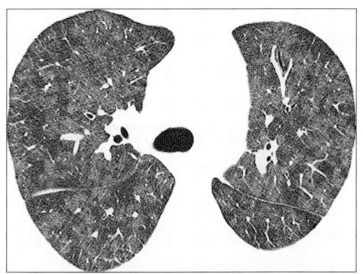

Figure 1. High-resolution CT shows extensive bilateral ground-glass opacities. The patient was a young man with pulmonary capillary hemangiomatosis. (Courtesy of Dr. Nicholas Screaton, Papworth Hospital, Cambridge, UK.)

Case 119

DEMOGRAPHICS/CLINICAL HISTORY

A 30-year-old woman who is an intravenous drug user with progressive shortness of breath, undergoing radiography and computed tomography (CT).

FINDINGS

Posteroanterior chest radiograph (Fig. 1) shows conglomerate masses in the perihilar regions, superior retraction of the hila, and numerous, well-defined, small nodules, mainly in the right lung. High-resolution CT (Fig. 2) shows numerous, well-defined, small nodules mainly in the right upper lobe; partial atelectasis of the left upper lobe; and conglomerate masses with associated distortion of the architecture in the right upper lobe and superior segment of left lower lobe. High-resolution CT using soft tissue windows (Fig. 3) shows foci of high signal attenuation within the conglomerate masses that are consistent with talc deposition.

DISCUSSION

Definition/Background

Talc embolism is seen almost invariably in chronic intravenous drug users. In most instances, the complication occurs with intravenous injection of medications intended solely for oral use, most commonly amphetamines, methylphenidate hydrochloride (Ritalin), and methadone.

Characteristic Clinical Features

Most patients are asymptomatic. Clinical symptoms include dyspnea and, less commonly, persistent cough.

Characteristic Radiologic Findings

The earliest radiologic manifestation of intravenous talcosis is the presence of widespread nodules ranging from barely visible to about 1 mm in diameter. In the early stages, the nodules are usually distributed diffusely and uniformly throughout the lungs. Over time, the upper lobe nodules often coalesce to form an almost homogeneous opacity of progressive, massive fibrosis that has characteristic high signal attenuation on CT due to accumulation of talc.

Less Common Radiologic Manifestations

Findings include diffuse ground-glass opacities, fibrosis, and enlarged central pulmonary arteries due to pulmonary arterial hypertension.

Differential Diagnosis

- Alveolar microlithiasis
- Miliary tuberculosis
- Silicosis
- Coal worker's pneumoconiosis

Discussion

In the early stages, the radiologic manifestations of intravenous talcosis may resemble alveolar microlithiasis or miliary tuberculosis. Talcosis is differentiated from miliary tuberculosis based on the clinical history of intravenous drug use and lack of fever or other systemic symptoms. In more advanced disease, the coalescent, upper lobe, large opacities resemble the progressive massive fibrosis of silicosis or coal worker's pneumoconiosis, except for the presence of characteristic high signal attenuation on CT due to the accumulation of talc.

Diagnosis

Talc embolism: talcosis

Suggested Readings

Nguyen ET, Silva CI, Souza CA, Müller NL: Pulmonary complications of illicit drug use: Differential diagnosis based on CT findings. J Thorac Imaging 22:199-206, 2007.

Ward S, Heyneman LE, Reittner P, et al: Talcosis associated with IV abuse of oral medications: CT findings. AJR Am J Roentgenol 174:789-793, 2000.

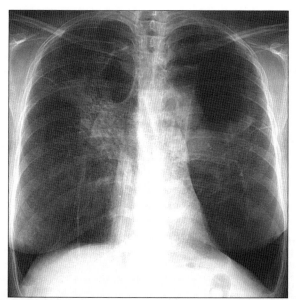

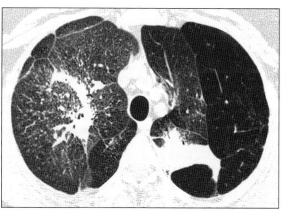

Figure 2. In the same patient, high-resolution CT shows numerous, well-defined, small nodules mainly in the right upper lobe; partial atelectasis of the left upper lobe; and conglomerate masses with associated distortion of the architecture in the right upper lobe and superior segment of the left lower lobe.

Figure 1. Posteroanterior chest radiograph shows conglomerate masses in the perihilar regions, superior retraction of the hila, and numerous, well-defined, small nodules mainly in the right lung. The patient was a 30-year-old intravenous drug user with pulmonary talcosis.

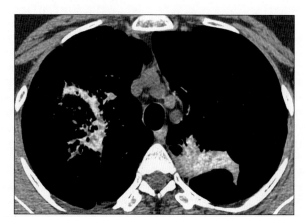

Figure 3. In the same patient, high-resolution CT using soft tissue windows shows foci of high signal attenuation within the conglomerate masses that are consistent with talc deposition.

Case 120

DEMOGRAPHICS/CLINICAL HISTORY

A 71-year-old woman, stridor and exertional dyspnea, had tracheostomy.

FINDINGS

Magnified view of the proximal trachea from a chest radiograph (Fig. 1) reveals focal narrowing of the trachea at the level of the second thoracic vertebra. CT image at the level of the second thoracic vertebra (Fig. 2) demonstrates anterior triangular soft tissue opacity projecting into the tracheal lumen. CT image at the level of the thoracic inlet (Fig. 3) shows narrowing of the tracheal lumen. Coronal reformation CT image (Fig. 4) shows focal narrowing of the trachea at the level of the thoracic inlet.

DISCUSSION

Definition/Background
Tracheal stenosis (i.e., narrowing of the tracheal lumen) may result from a variety of iatrogenic, inflammatory, infectious, and neoplastic processes. The most common causes are difficult or prolonged intubation and long-standing tracheostomy tube placement.

Characteristic Clinical Features
Dyspnea on exertion, stridor, and wheezing.

Characteristic Radiologic Findings
Post-intubation stenosis is characterized by concentric or eccentric tracheal wall thickening and associated luminal narrowing, most commonly in the subglottic region at the level of the endotracheal tube balloon (Figs. 1, 2, 3, and 4). The craniocaudad length of the stenosis usually ranges from 1.5 to 2.5 cm and is best assessed on multiplanar reformations of CT images obtained using thin sections (1 mm or less) (Fig. 4). In patients who have undergone tracheostomy tube placement, the stenosis occurs most commonly at the stoma site.

Less Common Radiologic Manifestations
Occasionally the tracheal stenosis may consist only of a thin membrane projecting into the tracheal lumen or may be long, extending over several centimeters.

Differential Diagnosis
- Tracheal stenosis post-intubation
- Tracheal stenosis post-tracheostomy
- Wegener granulomatosis
- Adenoid cystic carcinoma
- Relapsing polychondritis
- Tracheobronchial amyloidosis

Discussion
The diagnosis of tracheal stenosis following intubation or tracheostomy can usually be readily diagnosed based on clinical history, characteristic location, and focal nature of the stenosis. Wegener granulomatosis may result in focal subglottic stenosis. Adenoid cystic carcinoma may result in focal thickening of the tracheal wall and narrowing of the lumen. The tracheal narrowing is usually focal and asymmetric, unlike the more circumferential and symmetric narrowing seen in tracheal stenosis.

Relapsing polychondritis and tracheobronchial amyloidosis typically result in extensive tracheal wall thickening and luminal narrowing.

Diagnosis
Tracheal stenosis

Suggested Readings

Marom EM, Goodman PC, McAdams HP: Focal abnormalities of the trachea and bronchi. AJR Am J Roentgenol 176:707-711, 2001.

Prince JS, Duhamel DR, Levin DL, Harrel JH, Friedman P: Nonneoplastic lesions of the tracheobronchial wall: Radiographic findings with bronchoscopic correlation. Radiographics 22:S215-S230, 2002.

Sun M, Ernst A, Boiselle PM: MDCT of the central airways: Comparison with bronchoscopy in the evaluation of complications of endotracheal and tracheostomy tubes. J Thorac Imag 22:136-142, 2007.

Webb EM, Elicker BM, Webb WR: Using CT to diagnose nonneoplastic tracheal abnormalities. AJR Am J Roentgenol 174:1315-1321, 2000.

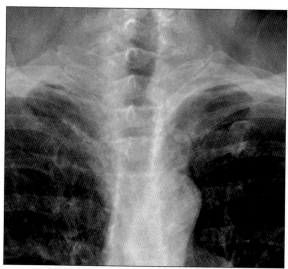

Figure 1. Magnified view of the proximal trachea from a chest radiograph reveals focal narrowing of the trachea at the level of the second thoracic vertebra. The patient was a 71-year-old woman with tracheal stenosis following intubation and tracheostomy.

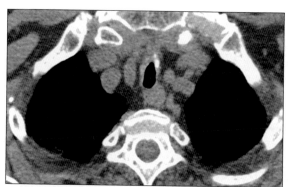

Figure 3. In the same patient, CT image at the level of the thoracic inlet shows narrowing of the tracheal lumen.

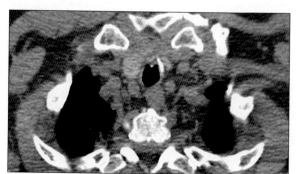

Figure 2. In the same patient, CT image at the level of the second thoracic vertebra demonstrates anterior triangular soft tissue opacity projecting into the tracheal lumen.

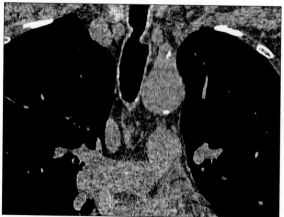

Figure 4. In the same patient, coronal reformation CT image shows focal narrowing of the trachea at the level of the thoracic inlet.

Case 121

DEMOGRAPHICS/CLINICAL HISTORY

A 58-year-old woman with wheezing and exertional dyspnea, undergoing computed tomography (CT).

FINDINGS

Inspiratory, high-resolution CT (Fig. 1) at the level of the aortic arch shows normal anatomy. High-resolution CT performed at maximal expiration (Fig. 2) shows marked narrowing of the trachea. The lumen of the narrowed trachea has the appearance of a frown.

DISCUSSION

Definition/Background

Tracheomalacia is characterized by increased compliance and excessive collapsibility of the trachea. It may be congenital or acquired. Common causes in the adult include chronic obstructive pulmonary disease (COPD), extrinsic compression (e.g., thyroid goiter, aortic aneurysm, vascular ring), prior intubation, and relapsing polychondritis.

Characteristic Clinical Features

Patients have cough, dyspnea on exertion, and wheezing.

Characteristic Radiologic Findings

Findings include a more than 50% reduction in the cross-sectional lumen of the trachea during expiration, as assessed on paired inspiratory-expiratory CT or preferably by imaging during forced expiration (i.e., dynamic expiratory CT or magnetic resonance imaging [MRI]). The tracheal lumen in tracheomalacia typically has a lunate configuration on inspiratory CT and a crescentic, frown-like configuration and less than 6 mm distance between the anterior and posterior walls on expiratory CT.

Less Common Radiologic Manifestations

Imaging may show tracheal wall thickening in patients with relapsing polychondritis.

Differential Diagnosis

- Asthma
- Tracheal stenosis
- Tracheal neoplasm

Discussion

The clinical symptoms of tracheomalacia can mimic those of asthma, partial tracheal obstruction by tumor, or tracheal stenosis. The diagnosis of tracheomalacia can be readily made on paired inspiratory–dynamic expiratory CT, dynamic MRI, fluoroscopy, or conventional bronchoscopy.

It should be noted that a greater than 50% reduction in the cross-sectional lumen of the trachea may also be seen on forced expiration in some healthy subjects. Therefore, clinical correlation is required in order not to overdiagnose tracheomalacia on expiratory CT.

Diagnosis

Tracheomalacia

Suggested Readings

Boiselle PM, Ernst A: Tracheal morphology in patients with tracheomalacia: Prevalence of inspiratory lunate and expiratory "frown" shapes. J Thorac Imaging 21:190-196, 2006.

Boiselle PM, Feller-Kopman D, Ashiku S, Ernst A: Tracheobronchomalacia: Evolving role of mutlislice helical CT. Radiol Clin North Am 41:627-636, 2003.

Boiselle PM, O'Donnell CR, Bankier AA, et al: Tracheal collapsibility in healthy volunteers during forced expiration: Assessment with multidetector CT. Radiology 252:255-262, 2009.

Carden K, Boiselle PM, Waltz D, Ernst A: Tracheomalacia and tracheobronchomalacia in children and adults: An in-depth review of a common disorder. Chest 127:984-1005, 2005.

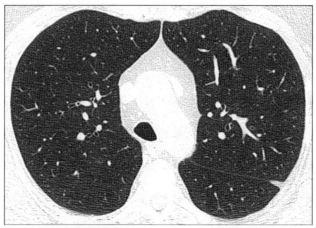

Figure 1. Inspiratory, high-resolution CT at the level of the aortic arch shows normal anatomy. The patient was a 58-year-old woman with tracheomalacia.

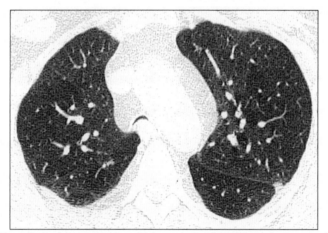

Figure 2. In the same patient, high-resolution CT performed at maximal expiration shows marked narrowing of the trachea. The lumen of the narrowed trachea has the appearance of a frown.

Case 122

DEMOGRAPHICS/CLINICAL HISTORY

A 54-year-old man with stridor and wheezing, undergoing computed tomography (CT).

FINDINGS

CT images of the trachea (Fig. 1) and tracheal carina (Fig. 2) show extensive thickening and calcification of the anterior and lateral walls of the trachea and normal posterior membranous portion. In another patient, CT using soft tissue windows shows thickening of the walls of the right and main bronchi affecting mainly the anterior and lateral portions (Fig. 3), and CT using lung windows shows marked narrowing of the lumen of the right main bronchus and slight narrowing of the left main bronchus (Fig. 4).

DISCUSSION

Definition/Background

Relapsing polychondritis is a rare autoimmune disease characterized by episodic inflammation of cartilaginous structures anywhere in the body but mainly the ears, nose, larynx, and trachea. Up to 30% of these patients have a concurrent connective tissue disease.

Characteristic Clinical Features

Respiratory symptoms include hoarseness, stridor, wheeze, cough, and dyspnea.

Characteristic Radiologic Findings

The chest radiograph is of limited value in the diagnosis. In patients with laryngeal chondritis, CT shows concentric subglottic stenosis. The characteristic CT manifestation of tracheal involvement consists of a smoothly thickened tracheal wall with sparing of the posterior membranous wall. The thickened wall may have increased attenuation ranging from subtle to frankly calcified. Tracheal stenosis may result from cartilaginous destruction. The stenosis in relapsing polychondritis is usually single and localized but can be multiple and may also involve the bronchi. Expiratory CT frequently shows collapse of the trachea due to tracheomalacia.

Less Common Radiologic Manifestations

The posterior membranous wall may be thickened. Cylindrical bronchiectasis is seen on high-resolution CT in up to 25% of patients. It is not clear whether the bronchiectasis is the result of cartilage inflammation or the indirect result of recurrent pneumonia.

Differential Diagnosis

- Amyloidosis
- Tracheobronchopathia osteochondroplastica

Discussion

The presence of a smoothly thickened tracheal wall with sparing of the posterior membranous wall on CT is virtually diagnostic of relapsing polychondritis. Tracheobronchial amyloidosis usually affects the airway circumferentially, and tracheopathia osteochondroplastica is characterized by multiple, calcified endoluminal airway nodules that do not typically cause circumferential tracheal narrowing.

Diagnosis

Relapsing polychondritis

Suggested Readings

Behar JV, Choi YW, Hartman TA, et al: Relapsing polychondritis affecting the lower respiratory tract. AJR Am J Roentgenol 178:173-177, 2002.

Gergely P Jr, Poor G: Relapsing polychondritis. Best Pract Res Clin Rheumatol 18:723-738, 2004.

Lee KS, Ernst A, Trentham DE, et al: Relapsing polychondritis: Prevalence of expiratory CT airway abnormalities. Radiology 240:565-573, 2006.

Marom EM, Goodman PC, McAdams HP: Diffuse abnormalities of the trachea and main bronchi. AJR Am J Roentgenol 176:713-717, 2001.

Marom EM, Goodman PC, McAdams HP: Focal abnormalities of the trachea and main bronchi. AJR Am J Roentgenol 176:707-711, 2001.

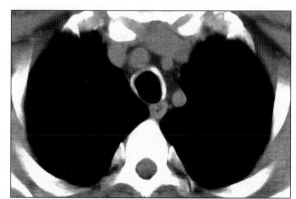

Figure 1. CT of the trachea shows extensive thickening and calcification of the anterior and lateral walls of the trachea and normal posterior membranous portion in a 54-year-old man with relapsing polychondritis.

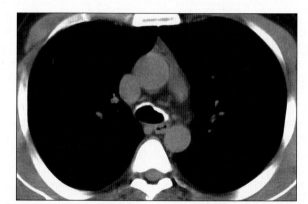

Figure 2. In the 54-year-old patient with relapsing polychondritis, CT of the tracheal carina shows extensive thickening and calcification of the anterior and lateral walls of the trachea and normal posterior membranous portion.

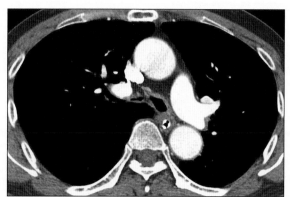

Figure 3. CT using soft tissue windows shows thickening of the walls of the right and main bronchi affecting mainly the anterior and lateral portions. The patient was a 68-year-old man with relapsing polychondritis.

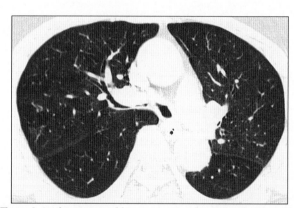

Figure 4. In the 68-year-old patient with relapsing polychondritis, CT using lung windows shows marked narrowing of the lumen of the right main bronchus and slight narrowing of the left main bronchus.

Case 123

DEMOGRAPHICS/CLINICAL HISTORY

A 48-year-old woman with stridor, undergoing computed tomography (CT).

FINDINGS

CT shows marked circumferential thickening of the tracheal wall (Fig. 1). In another patient, CT shows circumferential thickening and foci of calcification of the walls of the main bronchi (Fig. 2).

DISCUSSION

Definition/Background

Amyloidosis is a generic term used for a heterogeneous group of disorders characterized by accumulation of various insoluble fibrillar proteins (i.e., amyloid). Amyloidosis may involve the trachea, bronchi, or lung parenchyma.

Characteristic Clinical Features

Tracheobronchial amyloidosis usually manifests with dyspnea and cough.

Characteristic Radiologic Findings

For most patients with tracheobronchial amyloidosis, the chest radiograph is normal. CT manifestations of tracheobronchial amyloidosis consist of thickening of the airway wall, narrowing of the lumen, and in some cases, foci of calcification. The airway wall thickening may be focal or diffuse and nodular, plaquelike, or circumferential. Thickening usually is confined to the trachea but can extend to the main, lobar, and segmental bronchi.

Less Common Radiologic Manifestations

Bronchial involvement may be associated with distal air trapping, atelectasis, or bronchiectasis.

Differential Diagnosis

- Relapsing polychondritis
- Tracheobronchopathia osteochondroplastica

Discussion

The main differential diagnosis of diffuse tracheal wall thickening includes amyloidosis, relapsing polychondritis, and tracheobronchopathia osteochondroplastica. Tracheobronchial amyloidosis usually affects the airway circumferentially, whereas relapsing polychondritis typically spares the posterior membranous wall. Tracheopathia osteochondroplastica is characterized by multiple, calcified, endoluminal airway nodules that do not typically cause circumferential tracheal narrowing. The diagnosis of amyloidosis usually requires histologic confirmation by needle, bronchial, transbronchial, or surgical biopsy. The diagnosis is based on demonstration of amyloid by Congo red staining, which produces characteristic green birefringence under crossed polarized light.

Diagnosis

Tracheobronchial amyloidosis

Suggested Readings

Aylwin AC, Gishen P, Copley SJ: Imaging appearance of thoracic amyloidosis. J Thorac Imaging 20:41-46, 2005.

Chung MJ, Lee KS, Franquet T, et al: Metabolic lung disease: Imaging and histopathologic findings. Eur J Radiol 54:233-245, 2005.

O'Regan A, Fenlon HM, Beamis JF Jr, et al: Tracheobronchial amyloidosis. The Boston University experience from 1984 to 1999. Medicine (Baltimore) 79:69-79, 2000.

Utz JP, Swensen SJ, Gertz MA: Pulmonary amyloidosis. The Mayo Clinic experience from 1980 to 1993. Ann Intern Med 124:407-413, 1996.

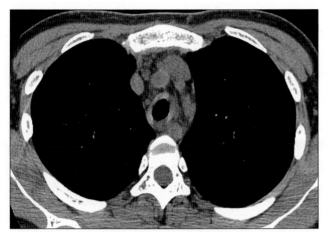

Figure 1. CT shows marked circumferential thickening of the tracheal wall in a 48-year-old woman with tracheal amyloidosis.

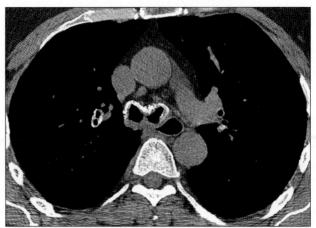

Figure 2. In a 53-year-old man with tracheobronchial amyloidosis, CT shows circumferential thickening and foci of calcification of the walls of the main bronchi and involvement of the right apical segmental bronchi.

Case 124

DEMOGRAPHICS/CLINICAL HISTORY

A 75-year-old man with chronic cough, undergoing radiography and computed tomography (CT).

FINDINGS

Posteroanterior (Fig. 1) and lateral (Fig. 2) chest radiographs show an increase in the caliber of the trachea and main bronchi. Notice the left lower lobe bronchiectasis. High-resolution CT at the level of the trachea (Fig. 3) shows tracheomegaly. High-resolution CT at the level of the main bronchi (Fig. 4) shows increased caliber of the main bronchi and protrusion of mucosal and submucosal tissue that is consistent with bronchial diverticulosis (*arrows*). CT also reveals mild emphysema.

DISCUSSION

Definition/Background

Tracheobronchomegaly (Mounier-Kuhn syndrome) is a rare condition characterized by dilation of the tracheobronchial tree that tends to involve the trachea and main bronchi but that may extend from the larynx to the periphery of the lungs. Most cases are congenital; a few cases are associated with diffuse pulmonary fibrosis, ankylosing spondylitis, or rheumatoid arthritis.

Characteristic Clinical Features

Patients have recurrent pneumonia and productive cough.

Characteristic Radiologic Findings

Tracheobronchomegaly can be diagnosed in women when the transverse and sagittal diameters of the trachea exceed 21 and 23 mm, respectively, and the transverse diameters of the right and left main bronchi exceed 19.8 and 17.4 mm, respectively. In men, it is diagnosed when the transverse and sagittal diameters of the trachea exceed 25 and 27 mm, respectively, and the transverse diameters of the right and left main bronchi exceed 21.1 and 18.4 mm, respectively.

Less Common Radiologic Manifestations

The trachea and major bronchi often have an irregular, corrugated appearance caused by the protrusion of mucosal and submucosal tissue between the cartilaginous rings, an appearance that has been called tracheal and bronchial diverticulosis.

Differential Diagnosis

- Bronchiectasis

Discussion

The radiologic findings of abnormal dilatation of the trachea and main bronchi are diagnostic. The abnormal intraparenchymal bronchial dilatation seen in tracheobronchomegaly can be distinguished from bronchiectasis by the very thin wall of the ectatic bronchi as compared with the thickened bronchial wall typically seen in bronchiectasis.

Diagnosis

Tracheobronchomegaly (Mounier-Kuhn syndrome)

Suggested Readings

Marom EM, Goodman PC, McAdams HP: Diffuse abnormalities of the trachea and main bronchi. AJR Am J Roentgenol 176:713-717, 2001.

Menon B, Aggarwal B, Iqbal A: Mounier-Kuhn syndrome: Report of 8 cases of tracheobronchomegaly with associated complications. South Med J 101:83-87, 2008.

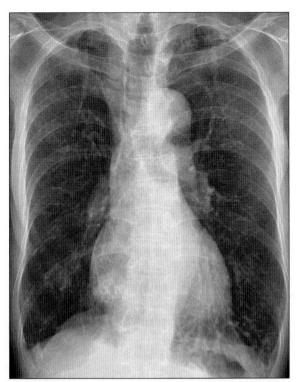

Figure 1. Posteroanterior chest radiograph shows an increase in the caliber of the trachea and main bronchi. Left lower lobe bronchiectasis also can be seen in the 75-year-old man with tracheobronchomegaly.

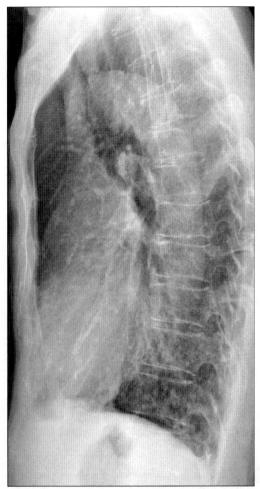

Figure 2. In the same patient, the lateral chest radiograph shows an increase in the caliber of the trachea and main bronchi. Notice the left lower lobe bronchiectasis.

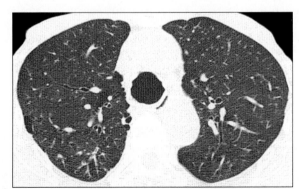

Figure 3. In the same patient, high-resolution CT at the level of the trachea shows tracheomegaly and mild emphysema.

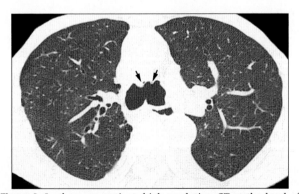

Figure 4. In the same patient, high-resolution CT at the level of the main bronchi shows increased caliber of the main bronchi and protrusion of mucosal and submucosal tissue that is consistent with bronchial diverticulosis (arrows). CT also reveals mild emphysema.

Case 125

DEMOGRAPHICS/CLINICAL HISTORY

A 67-year-old man with chronic cough and recurrent respiratory infections, undergoing computed tomography (CT).

FINDINGS

High-resolution CT (Fig. 1) shows cylindrical bronchiectasis in the anterior segment of the right upper lobe. Notice that the affected bronchi do not taper as they branch and extend into the lung periphery. In other patients, CT shows varicose bronchiectasis in the right upper lobe (Fig. 2), cystic bronchiectasis in the left lower lobe associated with left lower lobe atelectasis (Fig. 3), and extensive, bilateral bronchiectasis and bronchiolectasis (Fig. 4).

DISCUSSION

Definition/Background

Bronchiectasis is characterized by abnormal, irreversible dilatation of one or more bronchi, with or without associated thickening of the airway walls. It may be caused by congenital diseases (e.g., cystic fibrosis, immotile cilia syndrome) or acquired diseases (e.g., respiratory infection [most common]).

Characteristic Clinical Features

Patients are often asymptomatic. Symptoms include chronic cough with or without purulent sputum and intermittent hemoptysis.

Characteristic Radiologic Findings

Imaging often shows an internal diameter of the bronchus greater than that of the adjacent pulmonary artery (bronchoarterial diameter ratio > 1), lack of bronchial tapering, and a bronchus visualized within 1 cm of the costal pleura or abutting the mediastinal pleura. Bronchiectasis can be classified as cylindrical, varicose, or cystic, depending on the appearance of the affected bronchi.

Less Common Radiologic Manifestations

Bronchial wall thickening and filling of the ectatic bronchi with secretions are common. Patchy areas of decreased signal attenuation and vascularity (i.e., mosaic attenuation/perfusion pattern) are common and reflect the presence of associated bronchiolitis obliterans.

Differential Diagnosis

- Normal bronchi

Discussion

Identification of bronchiectasis requires the use of thin-section (≈1 mm) and helical CT; mild bronchiectasis is frequently missed on thicker sections and can be missed on high-resolution CT performed at 10-mm intervals. The diagnosis of severe bronchiectasis (i.e., varicose and cystic) is straightforward on CT. However, mild bronchiectasis (i.e., cylindrical bronchiectasis) may be difficult to distinguish from normal bronchi. A spurious increase in the bronchoarterial ratio may be seen when the accompanying pulmonary artery divides before the airway. In this situation, the bronchial diameter appears to be increased against the usual yardstick, the homologous arterial branch. Another consideration is that a bronchoarterial ratio greater than 1 is not always abnormal. The pulmonary artery may have a reduced diameter due to vasoconstriction or remodeling in areas of emphysema or bronchiolitis obliterans, resulting in an increased bronchoarterial diameter ratio even if the bronchus is normal. There is a normal but progressive increase in the internal diameter of the airways with age, with a bronchoarterial ratio exceeding 1 in more than 40% of asymptomatic persons older than 65 years.

Diagnosis

Bronchiectasis

Suggested Readings

Dodd JD, Souza CA, Müller NL: Conventional high-resolution CT versus helical high-resolution MDCT in the detection of bronchiectasis. AJR Am J Roentgenol 187:414-420, 2006.

McGuinness G, Naidich DP: CT of airways disease and bronchiectasis. Radiol Clin North Am 40:1-19, 2002.

Rosen MJ: Chronic cough due to bronchiectasis: ACCP evidence-based clinical practice guidelines. Chest 129(Suppl):122S-131S, 2006.

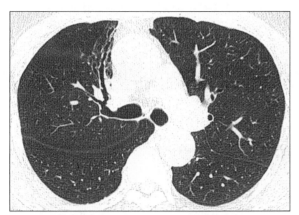

Figure 1. High-resolution CT shows cylindrical bronchiectasis in the anterior segment of the right upper lobe. Notice that the affected bronchi do not taper as they branch and extend into the lung periphery. The patient was a 67-year-old man.

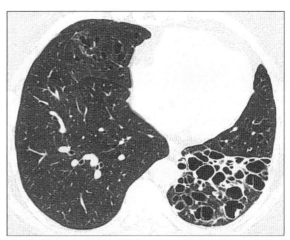

Figure 3. High-resolution CT shows cystic bronchiectasis in the left lower lobe associated with left lower lobe atelectasis. Bronchiectasis also is evident in the lingula and right middle lobe. The patient was a 52-year-old woman.

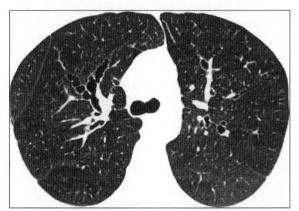

Figure 2. High-resolution CT shows varicose bronchiectasis in the right upper lobe. Notice that the affected bronchi are dilated and have a beaded or varicose appearance. Bronchiectasis also is evident in the left upper lobe. The patient was a 32-year-old woman.

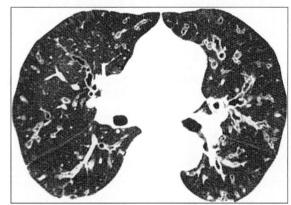

Figure 4. High-resolution CT shows extensive, bilateral bronchiectasis and bronchiolectasis. The affected airways have thick walls, and several of them are filled with secretions. The patient was a 52-year-old woman.

Case 126

DEMOGRAPHICS/CLINICAL HISTORY

A 27-year-old man with chronic productive cough and weight loss, undergoing radiography and computed tomography (CT).

FINDINGS

Posteroanterior chest radiograph (Fig. 1) shows increased lung volumes, bronchial wall thickening, bronchiectasis, and poorly defined nodular and linear opacities, mainly in the upper lobes. High-resolution CT at the level of the lung apices (Fig. 2), tracheal carina (Fig. 3), and right middle lobe bronchus (Fig. 4) shows extensive bilateral bronchiectasis and areas of decreased attenuation and vascularity. Notice the few centrilobular nodules and branching opacities (i.e., tree-in-bud pattern) (Fig. 4).

DISCUSSION

Definition/Background

Cystic fibrosis (CF) is an autosomal recessive disease characterized by the production of abnormal secretions from exocrine glands, such as the salivary and sweat glands, and from the pancreas, large bowel, and tracheobronchial tree. The main clinical manifestations are bronchiectasis, obstructive pulmonary disease, and pancreatic insufficiency.

Characteristic Clinical Features

Patients have recurrent respiratory infections associated with productive cough, wheezing, and dyspnea.

Characteristic Radiologic Findings

The chest radiograph shows bronchial wall thickening and bronchiectasis that is most severe in the upper lobes, increased lung volumes, poorly defined reticulonodular opacities, and, commonly, focal areas of consolidation. High-resolution CT shows diffuse bronchiectasis that is typically most severe in the upper lobes, mucoid impaction, centrilobular nodules, and areas of decreased signal attenuation and vascularity (i.e., mosaic perfusion and attenuation).

Less Common Radiologic Manifestations

Imaging may show areas of atelectasis, hilar or mediastinal lymph node enlargement, and enlargement of the central pulmonary arteries due to pulmonary hypertension.

Differential Diagnosis

- Bronchiectasis from other causes

Discussion

The radiologic findings of CF are relatively nonspecific and mimic those of other causes of bronchiectasis. The most characteristic features of bronchiectasis in CF are bilateral, symmetric distribution and upper lobe predominance. Similar findings, however, can be seen in patients with allergic bronchopulmonary aspergillosis, bronchiectasis due to prior tuberculosis, and several less common conditions. Although the diagnosis of CF may be suggested by a positive family history, persistent respiratory disease, or clinical evidence of pancreatic insufficiency, confirmation requires a positive sweat test result or identification of two abnormal copies of the CF gene.

Diagnosis

Cystic fibrosis, chest

Suggested Readings

Aziz ZA, Davies JC, Alton EW, et al: Computed tomography and cystic fibrosis: Promises and problems. Thorax 62:181-186, 2007.

Cleveland RH, Zurakowski D, Slattery DM, Colin AA: Chest radiographs for outcome assessment in cystic fibrosis. Proc Am Thorac Soc 4:302-305, 2007.

Robinson TE: Computed tomography scanning techniques for the evaluation of cystic fibrosis lung disease. Proc Am Thorac Soc 4:310-315, 2007.

Nick JA, Rodman DM: Manifestations of cystic fibrosis diagnosed in adulthood. Curr Opin Pulm Med 11:513-518, 2005.

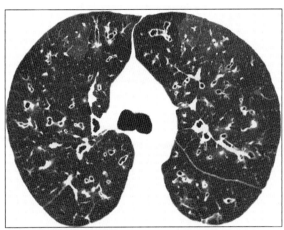

Figure 3. In the same patient, high-resolution CT at the level of the tracheal carina shows extensive bilateral bronchiectasis and areas of decreased signal attenuation and vascularity.

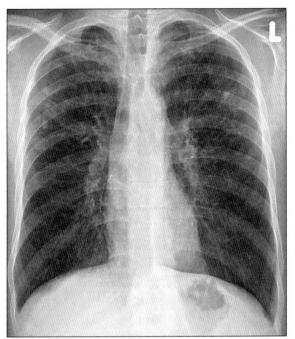

Figure 1. Posteroanterior chest radiograph shows bronchial wall thickening and poorly defined nodular and linear opacities mainly in the upper lobes. The patient was a 27-year-old man with cystic fibrosis.

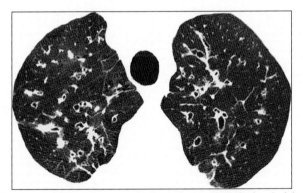

Figure 2. In the same patient, high-resolution CT at the level of the lung apices shows extensive bilateral bronchiectasis and areas of decreased signal attenuation and vascularity.

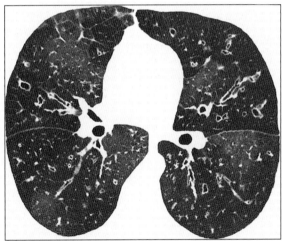

Figure 4. In the same patient, high-resolution CT at the level of the right middle lobe bronchus shows extensive, bilateral bronchiectasis and areas of decreased signal attenuation and vascularity. Notice the few centrilobular nodules and branching opacities (i.e. tree-in-bud pattern).

Case 127

DEMOGRAPHICS/CLINICAL HISTORY

An 88-year-old man with chronic cough and intermittent mild hemoptysis, undergoing computed tomography (CT).

FINDINGS

High-resolution CT images (Figs. 1 and 2) show a calcified opacity in the wall of the bronchus intermedius and projecting into the lumen.

DISCUSSION

Definition/Background

Broncholithiasis is an uncommon condition characterized by calcified or ossified material within the bronchial lumen. Most cases are caused by extrusion of calcified material from adjacent lymph nodes and erosion into the airways; the calcified nodes usually are caused by prior tuberculosis or histoplasmosis.

Characteristic Clinical Features

Patients have chronic cough, intermittent hemoptysis, and rarely, expectoration of calcific material (i.e., lithoptysis).

Characteristic Radiologic Findings

Thin-section, helical CT shows calcified endobronchial material or peribronchial calcification with airway distortion. The broncholithiasis is best visualized on multiplanar reformations obtained from thin-section, volumetric CT data (Figs. 3 and 4). Calcification of mediastinal and hilar lymph nodes is common.

Less Common Radiologic Manifestations

Imaging may show atelectasis and bronchiectasis distal to the bronchial obstruction.

Differential Diagnosis

- Endobronchial carcinoid
- Endobronchial hamartoma
- Foreign body

Discussion

Endobronchial carcinoid tumor and hamartomas may calcify and mimic a broncholith. Similarly, an endobronchial foreign body may mimic a broncholith. Unlike broncholithiasis, these conditions are not associated with calcified lymph nodes.

Diagnosis

Broncholithiasis

Suggested Readings

Seo JB, Song KS, Lee JS, et al: Broncholithiasis: Review of the causes with radiologic-pathologic correlation. Radiographics 22:S199-S213, 2002.

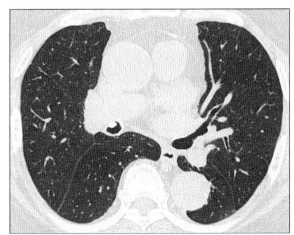

Figure 1. High-resolution CT using a multidetector scanner shows a dense, nodular opacity projecting into the lumen of the bronchus intermedius. The patient was an 88-year-old man with broncholithiasis related to prior tuberculosis.

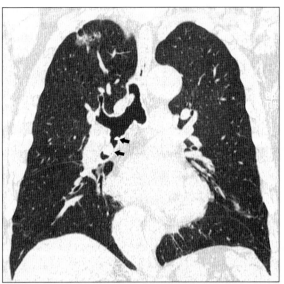

Figure 3. In the same patient, coronal reformation from volumetric, high-resolution CT of the chest shows two nodular opacities *(arrows)* within the bronchus intermedius and shows right upper lobe scarring due to prior tuberculosis.

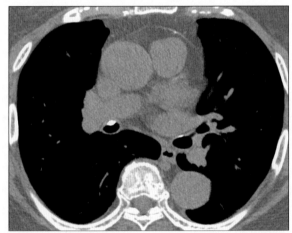

Figure 2. In the same patient, CT using soft tissue windows shows a calcified opacity in the wall of the bronchus intermedius and projecting into the lumen.

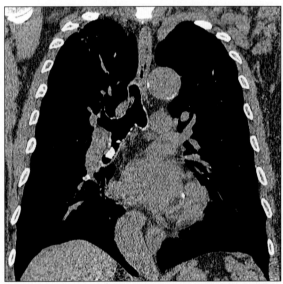

Figure 4. In the same patient, coronal reformation from volumetric, high-resolution CT using soft tissue windows shows two calcified nodules within the lumen of the bronchus intermedius.

Case 128

DEMOGRAPHICS/CLINICAL HISTORY

A 43-year-old man, smoker and asymptomatic, undergoing computed tomography (CT).

FINDINGS

High-resolution CT images at the level of the lung apices (Figs. 1 and 2) show bilateral centrilobular nodules with ground-glass attenuation. Minimal paraseptal emphysema is identified anteriorly in the left lung (Fig. 2). Centrilobular nodular opacities are better seen on maximum-intensity projection (MIP) CT image (Fig. 3).

DISCUSSION

Definition/Background
Respiratory bronchiolitis is characterized by the accumulation of pigmented macrophages in the lumen of respiratory bronchioles and adjacent alveoli. Respiratory bronchiolitis occurs almost exclusively in cigarette smokers.

Characteristic Clinical Features
By definition, respiratory bronchiolitis is not associated with symptoms. It is found incidentally on lung specimens of asymptomatic cigarette smokers.

Characteristic Radiologic Findings
Results of chest radiography and high-resolution CT are usually normal or show only centrilobular emphysema. When present, the high-resolution CT findings of respiratory bronchiolitis consist of poorly defined centrilobular nodules or patchy, bilateral ground-glass opacities, or both. The centrilobular nodules and ground-glass opacities can be diffuse but most commonly involve predominantly or exclusively the upper lobes.

Less Common Radiologic Manifestations
Imaging may show bronchial wall thickening due to chronic bronchitis.

Differential Diagnosis
- Respiratory bronchiolitis-associated interstitial lung disease (RBILD)
- Hypersensitivity pneumonitis (HP)

Discussion
Patients with respiratory bronchiolitis (RB) are by definition asymptomatic. A small number of smokers with RB develop associated symptoms and are classified as having RBILD. The high-resolution CT manifestations of RBILD are similar to those of RB, except that the findings tend to be more extensive. The differential diagnosis is based on the presence of clinical symptoms and combined restrictive and obstructive lung function abnormalities in patients with RBILD.

The main differential diagnosis of RB and RBILD is with HP. Similar to RB, HP usually manifests with poorly defined centrilobular nodules and ground-glass opacities. The abnormalities can be diffuse but tend to involve mainly the lower lung zones. Another common manifestation of HP is the presence of focal air trapping that is often restricted to secondary pulmonary lobules. Upper lobe predominance of centrilobular nodules and association with emphysema favors the diagnosis of RB, whereas diffuse parenchymal involvement associated with areas of lobular air trapping favors HP. However, more important are a clinical history of possible exposure to organic dust and a history of cigarette smoking. Cigarette smokers have a lower prevalence of HP than nonsmokers; only 6% of patients with HP are smokers.

Diagnosis
Respiratory bronchiolitis

Suggested Readings
Heyneman LE, Ward S, Lynch DA, et al: Respiratory bronchiolitis, respiratory bronchiolitis-associated interstitial lung disease, and desquamative interstitial pneumonia: Different entities or part of the spectrum of the same disease process? AJR Am J Roentgenol 173:1617-1622, 1999.

Hidalgo A, Franquet T, Giménez A, et al: Smoking-related interstitial lung diseases: Radiologic-pathologic correlation. Eur Radiol 16:2463-2470, 2006.

Pipavath SJ, Lynch DA, Cool C, et al: Radiologic and pathologic features of bronchiolitis. AJR Am J Roentgenol 185:354-363, 2005.

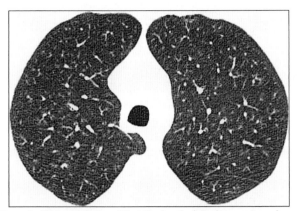

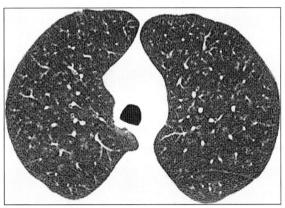

Figure 1. High-resolution CT at the level of the lung apices shows bilateral centrilobular nodules with ground-glass attenuation and minimal paraseptal emphysema anteriorly in the left lung. The patient was a 43-year-old male smoker with respiratory bronchiolitis.

Figure 2. In the same patient, high-resolution CT at the level of the lung apices shows bilateral centrilobular nodules with ground-glass attenuation.

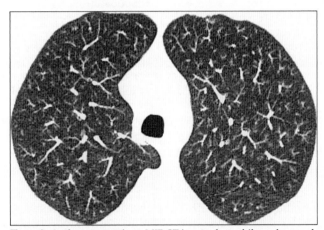

Figure 3. In the same patient, MIP CT image shows bilateral ground-glass centrilobular nodules.

Case 129

DEMOGRAPHICS/CLINICAL HISTORY

A 47-year-old man of Japanese descent with chronic cough and recurrent respiratory infections, undergoing computed tomography (CT).

FINDINGS

High-resolution CT shows centrilobular nodules and branching opacities resulting in a tree-in-bud pattern, extensive bronchiectasis, and localized areas of decreased attenuation (Fig. 1).

DISCUSSION

Definition/Background

Diffuse panbronchiolitis (DPB) is a disease of unknown origin, and its pathogenesis is associated with chronic inflammation of the respiratory bronchioles and paranasal sinuses. It is characterized histologically by a striking accumulation of foamy macrophages in the walls of respiratory bronchioles and alveolar ducts. It has been recognized almost exclusively in Asia, particularly in Japan.

Characteristic Clinical Features

Patients have panbronchiolitis, which manifests insidiously with cough, often with sputum production, and with progressive shortness of breath.

Characteristic Radiologic Findings

Radiographic abnormalities include diffuse, small (< 5 mm) nodules or a reticulonodular pattern, bronchial wall thickening, and mild to moderate hyperinflation. The characteristic manifestations on high-resolution CT consist of small centrilobular nodules and branching opacities (i.e., tree-in-bud pattern), bronchiolectasis, bronchiectasis, and areas of decreased parenchymal attenuation and vascularity.

Less Common Radiologic Manifestations

Imaging may show hilar and mediastinal lymphadenopathy.

Differential Diagnosis

- Infectious bronchiolitis (bacterial, fungal, viral)
- Tuberculosis (endobronchial spread of *Mycobacterium tuberculosis*)
- *Mycobacterium avium-intracellulare* complex infection
- Mucoid impaction distal to bronchiectasis

Discussion

DPB should be suspected in patients of East Asian descent who have a history of sinusitis and recurrent respiratory infections and have an extensive bilateral tree-in-bud pattern. The main differential diagnosis for these patients is between DPB and infectious bronchiolitis, endobronchial spread of *M. tuberculosis* or *M. avium-intracellulare* complex, or mucoid impaction distal to bronchiectasis. Panbronchiolitis typically results in a bilateral, symmetric tree-in-bud pattern that may be diffuse but tends to have lower lobe predominance and is commonly associated with air trapping and bronchiectasis. DPB is a common condition in East Asia, particularly in Japan but is uncommon in Europe and North America. The various forms of infectious bronchiolitis and endobronchial spread of mycobacterial infection tend to result in a focal or multifocal, unilateral or bilateral tree-in-bud pattern. Centrilobular nodules and a tree-in-bud pattern involving mainly the dependent regions suggest aspiration bronchiolitis.

Diagnosis

Diffuse panbronchiolitis

Suggested Readings

Akira M, Higashihara T, Sakatani M, Hara H: Diffuse panbronchiolitis: Follow-up CT examination. Radiology 189:559-562, 1993.

Collins J, Blankenbaker D, Stern EJ: CT patterns of bronchiolar disease: What is "tree-in-bud"? AJR Am J Roentgenol 171:365-370, 1998.

Rossi SE, Franquet T, Volpacchio M, et al: Tree-in-bud pattern at thin-section CT of the lungs: Radiologic-pathologic overview. Radiographics 25:789-801, 2005.

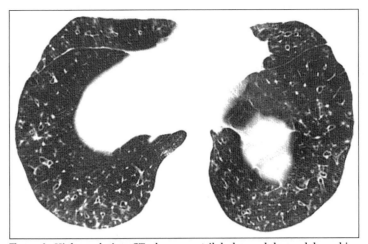

Figure 1. High-resolution CT shows centrilobular nodules and branching opacities resulting in a tree-in-bud pattern, extensive bronchiectasis, and localized areas of decreased attenuation. The patient was a 47-year-old man of Japanese descent with panbronchiolitis.

Case 130

DEMOGRAPHICS/CLINICAL HISTORY

A 23-year-old woman with progressive shortness of breath 2 years after hematopoietic stem cell transplantation, undergoing computed tomography (CT).

FINDINGS

High-resolution CT images (Figs. 1 and 2) show extensive areas of decreased attenuation and vascularity and adjacent areas of increased attenuation and vascularity resulting in a mosaic attenuation (perfusion) pattern.

DISCUSSION

Definition/Background

Bronchiolitis obliterans, also known as obliterative bronchiolitis, is characterized histologically by submucosal and peribronchiolar fibrosis, with resulting bronchiolar narrowing or obliteration of the bronchiolar lumen. The most common causes are previous infection (particularly tuberculosis and childhood viral and *Mycoplasma* pneumonia), connective tissue diseases (particularly rheumatoid arthritis), and transplantation (particularly lung transplantation).

Characteristic Clinical Features

Patients have dry cough, progressive shortness of breath, and obstructive lung function.

Characteristic Radiologic Findings

The chest radiograph is often normal for patients with mild to moderate disease. The main radiographic manifestations of bronchiolitis obliterans are peripheral attenuation of the vascular markings and hyperinflation. The characteristic high-resolution CT findings consist of sharply defined areas of decreased lung attenuation and vascularity on inspiratory CT and air trapping on expiratory CT.

Less Common Radiologic Manifestations

Imaging may show bronchiectasis or branching nodular opacities (i.e., tree-in-bud opacities).

Differential Diagnosis

- Normal lung
- Asthma

Discussion

Some air trapping is common in normal individuals and patients with collagen vascular disease and normal lungs. The air trapping in normal subjects usually involves a small proportion of lung (<25% of the cross-sectional area of one lung at one scan level) and is typically seen in the superior segments of the lower lobes, the anterior middle lobe or lingula, or involving individual pulmonary lobules, particularly in the dependent regions of the lower lobes. Areas of decreased attenuation and vascularity and air trapping can be considered abnormal when they affect a volume of lung equal to or greater than a pulmonary segment and are not limited to the superior segment of the lower lobe or the lingula tip.

Asthma may result in patchy areas of decreased attenuation and vascularity on inspiratory CT and air trapping on expiratory CT. The diagnosis of asthma is based on the characteristic clinical findings. Some patients with long-standing asthma can develop irreversible airflow obstruction due to the development of bronchiolitis obliterans.

Diagnosis

Obliterative bronchiolitis

Suggested Readings

Lynch DA: Imaging of small airways disease and chronic obstructive pulmonary disease. Clin Chest Med 29:165-179, vii, 2008.

Pipavath SJ, Lynch DA, Cool C, et al: Radiologic and pathologic features of bronchiolitis. AJR Am J Roentgenol 185:354-363, 2005.

Silva CI, Colby TV, Müller NL: Asthma and associated conditions: High-resolution CT and pathologic findings. AJR Am J Roentgenol 183:817-824, 2004.

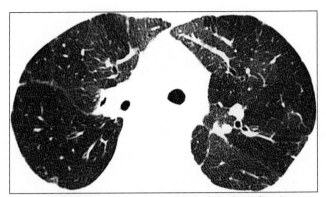

Figure 1. High-resolution CT at the level of the bronchus intermedius shows extensive areas of decreased attenuation and vascularity and adjacent areas of increased attenuation and vascularity resulting in a mosaic attenuation (perfusion) pattern. The patient was a 23-year-old woman with bronchiolitis obliterans resulting from chronic graft-versus-host disease 2 years after hematopoietic stem cell transplantation.

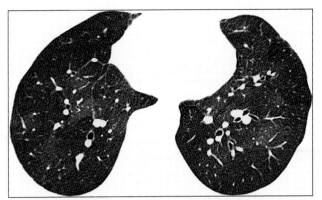

Figure 2. In the same patient, high-resolution CT at the level of the lower lobes shows extensive areas of decreased attenuation and vascularity and adjacent areas of increased attenuation and vascularity resulting in a mosaic attenuation (perfusion) pattern.

Case 131

DEMOGRAPHICS/CLINICAL HISTORY

A 47-year-old woman with progressive shortness of breath, undergoing radiography.

FINDINGS

Posteroanterior (Fig. 1) and lateral (Fig. 2) chest radiographs show large bullae in the lower lobes. The bullae are seen as lucent spaces outlined by hair-thin, curved lines. Lateral view (Fig. 2) shows flattening of the diaphragm. In another patient, radiographs show large lung volumes, with the diaphragm below the level of the anterior aspect of the seventh rib (Fig. 3) and increased retrosternal air space and flattening of the diaphragm, which is consistent with hyperinflation (Fig. 4)

DISCUSSION

Definition/Background

Emphysema is characterized by abnormal, permanent enlargement of the lung's air spaces distal to the terminal bronchiole and accompanied by destruction of their walls.

Characteristic Clinical Features

Patients, typically smokers, may be asymptomatic or present with cough and progressive shortness of breath.

Characteristic Radiologic Findings

The only direct sign of emphysema on radiographs is the presence of bullae. The main indirect and therefore nonspecific findings include focal absence of pulmonary vessels, the reduction of vessel caliber with tapering toward the lung periphery, bilateral hyperlucency, and overinflation with associated flattening of the diaphragm and increase in the retrosternal air space.

Less Common Radiologic Manifestations

Imaging may show compressive atelectasis of the adjacent lung.

Differential Diagnosis

- Asthma
- Bronchiolitis obliterans

Discussion

Emphysema is the most common cause of generalized bilateral hyperlucency and overinflation of both lungs seen on chest radiographs. However, the only direct sign of emphysema seen on a radiograph is the presence of bullae. Hyperlucency and overinflation can be seen in patients with severe asthma and bronchiolitis obliterans. The differential diagnosis for these various conditions typically can be made by a combination of clinical history, physical findings, pulmonary function test results, and when indicated, high-resolution CT.

Diagnosis

Emphysema: radiographic findings

Suggested Readings

Miniati M, Monti S, Stolk J, et al: Value of chest radiography in phenotyping chronic obstructive pulmonary disease. Eur Respir J 31:509-515, 2008.

Thurlbeck WM, Müller NL: Emphysema: Definition, imaging, and quantification. AJR Am J Roentgenol 163:1017-1025, 1994.

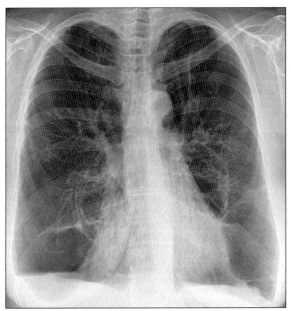

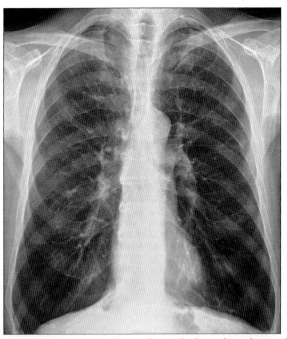

Figure 1. Posteroanterior chest radiograph shows large bullae in the lower lobes. The bullae are seen as lucent spaces outlined by hair-thin curved lines. The patient was a 47-year-old woman with bullous emphysema.

Figure 3. Posteroanterior chest radiograph shows large lung volumes, with the diaphragm below the level of the anterior aspect of the seventh rib. The patient was a 60-year-old man with emphysema.

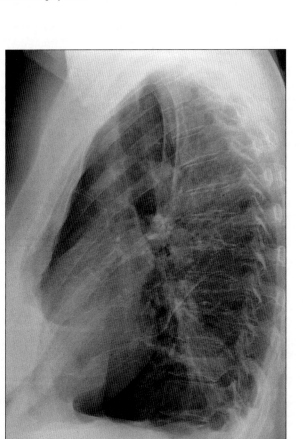

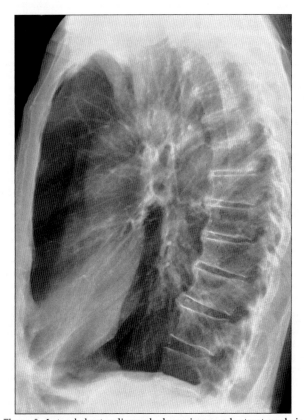

Figure 2. In the same patient, lateral chest radiograph shows large bullae immediately above the level of the diaphragm. The bullae are seen as lucent spaces outlined by hair-thin, curved lines. Notice the flattening of the diaphragm, which is consistent with hyperinflation.

Figure 4. Lateral chest radiograph shows increased retrosternal air space and flattening of the diaphragm, which is consistent with hyperinflation, in a 60-year-old man with emphysema.

Case 132

DEMOGRAPHICS/CLINICAL HISTORY

A 78-year-old female smoker with a chronic cough, undergoing computed tomography (CT).

FINDINGS

High-resolution CT images at the levels of the great vessels (Fig. 1) and aortic arch (Fig. 2) show numerous bilateral focal areas of decreased attenuation. These focal areas are a few millimeters away from the pleura and large intraparenchymal vessels, consistent with a centrilobular distribution. In other patients, high-resolution CT at the level of the lung apices shows numerous bilateral focal areas of decreased attenuation without walls (Fig. 3), and at the level of the aortic arch, CT shows bilateral, small focal areas of decreased attenuation and more confluent areas of low attenuation in the right upper lobe (Fig. 4).

DISCUSSION

Definition/Background

Emphysema is characterized by abnormal, permanent enlargement of the lung's air spaces distal to the terminal bronchiole, accompanied by destruction of their walls. Centrilobular (centriacinar) emphysema is characterized by dilatation or destruction of the respiratory bronchioles and associated alveoli. It is the type of emphysema most closely associated with cigarette smoking.

Characteristic Clinical Features

The patients, typically smokers, may be asymptomatic or present with cough and progressive shortness of breath.

Characteristic Radiologic Findings

Centrilobular emphysema is characterized on high-resolution CT by the presence of multiple rounded areas of low attenuation measuring several millimeters in diameter that typically have upper lobe predominance. The lesions have no walls, commonly have small vessels coursing within them, and often are grouped around the center of secondary pulmonary lobules. With increased severity, the areas of centrilobular emphysema become confluent and may affect large areas of the lung.

Less Common Radiologic Manifestations

Imaging may show bullae, which are air spaces measuring more than 1 cm (usually several centimeters) in diameter and sharply demarcated by a thin wall that is no more than 1 mm thick.

Differential Diagnosis

- Panacinar emphysema

Discussion

The presence of multiple, rounded areas of low attenuation measuring several millimeters in diameter without walls and grouped around the center of secondary pulmonary lobules on high-resolution CT is diagnostic for centrilobular emphysema. Panacinar (panlobular) emphysema is characterized by widespread and relatively homogeneous low attenuation that may be diffuse but tends to involve mainly the lower lobes. Although mild to moderate centrilobular emphysema is readily recognized on CT, severe confluent centrilobular emphysema may be indistinguishable from panacinar emphysema.

Diagnosis

Centrilobular emphysema: CT findings

Suggested Readings

Hartman TE, Tazelaar HD, Swensen SJ, Müller NL: Cigarette smoking: CT and pathologic findings of associated pulmonary diseases. Radiographics 17:377-390, 1997.

Lynch DA: Imaging of small airways disease and chronic obstructive pulmonary disease. Clin Chest Med 29:165-179, vii, 2008.

Müller NL, Coxson H: Chronic obstructive pulmonary disease. 4. Imaging the lungs in patients with chronic obstructive pulmonary disease. Thorax 57:982-985, 2002.

Thurlbeck WM, Müller NL: Emphysema: Definition, imaging, and quantification. AJR Am J Roentgenol 163:1017-1025, 1994.

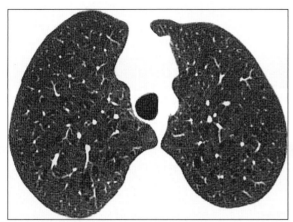

Figure 1. High-resolution CT at the level of the great vessels shows numerous bilateral focal areas of decreased attenuation. These focal areas are a few millimeters away from the pleura and large intraparenchymal vessels, consistent with a centrilobular distribution. The patient was a 78-year-old woman with centrilobular emphysema.

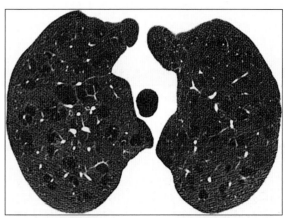

Figure 3. High-resolution CT at the level of the lung apices shows numerous, bilateral focal areas of decreased attenuation without walls. Small pulmonary vessels, corresponding to centrilobular arteries, can be seen in several of these areas. The patient was a 48-year-old man with centrilobular emphysema.

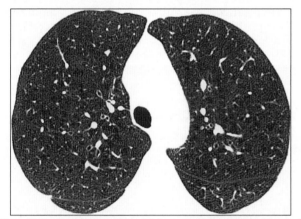

Figure 2. In the same patient, high-resolution CT at the level of the aortic arch shows numerous, bilateral focal areas of decreased attenuation. These focal areas are a few millimeters away from the pleura and large intraparenchymal vessels, consistent with a centrilobular distribution.

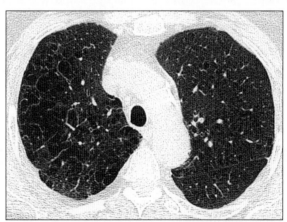

Figure 4. High-resolution CT at the level of the aortic arch shows bilateral, small focal areas of decreased attenuation and more confluent areas of low attenuation in the right upper lobe. The patient was a 65-year-old woman with centrilobular emphysema.

Case 133

DEMOGRAPHICS/CLINICAL HISTORY

A 63-year-old man with progressive shortness of breath, undergoing computed tomography (CT).

FINDINGS

High-resolution CT at the level of the inferior pulmonary veins (Fig. 1) shows extensive bilateral areas of decreased attenuation with an appearance consistent with involvement of the entire secondary lobule. The linear opacities represent displaced interlobular septa and pulmonary vessels. Coronal, reformatted, high-resolution CT (Fig. 2) shows diffuse involvement of the lung bases and less severe involvement of the upper lung zones.

DISCUSSION

Definition/Background

Panacinar (panlobular) emphysema is characterized by uniform destruction of the secondary pulmonary lobule. It is the form of emphysema associated with α_1-antitrypsin deficiency, and it typically involves mainly the lower lobes.

Characteristic Clinical Features

Patients may be asymptomatic or present with cough and progressive shortness of breath.

Characteristic Radiologic Findings

Panacinar emphysema is characterized on high-resolution CT by generalized decreased attenuation and vascularity of the affected parenchyma, typically predominantly or exclusively the lower lobes.

Less Common Radiologic Manifestations

Bronchiectasis occurs in 30% to 40% of patients with α_1-antitrypsin deficiency. Because most patients are smokers, findings of centrilobular emphysema, mainly in the upper lobes, are common. Severe panacinar emphysema may merge with severe centrilobular emphysema.

Differential Diagnosis

- Centrilobular emphysema
- Obliterative bronchiolitis

Discussion

The presence of multiple rounded areas of low attenuation measuring several millimeters in diameter without walls and grouped around the center of secondary pulmonary lobules on high-resolution CT is diagnostic of centrilobular emphysema. Panacinar (panlobular) emphysema is characterized by widespread and relatively homogeneous low attenuation that may be diffuse but tends to involve mainly the lower lobes and therefore can usually be distinguished from centrilobular emphysema. However, the findings of widespread and relatively homogeneous low attenuation and vascularity may be indistinguishable from severe bronchiolitis obliterans (i.e., obliterative bronchiolitis).

Diagnosis

Panacinar emphysema, CT findings

Suggested Readings

Hansell DM, Bankier AA, MacMahon H, et al: Fleischner Society: Glossary of terms for thoracic imaging. Radiology 246:697-722, 2008.

Hartman TE, Tazelaar HD, Swensen SJ, Müller NL: Cigarette smoking: CT and pathologic findings of associated pulmonary diseases. Radiographics 17:377-390, 1997.

Lynch DA: Imaging of small airways disease and chronic obstructive pulmonary disease. Clin Chest Med 29:165-179, vii, 2008.

Thurlbeck WM, Müller NL: Emphysema: Definition, imaging, and quantification. AJR Am J Roentgenol 163:1017-1025, 1994.

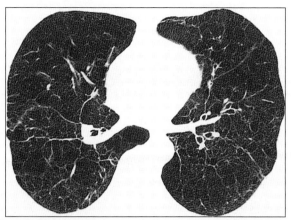

Figure 1. High-resolution CT at the level of the inferior pulmonary veins shows extensive bilateral areas of decreased attenuation and vascularity with an appearance consistent with involvement of the entire secondary lobule. The linear opacities represent displaced interlobular septa and pulmonary vessels. The patient was a 63-year-old male smoker with α_1-antitrypsin deficiency and panacinar emphysema.

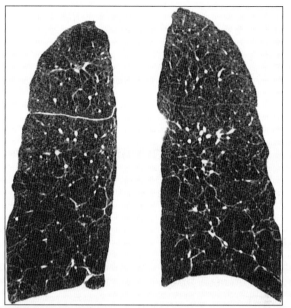

Figure 2. In the same patient, coronal, reformatted, high-resolution CT shows confluent areas of decreased attenuation and vascularity in the lung bases, characteristic of panacinar emphysema. Small, focal areas of decreased attenuation consistent with centrilobular emphysema are present in the upper lobes.

Case 134

DEMOGRAPHICS/CLINICAL HISTORY

A 44-year-old man with recurrent pneumothorax, undergoing computed tomography (CT).

FINDINGS

Cross-sectional (Fig. 1) and coronal, reformatted (Fig. 2), high-resolution CT images show subpleural emphysema.

DISCUSSION

Definition/Background

Paraseptal (distal acinar) emphysema is characterized by predominant involvement of the distal alveoli and their ducts and sacs and is therefore characteristically bounded by interlobular septa and any pleural surface. Paraseptal emphysema can be associated with centrilobular emphysema in smokers or occur as an isolated phenomenon in smokers and nonsmokers.

Characteristic Clinical Features

Patients may be asymptomatic or present with cough and progressive shortness of breath or pneumothorax.

Characteristic Radiologic Findings

Paraseptal emphysema is characterized on high-resolution CT by regions of low attenuation in the subpleural and peribronchovascular regions that are separated by intact interlobular septa. It may be associated with bullae, which are localized air spaces measuring more than 1 cm in diameter and sharply demarcated by thin walls that are 1 mm thick or less.

Less Common Radiologic Manifestations

Imaging may show associated centrilobular emphysema in smokers.

Differential Diagnosis

- Pulmonary Langerhans cell histiocytosis
- Birt-Hogg-Dubé syndrome

Discussion

The characteristic distribution of paraseptal emphysema and the common association with centrilobular emphysema usually allow ready differentiation from cystic lung diseases on high-resolution CT. The characteristic findings of Langerhans cell histiocytosis on high-resolution CT consist of cysts (in approximately 80% of patients) and nodules (in 60% to 80%). Because most patients are cigarette smokers, they may also have paraseptal emphysema and bullae. Distinct from bullae, the cysts in Langerhans histiocytosis have a random distribution and commonly have bizarre shapes, with a bilobed, cloverleaf, and branching configuration.

Birt-Hogg-Dubé syndrome is a rare, autosomal dominant disorder characterized by the presence of facial papules, which represent fibrofolliculomas; multiple, thin-walled cystic spaces; and commonly, renal tumors. The thin-walled cystic spaces resemble bullae, but distinct from paraseptal emphysema, they involve mainly the lower lobes.

Diagnosis

Paraseptal emphysema, CT findings

Suggested Readings

Hansell DM, Bankier AA, MacMahon H, et al: Fleischner Society: Glossary of terms for thoracic imaging. Radiology 246:697-722, 2008.

Satoh K, Kobayashi T, Misao T, et al: CT assessment of subtypes of pulmonary emphysema in smokers. Chest 120:725-729, 2001.

Thurlbeck WM, Müller NL: Emphysema: Definition, imaging, and quantification. AJR Am J Roentgenol 163:1017-1025, 1994.

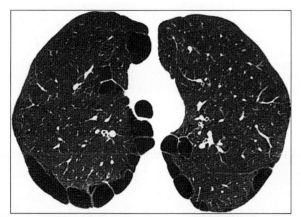

Figure 1. High-resolution CT at the level of the lung apices shows bilateral subpleural emphysema. Notice the two bullae adjacent to an interlobular septum in the right upper lobe. The patient was a 44-year-old smoker with paraseptal emphysema.

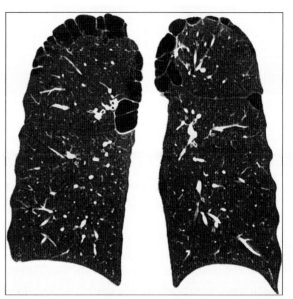

Figure 2. In the same patient, coronal, reformatted, high-resolution CT demonstrates bilateral subpleural emphysema, mainly at the lung apices.

Case 135

DEMOGRAPHICS/CLINICAL HISTORY

A 44-year-old man with acute shortness of breath after hematopoietic stem cell transplantation, undergoing radiography.

FINDINGS

Posteroanterior chest radiograph (Fig. 1) shows bilateral septal (Kerley B) lines, prominence of the pulmonary vessels, and blunting of the costophrenic sulci. The lateral radiograph (Fig. 2) confirms the presence of small, bilateral pleural effusions and shows thickening of the interlobar fissures. In another patient, the anteroposterior chest radiograph shows enlarged and poorly defined pulmonary vessels, perihilar haze in the right lung, and perihilar haze and consolidation in the left lung (Fig. 3).

DISCUSSION

Definition/Background

Hydrostatic pulmonary edema is an abnormal accumulation of fluid in the extravascular compartments (interstitial and air spaces) of the lung that is caused by a rise in pulmonary venous pressure. It most frequently results from disease of the left side of the heart, most often from a failing left ventricle or obstruction to left atrial outflow. Other common causes of hydrostatic pulmonary edema are renal disease, hypervolemia, and liver failure.

Characteristic Clinical Features

Patients have acute or chronic dyspnea, tachypnea, and orthopnea.

Characteristic Radiologic Findings

Pulmonary venous hypertension usually is evidenced by redistribution of blood flow from lower to upper lung zones, resulting in an increase in caliber of the upper zone vessels. Interstitial pulmonary edema typically results in loss of definition of segmental and subsegmental pulmonary vessels, thickening of the interlobular septa (Kerley A and B lines), thickening of the interlobar fissures, peribronchial cuffing, and small pleural effusions. Air-space hydrostatic pulmonary edema is characterized by patchy or confluent bilateral areas of consolidation that tend to be symmetric and to involve mainly the perihilar regions and the lower lung zones.

Less Common Radiologic Manifestations

Imaging may show atypical distribution in patients with underlying lung disease.

Differential Diagnosis

- Lymphangitic carcinomatosis
- Permeability pulmonary edema
- Diffuse pulmonary hemorrhage

Discussion

Extensive bilateral septal thickening may result from several acute or chronic conditions. The most important considerations are hydrostatic pulmonary edema and lymphangitic carcinomatosis. Lymphangitic carcinomatosis should be suspected in patients with associated lung nodules and in patients with known malignancy, particularly carcinoma of the breast, lung, stomach, pancreas, or colon. Definitive diagnosis requires lung biopsy.

Hydrostatic pulmonary edema is characterized by prominence of the pulmonary vessels, predominant perihilar distribution, presence of septal lines, and pleural effusions. Radiographic features that suggest permeability edema include diffuse or predominantly peripheral distribution, presence of air bronchograms, and lack of septal lines. However, there can be considerable overlap between the clinical and radiologic manifestations of hydrostatic and permeability pulmonary edema, and many patients with acute respiratory distress syndrome have associated fluid overload or left heart failure.

Diffuse pulmonary hemorrhage may result in bilateral ground-glass opacities and consolidation in a predominantly perihilar distribution. Most patients with diffuse alveolar hemorrhage present with hemoptysis; however, in some cases, the diagnosis is first suspected based on the presence of blood cells on tracheal aspirates or bronchoalveolar lavage fluid.

Diagnosis

Hydrostatic pulmonary edema: radiographic findings

Suggested Readings

Gluecker T, Capasso P, Schnyder P, et al: Clinical and radiologic features of pulmonary edema. Radiographics 19:1507-1531, 1999.

Ware LB, Matthay MA: Clinical practice. Acute pulmonary edema. N Engl J Med 353:2788-2796, 2005.

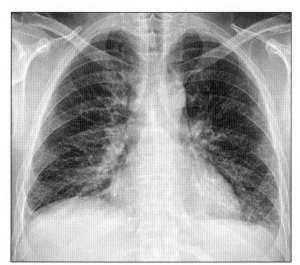

Figure 1. Posteroanterior chest radiograph shows bilateral septal (Kerley B) lines, prominence of the pulmonary vessels, and blunting of the costophrenic sulci. The patient was a 44-year-old man with interstitial pulmonary edema and bilateral pleural effusions due to fluid overload.

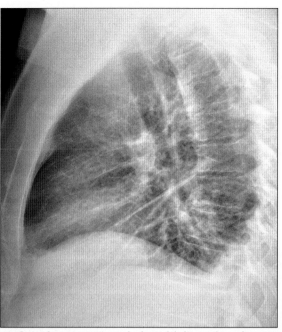

Figure 2. In the same patient, the lateral radiograph confirms presence of small, bilateral pleural effusions and shows thickening of the interlobar fissures.

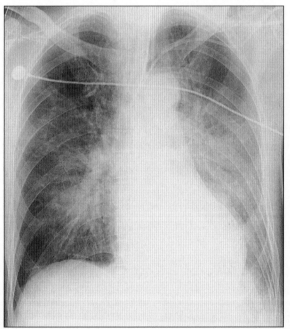

Figure 3. Anteroposterior chest radiograph shows enlarged and poorly defined pulmonary vessels, perihilar haze in the right lung, and perihilar haze and consolidation in the left lung. An endotracheal tube and central venous line are in place. The patient was a 76-year-old man with acute hydrostatic pulmonary edema due to left heart failure.

Case 136

DEMOGRAPHICS/CLINICAL HISTORY

A 23-year-old woman with shortness of breath after hematopoietic stem cell transplantation, undergoing computed tomography (CT).

FINDINGS

High-resolution CT (Fig. 1) shows bilateral, smooth thickening of the interlobular septa; mild, patchy ground-glass opacities in the lower lobes; and small, bilateral pleural effusions. In another female patient, CT shows bilateral, smooth thickening of the interlobular septa; peribronchial cuffing; ground-glass opacities in the lower lobes; and small, bilateral pleural effusions (Fig. 2). In a male patient, CT shows consolidation and ground-glass opacities in the lower lobes (Fig. 3) and a predominantly perihilar distribution of the consolidation and ground-glass opacities (Fig. 4).

DISCUSSION

Definition/Background

Hydrostatic pulmonary edema is defined as an abnormal accumulation of fluid in the extravascular compartments (interstitial and air space) of the lung that results from a rise in pulmonary venous pressure. Although a diagnosis of hydrostatic pulmonary edema is usually based on clinical information and findings on conventional chest radiography, it is important to recognize its appearance on CT, because it can mimic other diseases and because it is seen occasionally in patients not suspected clinically to have edema.

Characteristic Clinical Features

Patients have acute or chronic dyspnea, tachypnea, and orthopnea.

Characteristic Radiologic Findings

The manifestations of interstitial pulmonary edema on high-resolution CT typically consist of smooth septal thickening and perihilar opacities. Other common findings include increased vascular caliber, thickening of the perihilar peribronchovascular interstitium (i.e., peribronchial cuffing), interlobar fissures, prominence of the centrilobular structures due to interstitial edema, and small pleural effusions. Air-space pulmonary edema results in ground-glass opacities and consolidation, which, similar to the interstitial changes, tend to involve mainly the perihilar and dependent lung regions.

Less Common Radiologic Manifestations

Patients with chronic hydrostatic pulmonary edema often have slightly enlarged mediastinal lymph nodes and hazy opacification of the mediastinal fat.

Differential Diagnosis

- Lymphangitic carcinomatosis
- Churg-Strauss syndrome
- Acute lung rejection
- Pulmonary veno-occlusive disease

Discussion

Extensive, bilateral septal thickening may result from several acute or chronic conditions. The most important considerations are hydrostatic pulmonary edema and lymphangitic carcinomatosis. In interstitial pulmonary edema, the interlobular septal thickening is smooth and uniform, except for a focal nodular appearance due to prominent septal veins. In lymphangitic carcinomatosis, the septal thickening may be nodular or associated with lung nodules and extensive lymphadenopathy. However, the septal thickening in lymphangitic carcinomatosis is also commonly smooth and therefore indistinguishable from that of pulmonary edema. Lymphangitic carcinomatosis should be suspected in patients with associated lung nodules and in patients with known malignancy, particularly carcinoma of the breast, lung, stomach, pancreas, or colon. Definitive diagnosis requires lung biopsy.

Less common causes of smooth septal thickening include lymphoma, leukemia, Churg-Strauss syndrome, acute lung rejection, pulmonary veno-occlusive disease, congenital lymphangiectasia, and Niemann-Pick syndrome.

Diagnosis

Hydrostatic pulmonary edema: CT findings

Suggested Readings

Gluecker T, Capasso P, Schnyder P, et al: Clinical and radiologic features of pulmonary edema. Radiographics 19:1507-1531, 1999.

Ware LB, Matthay MA: Clinical practice. Acute pulmonary edema. N Engl J Med 353:2788-2796, 2005.

Webb WR: Thin-section CT of the secondary pulmonary lobule: Anatomy and the image—the 2004 Fleischner lecture. Radiology 239:322-338, 2006.

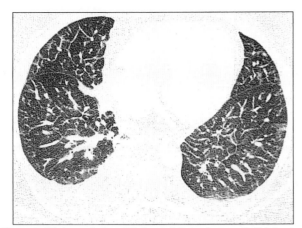

Figure 1. High-resolution CT shows bilateral, smooth thickening of the interlobular septa; mild, patchy ground-glass opacities in the lower lobes; and small, bilateral pleural effusions. The patient was a 23-year-old woman with acute interstitial pulmonary edema due to fluid overload.

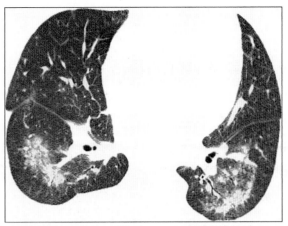

Figure 3. High-resolution CT shows consolidation and ground-glass opacities in the lower lobes. Notice the mild, interlobular septal thickening and small pleural effusions. The patient was a 45-year-old man with acute hydrostatic pulmonary edema due to left heart failure.

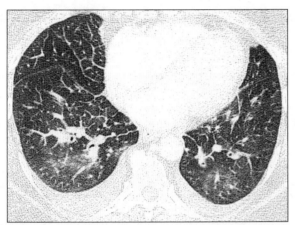

Figure 2. High-resolution CT shows bilateral, smooth thickening of the interlobular septa; peribronchial cuffing; ground-glass opacities in the lower lobes; and small, bilateral pleural effusions. The patient was a 64-year-old woman with acute interstitial pulmonary edema due left heart failure.

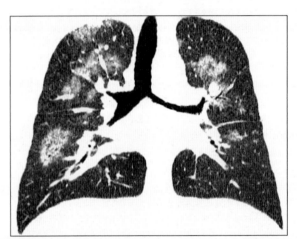

Figure 4. Coronal, reformatted, high-resolution CT shows predominantly perihilar (batwing) distribution of the consolidation and ground-glass opacities in a 45-year-old man with acute hydrostatic pulmonary edema due to left heart failure.

Case 137

DEMOGRAPHICS/CLINICAL HISTORY

A 31-year-old man with acute shortness of breath and hypoxemia, undergoing radiography.

FINDINGS

Chest radiograph (Fig. 1) shows diffuse, bilateral consolidation and a hazy increase in density (i.e., ground-glass opacity). Patent bronchi (i.e., air bronchograms) can be seen within the areas of consolidation, and a nasogastric tube and central venous line are in place. The tip of the endotracheal tube is just above the level of the carina and should be pulled back 2 to 3 cm. In another patient, the anteroposterior chest radiograph shows extensive bilateral areas of consolidation (Fig. 2).

DISCUSSION

Definition/Background

Acute respiratory distress syndrome (ARDS) is characterized clinically by acute onset of shortness of breath, refractory hypoxemia, bilateral opacities on chest radiography, and no evidence of left ventricular dysfunction; physiologically by increased permeability pulmonary edema; and histologically by the presence of diffuse alveolar damage (DAD). It may result from pulmonary causes (e.g., severe pneumonia, aspiration of gastric contents) or extrapulmonary causes (e.g., sepsis, major trauma, multiple transfusions).

Characteristic Clinical Features

Patients have acute onset of shortness of breath, bilateral parenchymal opacities on chest radiography, refractory hypoxemia, and no evidence of left heart failure.

Characteristic Radiologic Findings

Characteristic radiographic manifestations consist of extensive bilateral ground-glass opacities or consolidation or both. The areas of consolidation are relatively symmetric, are diffuse or involve mainly the peripheral lung regions, and are usually associated with air bronchograms and a lack of septal lines and pleural effusion.

Less Common Radiologic Manifestations

Asymmetric bilateral consolidation

Differential Diagnosis

- Acute interstitial pneumonia (AIP)
- Diffuse pulmonary hemorrhage
- Hydrostatic pulmonary edema

Discussion

AIP is essentially idiopathic ARDS. The patients have clinical, imaging, and histologic findings that are identical to those of patients with ARDS, but no cause is identified.

Most patients with diffuse alveolar hemorrhage present with hemoptysis. However, in some cases, the diagnosis is first suspected based on the presence of blood cells on tracheal aspirates or bronchoalveolar lavage fluid.

Hydrostatic pulmonary edema is characterized by prominence of the pulmonary vessels, blood flow redistribution (i.e., upper lobe vessel size greater than lower lobe vessel size), predominant perihilar distribution, presence of septal lines, and pleural effusions evident on the chest radiograph. Radiographic features most suggestive of permeability edema include inhomogeneous or predominantly peripheral distribution of the edema, presence of air bronchograms, and lack of septal lines and pleural effusion. However, there can be considerable overlap between the clinical and radiologic manifestations of hydrostatic and permeability pulmonary edema, and many patients with ARDS have associated fluid overload or left heart failure. In clinical practice, the differential diagnosis often requires measurements of pulmonary capillary wedge pressure with a Swan-Ganz catheter.

Diagnosis

Acute respiratory distress syndrome (ARDS): radiographic findings

Suggested Readings

Bernard GR: Acute respiratory distress syndrome. A historical perspective. Am J Respir Crit Care Med 172:798-806, 2005.

Caironi P, Carlesso E, Gattinoni L: Radiological imaging in acute lung injury and acute respiratory distress syndrome. Semin Respir Crit Care Med 27:404-415, 2006.

Desai SR: Acute respiratory distress syndrome: Imaging of the injured lung. Clin Radiol 57:8-17, 2002.

Goodman PC: Radiographic findings in patients with acute respiratory distress syndrome. Clin Chest Med 21:419-433, 2000.

Rubenfeld GD, Caldwell E, Peabody E, et al: Incidence and outcomes of acute lung injury. N Engl J Med 353:1685-1693, 2005.

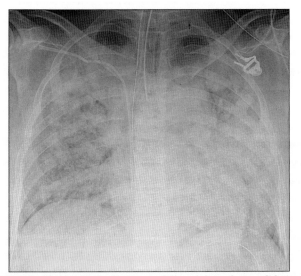

Figure 1. Chest radiograph shows diffuse bilateral consolidation and a hazy increase in density (i.e., ground-glass opacity). Patent bronchi (i.e., air bronchograms) can be seen within the areas of consolidation. A nasogastric tube and central venous line are in place. The tip of the endotracheal tube is just above the level of the carina and should be pulled back 2 to 3 cm. The patient was a 31-year-old man with ARDS.

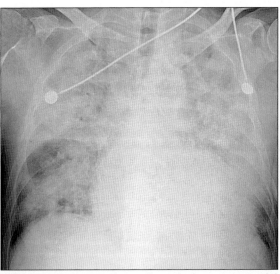

Figure 2. Anteroposterior chest radiograph shows extensive bilateral areas of consolidation in a 71-year-old man with ARDS.

Case 138

DEMOGRAPHICS/CLINICAL HISTORY

A 71-year-old man with acute shortness of breath and hypoxemia, undergoing computed tomography (CT).

FINDINGS

High-resolution CT images at the level of the upper (Fig. 1) and lower (Fig. 2) lung zones show extensive, bilateral ground-glass opacities and dependent areas of consolidation. Smooth, interlobular and intralobular, linear opacities can be seen superimposed on the ground-glass opacities mainly in the upper lobes. Notice the areas of relatively normal lung, mainly in the anterior aspects of the upper lobes and in the right middle and lower lobes. In another patient, high-resolution CT shows extensive, bilateral ground-glass opacities with superimposed smooth, interlobular and intralobular, linear opacities (Fig. 3).

DISCUSSION

Definition/Background

Acute respiratory distress syndrome (ARDS) is characterized clinically by acute onset of shortness of breath, refractory hypoxemia, bilateral opacities on chest radiography, and no evidence of left ventricular dysfunction; physiologically by increased permeability pulmonary edema; and histologically by the presence of diffuse alveolar damage (DAD). CT helps to establish the cause in selected cases and is a problem-solving tool for patients with complex appearances on the chest radiograph and patients with suspected complications.

Characteristic Clinical Features

Patients have an acute onset of shortness of breath, bilateral parenchymal opacities on chest radiography, refractory hypoxemia, and no evidence of left heart failure.

Characteristic Radiologic Findings

Characteristic CT manifestations consist of extensive, bilateral ground-glass opacities that may be diffuse but most commonly are patchy, sparing up to one third of the lung parenchyma. Areas of consolidation usually are bilateral and mainly in the dependent lung regions. Interlobular and intralobular septal thickening is frequently seen on high-resolution CT superimposed on the ground-glass opacities, resulting in a crazy-paving pattern.

Less Common Radiologic Manifestations

Traction bronchiectasis and bronchiolectasis and reticulation are present on CT in the late proliferative and fibrotic phases of diffuse alveolar damage.

Differential Diagnosis

- Acute interstitial pneumonia (AIP)
- Diffuse pulmonary hemorrhage
- Hydrostatic pulmonary edema

Discussion

AIP is essentially idiopathic acute respiratory distress syndrome (ARDS). The patients have clinical, imaging, and histologic findings identical to those of patients with ARDS, but no cause is identified.

Most patients with diffuse alveolar hemorrhage present with hemoptysis. However, in some cases, the diagnosis is first suspected based on the presence of blood cells on tracheal aspirates or bronchoalveolar lavage fluid.

Hydrostatic pulmonary edema is characterized by prominence of the pulmonary vessels, predominant perihilar distribution, presence of septal lines, and pleural effusions. Radiographic features most suggestive of permeability edema include diffuse or predominantly peripheral distribution, presence of air bronchograms, and lack of septal lines. However, there can be considerable overlap between the clinical and radiologic manifestations of hydrostatic and permeability pulmonary edema, and many patients with ARDS have associated fluid overload or left heart failure. In clinical practice, the differential diagnosis often requires measurements of pulmonary capillary wedge pressure with a Swan-Ganz catheter.

Diagnosis

Acute respiratory distress syndrome (ARDS): computed tomography

Suggested Readings

Desai SR: Acute respiratory distress syndrome: Imaging of the injured lung. Clin Radiol 57:8-17, 2002.

Gattinoni L, Caironi P, Valenza F, Carlesso E: The role of CT-scan studies for the diagnosis and therapy of acute respiratory distress syndrome. Clin Chest Med 27:559-570, 2006.

Rubenfeld GD, Caldwell E, Peabodt E, et al: Incidence and outcomes of acute lung injury. N Engl J Med 353:1685-1693, 2005.

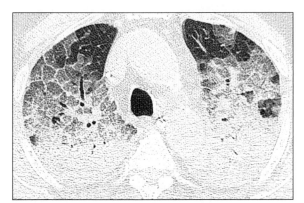

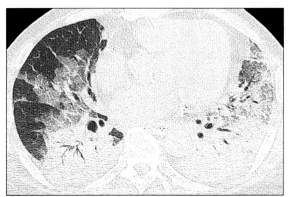

Figure 1. High-resolution CT at the level of the upper lung zones shows extensive, bilateral ground-glass opacities and dependent areas of consolidation. Smooth, interlobular and intralobular, linear opacities can be seen superimposed on the ground-glass opacities (i.e., crazy-paving pattern). Notice the areas of relatively normal lung in the anterior aspects of the upper lobes. The patient was a 71-year-old man with ARDS.

Figure 2. In the same patient high-resolution CT at the level of the lower lung zones shows extensive, bilateral ground-glass opacities and dependent areas of consolidation. Areas of relatively normal lung can be seen in the right middle and lower lobes.

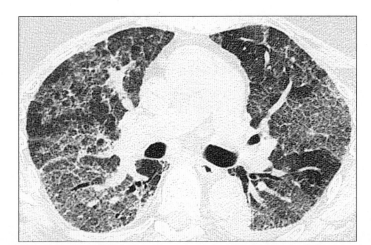

Figure 3. High-resolution CT shows extensive bilateral ground-glass opacities with superimposed smooth, interlobular and intralobular, linear opacities (i.e., crazy-paving pattern). The patient was a 58-year-old woman with ARDS.

Case 139

DEMOGRAPHICS/CLINICAL HISTORY

A 59-year-old man who is asymptomatic, undergoing radiography.

FINDINGS

Posteroanterior chest radiograph (Fig. 1) shows bilateral, large opacities immediately above the level of the hila and multiple, bilateral, small nodules in the middle and upper lung zones. Notice the increased lucency of the left lung apex due to emphysema. Chest radiograph obtained 11 years earlier (Fig. 2) shows multiple, small nodules in the middle and upper lung zones.

DISCUSSION

Definition/Background

Silicosis is an occupational lung disease caused by continued exposure to excessive amounts of dust containing crystalline silica. It occurs most commonly in coal miners, sandblasters, and quarry workers.

Characteristic Clinical Features

Patients are often asymptomatic. The main symptom is slowly progressing shortness of breath.

Characteristic Radiologic Findings

The characteristic radiographic manifestations of silicosis consist of small (1 to 10 mm in diameter), well-defined nodules that may be diffuse but tend to involve predominantly or exclusively the upper lung zones. The nodules may conglomerate and form large opacities (i.e., progressive massive fibrosis) in the upper zones of the lungs with smooth or irregular borders, initially at the outer two thirds of the lung but with slow migration toward the hilum and progressive volume loss.

Less Common Radiologic Manifestations

Imaging commonly shows lymphadenopathy and calcification of hilar and mediastinal lymph nodes; the calcification may involve mainly the periphery of the nodes (i.e., eggshell calcification), a finding that strongly suggests silicosis. Nodule calcification is evident on the radiograph in up to 20% of cases.

Differential Diagnosis

- Coal worker's pneumoconiosis
- Sarcoidosis
- Tuberculosis
- Fungal infection

Discussion

Coal worker's pneumoconiosis results in lung nodules with a pattern and distribution identical to those seen in silicosis, and like silicosis, it may result in progressive massive fibrosis. The differential diagnosis is based on clinical history.

Sarcoidosis frequently results in a small nodular pattern that may be diffuse but also tends to involve mainly the upper lung zones. In most cases, the small nodular pattern in sarcoidosis is associated with bilateral symmetric hilar and paratracheal lymphadenopathy, a finding that strongly suggests the diagnosis.

Tuberculosis and fungal infection may result in diffuse nodular pattern, but the patients tend to present with more acute symptoms and are often febrile.

Diagnosis

Silicosis, radiographic findings

Suggested Readings

Chong S, Lee KS, Chung MJ, et al: Pneumoconiosis: Comparison of imaging and pathologic findings. Radiographics 26:59-77, 2006.
Fujimura N: Pathology and pathophysiology of pneumoconiosis. Curr Opin Pulm Med 6:140-144, 2000.
Kim KI, Kim CW, Lee MK, et al: Imaging of occupational lung disease. Radiographics 21:1371-1391, 2001.

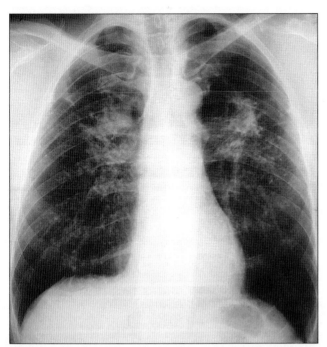

Figure 1. Posteroanterior chest radiograph shows bilateral, large opacities immediately above the level of the hila and multiple, bilateral, small nodules in the middle and upper lung zones. Notice the increased lucency of the left lung apex due to emphysema. The patient was a 59-year-old man with silicosis.

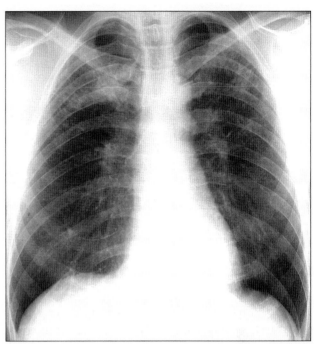

Figure 2. In the same patient, a posteroanterior chest radiograph, performed 11 years earlier than the one in Figure 1, shows multiple, bilateral, small nodules in the middle and upper lung zones.

Case 140

DEMOGRAPHICS/CLINICAL HISTORY

A 73-year-old man with chronic cough, undergoing computed tomography (CT).

FINDINGS

High-resolution CT at the level of the lung apices (Fig. 1) shows bilateral, large opacities and multiple, well-defined centrilobular and subpleural nodules. Notice the emphysema. High-resolution CT at the level of the right upper lobe bronchus (Fig. 2) shows bilateral centrilobular and subpleural nodules, mild scarring, and emphysema. In another patient, CT shows bilateral hilar and subcarinal lymph nodes, most of which have eggshell calcification (Fig. 3).

DISCUSSION

Definition/Background
Silicosis is an occupational lung disease caused by continued exposure to excessive amounts of dust containing crystalline silica. It occurs most commonly in coal miners, sandblasters, and quarry workers.

Characteristic Clinical Features
Patients are often asymptomatic. The main symptom is slowly progressing shortness of breath.

Characteristic Radiologic Findings
The characteristic high-resolution CT manifestations of silicosis consist of small (1 to 10 mm in diameter), well-defined nodules that may be diffuse but tend to involve predominantly or exclusively the upper lung zones. The nodules have a predominantly centrilobular and subpleural distribution. The nodules may progress to bilateral upper lobe conglomerate masses (i.e., progressive massive fibrosis), usually with irregular margins and associated with adjacent paracicatricial emphysema and lung parenchymal architectural distortion.

Less Common Radiologic Manifestations
Imaging may show lymphadenopathy and calcification of hilar and mediastinal lymph nodes; the calcification may involve mainly the periphery of the nodes (i.e., eggshell calcification), a finding that strongly suggests silicosis. Calcification of silicotic nodules and conglomerate masses is often evident on CT.

Differential Diagnosis
- Coal worker's pneumoconiosis
- Sarcoidosis
- Tuberculosis
- Fungal infection

Discussion
Coal worker's pneumoconiosis results in lung nodules with a pattern and distribution identical to those seen in silicosis, and like silicosis, it may result in progressive massive fibrosis. Unlike silicosis, calcification of nodules, conglomerate masses, and lymph nodes are seldom present in coal worker's pneumoconiosis.

Sarcoidosis frequently results in a small nodular pattern that may be diffuse but tends to involve mainly the upper lung zones. However, on high-resolution CT, the nodules in sarcoidosis typically have a perilymphatic distribution along the bronchi, vessels, and interlobular septa, whereas the nodules in silicosis and coal worker's pneumoconiosis have a predominantly centrilobular distribution. All three conditions may be associated with subpleural nodules. In most cases, the small nodular pattern in sarcoidosis is associated with bilateral, symmetric hilar and paratracheal lymphadenopathy, a finding that strongly suggests the diagnosis.

Diagnosis
Silicosis, CT findings

Suggested Readings
Chong S, Lee KS, Chung MJ, et al: Pneumoconiosis: Comparison of imaging and pathologic findings. Radiographics 26:59-77, 2006.
Fujimura N: Pathology and pathophysiology of pneumoconiosis. Curr Opin Pulm Med 6:140-144, 2000.
Kim KI, Kim CW, Lee MK, et al: Imaging of occupational lung disease. Radiographics 21:1371-1391, 2001.

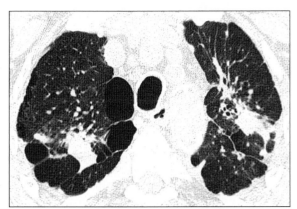

Figure 1. High-resolution CT at the level of the lung apices shows bilateral, large opacities and multiple, well-defined centrilobular and subpleural nodules. Notice the emphysema. The patient was a 73-year-old man with silicosis and emphysema.

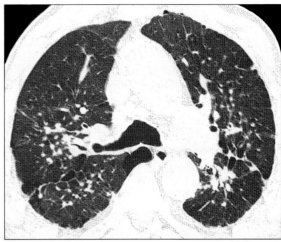

Figure 2. In the same patient, high-resolution CT at the level of the right upper lobe bronchus shows bilateral centrilobular and subpleural nodules, mild scarring, and emphysema.

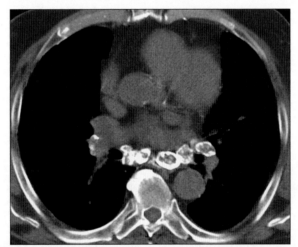

Figure 3. CT (5-mm section thickness) using soft tissue windows shows bilateral hilar and subcarinal lymph nodes, most of which have eggshell calcification. The patient was an 82-year-old man with silicosis.

Case 141

DEMOGRAPHICS/CLINICAL HISTORY

A 65-year-old male, asymptomatic, miner, nonsmoker.

FINDINGS

High-resolution CT images at the level of aortic arch (Fig. 1) and carina (Fig. 2) show bilateral, poorly defined, centrilobular nodules.

DISCUSSION

Definition/Background

Coalworker's pneumoconiosis (CWP) is an occupational lung disease caused by continued exposure to excessive amounts of coal dust (anthracosis).

Characteristic Clinical Features

The patients are usually asymptomatic. The main symptom is chronic cough.

Characteristic Radiologic Findings

The characteristic high-resolution CT manifestations of coalworker's pneumoconiosis consist of small (1–5 mm in diameter) well-defined or poorly defined centrilobular nodules that may be diffuse but that tend to predominantly or exclusively involve the upper lung zones (Figs. 1 and 2). The nodules may progress to bilateral upper lobe conglomerate masses (progressive massive fibrosis), usually with irregular margins and associated with adjacent paracicatricial emphysema and lung parenchymal architectural distortion.

Less Common Radiologic Manifestations

Small branching lines or ill-defined punctate areas of soft tissue attenuation.

Differential Diagnosis

- Silicosis
- Sarcoidosis
- Hypersensitivity pneumonitis
- Respiratory bronchiolitis

Discussion

Silicosis results in lung nodules with identical pattern and distribution to those seen in coalworker's pneumoconiosis and, like CWP, may result in progressive massive fibrosis. Unlike silicosis, calcification of nodules, conglomerate masses, or lymph nodes is seldom present in coalworker's pneumoconiosis.

Sarcoidosis also frequently results in a small nodular pattern that may be diffuse but that also tends to involve mainly the upper lung zones. However, on high-resolution CT, the nodules in sarcoidosis typically have a perilymphatic distribution along the bronchi, vessels, and interlobular septa, whereas the nodules in silicosis and coalworker's pneumoconiosis have a predominantly centrilobular distribution. In the vast majority of cases, the small nodular pattern in sarcoidosis is associated with bilateral symmetric hilar and paratracheal lymphadenopathy, a finding highly suggestive of the diagnosis.

Hypersensitivity pneumonitis (HP), like CWP, often results in centrilobular nodules. The nodules in HP typically have ground-glass attenuation, whereas those of CWP have soft tissue attenuation. Furthermore, HP is usually associated with patchy ground-glass opacities and lobular areas of decreased attenuation and vascularity. Respiratory bronchiolitis also manifests with poorly defined centrilobular nodules, predominantly in the upper lobes. The diagnosis is based on the history of cigarette smoking and lack of other environmental exposure.

Diagnosis

Coalworker's pneumoconiosis

Suggested Readings

Chong S, Lee KS, Chung MJ, Han J, Kwon OJ, Kim TS: Pneumoconiosis: Comparison of imaging and pathologic findings. Radiographics 26:59-77, 2006.

Kim KI, Kim CW, Lee MK, et al: Imaging of occupational lung disease. Radiographics 21:1371-91.

Fujimura N: Pathology and pathophysiology of pneumoconiosis. Curr Opin Pulm Med 6:140-144, 2000.

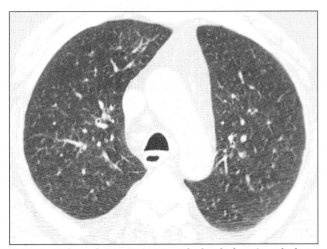

Figure 1. High-resolution CT image at the level of aortic arch shows bilateral poorly defined centrilobular nodules. The patient was a 65-year-old male with coalworker's pneumoconiosis.

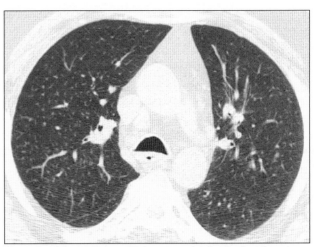

Figure 2. High-resolution CT image at the level of carina shows bilateral poorly defined centrilobular nodules. The patient was a 65-year-old male with coalworker's pneumoconiosis.

Case 142

DEMOGRAPHICS/CLINICAL HISTORY

A 76-year-old man who was a shipyard worker with progressive shortness of breath, undergoing computed tomography (CT).

FINDINGS

High-resolution CT (Fig. 1) shows bilateral, predominantly subpleural intralobular lines and irregular thickening of interlobular septa. The image also shows nondependent ground-glass opacities and architectural distortion in the anterolateral aspect of the left upper lobe. CT using soft tissue windows (Fig. 2) shows calcified, bilateral pleural plaques and diffuse, irregular, left pleural thickening. Coronal (Fig. 3) and sagittal (Fig. 4) reformation images show the predominant distribution of the fibrosis in the subpleural regions.

DISCUSSION

Definition/Background

Asbestosis is interstitial pulmonary fibrosis caused by the inhalation of excessive amounts of asbestos fibers. It is an occupational lung disease that is seen most commonly in workers exposed to asbestos in insulation materials, brake pads and linings, floor tiles, electric wiring, and cements.

Characteristic Clinical Features

Patients are usually asymptomatic. The main clinical manifestations are dry cough and slowly progressing shortness of breath, typically occurring 20 to 30 years after asbestos exposure.

Characteristic Radiologic Findings

The radiograph may be normal or show small, irregular, linear opacities (i.e., reticular pattern, s and t opacities in the International Labor Office [ILO] classification) mainly in the lower lung zones. The most common high-resolution CT manifestations of asbestosis are intralobular, linear opacities (i.e., reticular pattern); irregular thickening of the interlobular septa; nondependent ground-glass opacities; subpleural, small, rounded or branching opacities; subpleural, curvilinear opacities; and parenchymal bands. The abnormalities involve mainly the peripheral and dorsal regions of the lung bases. Most patients have pleural plaques or diffuse pleural thickening.

Less Common Radiologic Manifestations

Honeycombing may be seen in some patients.

Differential Diagnosis

- Idiopathic pulmonary fibrosis
- Nonspecific interstitial pneumonia

Discussion

The diagnosis of asbestosis requires the presence of pulmonary fibrosis and history of exposure of sufficient duration, latency, and intensity to be causal. The abnormal chest radiograph and its interpretation remain the most important factors in establishing the presence of pulmonary fibrosis. When the chest radiograph or lung function abnormalities are indeterminate, high-resolution CT scanning is often helpful in demonstrating the presence of fibrosis and the pleural changes that strongly suggest asbestos exposure. Clinically and radiologically, asbestosis resembles other interstitial lung diseases, particularly idiopathic pulmonary fibrosis. The differential diagnosis is based mainly on the history of asbestos exposure and on the radiologic demonstration of pleural abnormalities consistent with asbestos exposure. In some cases, definitive diagnosis may require lung biopsy.

Diagnosis

Asbestosis

Suggested Readings

American Thoracic Society: Diagnosis and initial management of non-malignant diseases related to asbestos. Am J Respir Crit Care Med 170:691-715, 2004.

Chong S, Lee KS, Chung MJ, et al: Pneumoconiosis: Comparison of imaging and pathologic findings. Radiographics 26:59-77, 2006.

Roach HD, Davies GJ, Attanoos R, et al: Asbestos: When the dust settles an imaging review of asbestos-related disease. Radiographics 22:S167-S184, 2002.

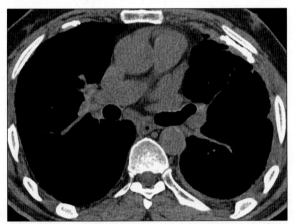

Figure 1. High-resolution CT shows bilateral, predominantly sub-pleural, intralobular lines and irregular thickening of interlobular septa. The image also shows nondependent ground-glass opacities and architectural distortion in the anterolateral aspect of the left upper lobe. The patient was a 76-year-old man with asbestosis after many years of asbestos exposure as a shipyard worker.

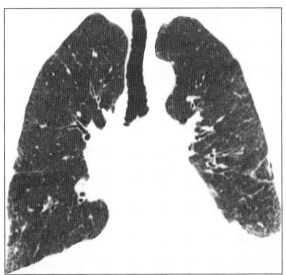

Figure 3. In the same patient, coronal, reformatted, high-resolution CT shows the predominant distribution of the fibrosis in the subpleural regions.

Figure 2. In the same patient, high-resolution CT using soft tissue windows shows calcified, bilateral pleural plaques, and diffuse, irregular, left pleural thickening.

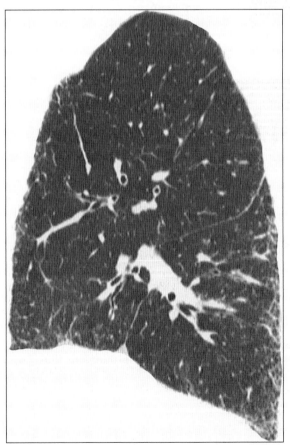

Figure 4. In the same patient, sagittal, high-resolution CT shows the predominant distribution of the fibrosis in the subpleural regions.

Case 143

DEMOGRAPHICS/CLINICAL HISTORY

A 51-year-old man who is asymptomatic, undergoing radiography and compared with computed tomography (CT).

FINDINGS

Posteroanterior chest radiograph (Fig. 1) shows multiple, focal, pleural-based opacities along the chest wall and diaphragm. In another patient, a radiograph shows numerous, bilateral, calcified pleural plaques (Fig. 2). In other patients, CT shows bilateral, circumscribed areas of pleural thickening and calcification that are characteristic of pleural plaques (Fig. 3 and Fig. 4).

DISCUSSION

Definition/Background

Pleural plaques are the most common form of asbestos-related pleuropulmonary disease. They consist of well-defined, pearly white foci of firm, fibrous tissue, usually 2 to 5 mm thick and up to 10 cm in diameter, and they are usually first seen 20 to 30 years after exposure. Asbestos exposure occurs most commonly in individuals working with insulation materials, brake pads and linings, floor tiles, electric wiring, and cements.

Characteristic Clinical Features

Pleural plaques typically do not result in any clinical symptoms.

Characteristic Radiologic Findings

The characteristic findings on the chest radiograph consist of focal, bilateral, pleural-based opacities that have irregular margins when seen in profile and sharp, often foliate borders when seen face on. The characteristic presentation of pleural plaques on high-resolution CT consists of circumscribed areas of pleural thickening separated from the underlying ribs and extrapleural soft tissues by a thin layer of fat.

Less Common Radiologic Manifestations

Calcification of pleural plaques is seen in 10% to 15% of cases.

Differential Diagnosis

- Extrapleural fat
- Tuberculosis
- Talc deposition

Discussion

Noncalcified pleural plaques may be indistinguishable from extrapleural fat on the radiograph. The distinction can be readily made on CT. Bilateral pleural plaques are almost invariably associated with asbestos exposure. However, isolated plaques may be caused by tuberculosis, trauma, hemothorax, or talc deposition.

Diagnosis

Asbestos-related pleural plaques

Suggested Readings

American Thoracic Society: Diagnosis and initial management of non-malignant diseases related to asbestos. Am J Respir Crit Care Med 170:691-715, 2004.

Chong S, Lee KS, Chung MJ, et al: Pneumoconiosis: Comparison of imaging and pathologic findings. Radiographics 26:59-77, 2006.

Roach HD, Davies GJ, Attanoos R, et al: Asbestos: When the dust settles an imaging review of asbestos-related disease. Radiographics 22:S167-S184, 2002.

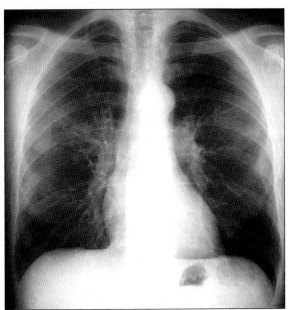

Figure 1. Posteroanterior chest radiograph shows multiple, focal, pleural-based opacities along the chest wall and diaphragm that are characteristic of pleural plaques. The patient was a 51-year-old shipyard worker with asbestos-related pleural plaques.

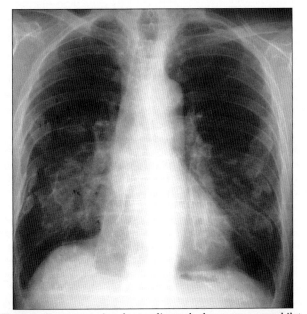

Figure 2. Posteroanterior chest radiograph shows numerous bilateral, calcified pleural plaques. The patient was an 82-year-old man with asbestos-related pleural plaques.

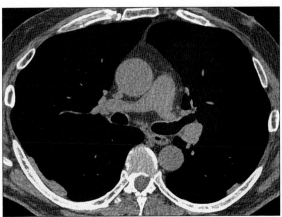

Figure 3. High-resolution CT shows bilateral, circumscribed areas of pleural thickening that are characteristic of pleural plaques. The patient was a 65-year-old man.

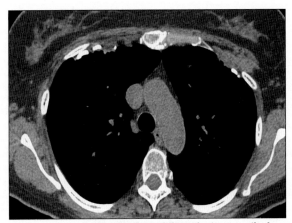

Figure 4. High-resolution CT shows bilateral, circumscribed areas of pleural thickening and calcification characteristic of pleural plaques. The patient was a 60-year-old woman.

Case 144

DEMOGRAPHICS/CLINICAL HISTORY

A 60-year-old man who had been a shipyard worker and now has progressive shortness of breath, undergoing computed tomography (CT).

FINDINGS

CT (Fig. 1) shows diffuse bilateral pleural thickening with small foci of calcification on the right. Notice that the thickening involves the paraspinal and costal pleura but spares the mediastinal pleura.

DISCUSSION

Definition/Background

Diffuse pleural thickening is diagnosed when there is a smooth, uninterrupted pleural thickening extending over at least one fourth of the chest wall. The revised 2000 International Labor Office (ILO) classification recognizes pleural thickening as diffuse "only in the presence of and in continuity with an obliterated costophrenic angle." Diffuse pleural thickening is seen in 9% to 22% of asbestos-exposed workers with pleural disease, and it has a latency period of 10 to 40 years after initial exposure.

Characteristic Clinical Features

Patients may be asymptomatic or may present with slowly progressing shortness of breath.

Characteristic Radiologic Findings

Smooth, uninterrupted pleural density extending over at least one fourth of the chest wall can be seen on the chest radiograph. Diffuse pleural thickening is defined on CT by the presence of a sheet of thickened pleura at least 5 cm in the lateral dimension and 8 cm in the craniocaudal dimension.

Less Common Radiologic Manifestations

Diffuse pleural thickening may be associated with ipsilateral or bilateral pleural plaques. Calcification may occur.

Differential Diagnosis

- Extrapleural fat
- Fibrothorax from other causes

Discussion

The main radiographic differential diagnosis of diffuse pleural thickening is extrapleural fat, which typically occurs bilaterally and symmetrically along the mid-lateral chest wall from the 4th to 8th ribs. The distinction is readily made in patients with blunting of the costophrenic angles or pleural calcification; in the remaining cases, confident diagnosis often requires CT.

Diffuse pleural thickening is commonly seen as a manifestation of fibrothorax after tuberculosis, empyema, or hemothorax. The diagnosis of asbestos-related diffuse pleural thickening is based on the clinical history of exposure and finding of associated pleural plaques.

Diagnosis

Asbestos-related diffuse pleural thickening

Suggested Readings

American Thoracic Society: Diagnosis and initial management of nonmalignant diseases related to asbestos. Am J Respir Crit Care Med 170:691-715, 2004.

Chong S, Lee KS, Chung MJ, et al: Pneumoconiosis: Comparison of imaging and pathologic findings. Radiographics 26:59-77, 2006.

Roach HD, Davies GJ, Attanoos R, et al: Asbestos: When the dust settles an imaging review of asbestos-related disease. Radiographics 22:S167-S184, 2002.

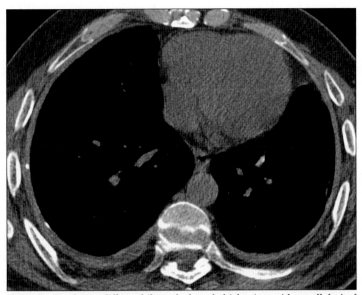

Figure 1. CT shows diffuse, bilateral pleural thickening with small foci of calcification on the right. Notice that the thickening involves the paraspinal and costal pleura but spares the mediastinal pleura. The patient was a 60-year-old man with bilateral, diffuse pleural thickening related to asbestos exposure when he was a shipyard worker.

Case 145

DEMOGRAPHICS/CLINICAL HISTORY

A 34-year-old male machinist with a 2-year history of cough and progressive shortness of breath, undergoing computed tomography (CT).

FINDINGS

High-resolution CT images at the level of the aortic arch (Fig. 1) and inferior pulmonary veins (Fig. 2) show bilateral, patchy ground-glass opacities and poorly defined centrilobular nodules. CT using soft tissue windows (Fig. 3) shows calcified, bilateral hilar and subcarinal lymph nodes.

DISCUSSION

Definition/Background

Hard metal lung disease is a rare occupational lung disease that can occur in workers engaged in the manufacture, use, or maintenance of tools composed of hard metal. Hard metal is an alloy of tungsten carbide and cobalt.

Characteristic Clinical Features

Exposure to hard metal may result in three main respiratory complications: asthma, hypersensitivity pneumonitis, and pulmonary fibrosis. Patients with pulmonary fibrosis usually present with dry cough and slowly progressing shortness of breath.

Characteristic Radiologic Findings

The chest radiograph may be normal or show small, irregular opacities resulting in a reticular or reticulonodular pattern, predominantly in the middle and lower lung zones. The high-resolution CT findings consist of bilateral, patchy ground-glass opacities, reticulation, and occasionally, honeycombing. Centrilobular nodules and consolidation may be seen.

Less Common Radiologic Manifestations

Imaging may show predominantly upper lobe fibrosis and calcified lymph nodes.

Differential Diagnosis
- Nonspecific interstitial pneumonia (NSIP)
- Idiopathic pulmonary fibrosis
- Other types of pneumoconiosis (e.g. silicosis, aluminum)

Discussion

The findings of ground-glass opacities and reticulation involving mainly the lower lung zones mimic those of NSIP. In patients with predominantly lower lung zone reticulation and honeycombing, the appearance is identical to that of idiopathic pulmonary fibrosis.

The diagnosis of hard metal lung disease is based on a careful history of exposure. The diagnosis can be confirmed by biopsy. Histologic findings of giant cell interstitial pneumonia are pathognomonic for hard metal lung disease. Tungsten particles usually can be demonstrated by energy-dispersive x-ray spectroscopy, and their presence confirms the diagnosis.

Diagnosis

Hard metal lung disease

Suggested Readings

Akira M: High-resolution CT in the evaluation of occupational and environmental disease. Radiol Clin North Am 40:43-59, 2002.

Chong S, Lee KS, Chung MJ, et al: Pneumoconiosis: Comparison of imaging and pathologic findings. Radiographics 26:59-77, 2006.

Dunlop P, Müller NL, Wilson J, et al: Hard metal lung disease: High resolution CT and histologic correlation of the initial findings and demonstration of interval improvement. J Thorac Imaging 20:301-304, 2005.

Nemery B, Verbeken EK, Demedts M: Giant cell interstitial pneumonia (hard metal lung disease, cobalt lung). Semin Respir Crit Care Med 22:435-448, 2001.

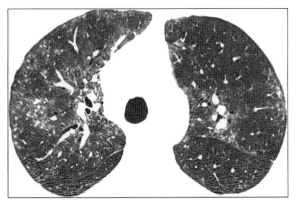

Figure 1. High-resolution CT at the level of the aortic arch shows bilateral, patchy ground-glass opacities and poorly defined centrilobular nodules. The patient was a 34-year-old man with hard metal lung disease resulting from 15 years of exposure to tungsten carbide dust as a machinist sharpening tungsten carbide blades.

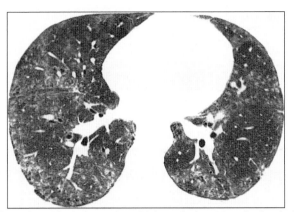

Figure 2. In the same patient, high-resolution CT at the level of the inferior pulmonary veins shows bilateral, patchy ground-glass opacities and poorly defined centrilobular nodules.

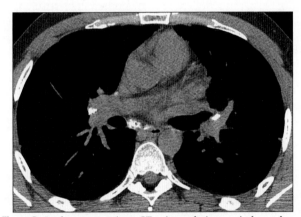

Figure 3. In the same patient, CT using soft tissue windows shows calcified, bilateral hilar and subcarinal lymph nodes.

Case 146

DEMOGRAPHICS/CLINICAL HISTORY

A 32-year-old woman with sudden onset of dyspnea 1 day after a motor vehicle accident and head injury, undergoing radiography and computed tomography (CT).

FINDINGS

Anteroposterior chest radiograph (Fig. 1) shows poorly defined areas of consolidation in the lower lobes. Contrast-enhanced CT images using lung windows (Fig. 2) and soft tissue windows (Fig. 3) show areas of dense consolidation in the lower lobes. CT also shows bilateral, small, centrilobular nodular opacities in the dependent regions of the right middle lobe and lingula and in the lower lobes.

DISCUSSION

Definition/Background
Aspiration is inhalation of oropharyngeal or gastric contents into the lower airways. Inhalation of these contents can lead to aspiration pneumonitis (i.e., chemical damage to the parenchyma caused by inhalation of regurgitated gastric contents) and aspiration pneumonia (i.e., inhalation of oropharyngeal secretions colonized with various bacteria and resulting in pulmonary infection). In clinical practice, these two entities are often interchangeably referred to as aspiration pneumonia. Common predisposing factors include alcoholism, drug intoxication or overdose, seizures, cerebrovascular accident, head trauma, and structural abnormalities of the pharynx and esophagus.

Characteristic Clinical Features
Patients have cough, fever, and shortness of breath, and they typically have a history of decreased consciousness.

Characteristic Radiologic Findings
Unilateral or bilateral, patchy or confluent air-space consolidations involve mainly the dependent lung regions. The location of the areas of consolidation depends on the position of the patient when aspiration occurs. In recumbent patients, aspiration involves mainly the posterior segments of the upper lobes or superior segments of the lower lobes, resulting in the perihilar consolidation seen on the chest radiograph; in upright patients, consolidation is seen mainly in the basal segments of the lower lobes.

Less Common Radiologic Manifestations
Massive aspiration of gastric contents (i.e., Mendelson syndrome) may result in diffuse, bilateral areas of consolidation. Aspiration pneumonia may result in abscess formation, cavitation, empyema, and lymphadenopathy.

Differential Diagnosis
- Bacterial pneumonia
- Pulmonary hemorrhage
- Pulmonary edema
- Organizing pneumonia
- Bronchioloalveolar cell carcinoma
- Lymphoma

Discussion
Aspiration pneumonia should be suspected in patients with consolidation involving mainly the dependent lung regions, particularly when there is a history of decreased consciousness. The radiologic differential diagnosis is broad and includes viral, bacterial, and fungal pneumonia; pulmonary edema; hemorrhage; organizing pneumonia; bronchioloalveolar cell carcinoma; and lymphoma.

Diagnosis
Aspiration pneumonia

Suggested Readings
Franquet T, Gimenez A, Roson N, et al: Aspiration diseases: Findings, pitfalls, and differential diagnosis. Radiographics 20:673-685, 2000.
Marik PE: Aspiration pneumonitis and aspiration pneumonia. N Engl J Med 344:665-671, 2001.

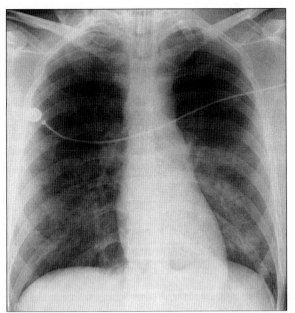

Figure 1. Anteroposterior chest radiograph shows poorly defined areas of consolidation in the lower lobes. The patient was a 32-year-old woman with aspiration pneumonia.

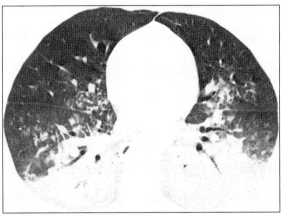

Figure 2. In the same patient, CT using lung windows shows dense consolidation in the lower lobes and bilateral, small, centrilobular nodular opacities in the dependent regions of the right middle lobe and lingula and in the lower lobes.

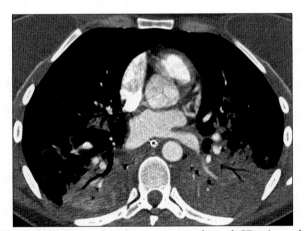

Figure 3. In the same patient, contrast-enhanced CT using soft tissue windows shows dense consolidation in the lower lobes.

Case 147

DEMOGRAPHICS/CLINICAL HISTORY

A 57-year-old man with persistent focal opacity on the chest radiograph, undergoing radiography and computed tomography (CT).

FINDINGS

Posteroanterior chest radiograph (Fig. 1) shows a focal opacity in the right upper lobe. CT using lung windows (Fig. 2) shows a spiculated nodule with adjacent ground-glass opacities and a pleural tag. CT using soft tissue windows (Fig. 3) shows an inhomogeneous appearance of the spiculated nodule with focal areas of low attenuation, which measured −30 Hounsfield units, which is consistent with fat. In another patient, high-resolution CT shows an extensive ground-glass opacity in the right upper lobe with superimposed smooth thickening of the interlobular septa (Fig. 4).

DISCUSSION

Definition/Background

Chronic exogenous lipoid pneumonia is an uncommon pulmonary disorder that results from repetitive aspiration or inhalation of mineral oil or a similar material into the distal lung. In adults, the most common causes of exogenous lipoid pneumonia are the use of mineral oil for the treatment of constipation and the use of oily nose drops for chronic rhinitis.

Characteristic Clinical Features

Patients are commonly asymptomatic. Symptoms include cough and low-grade fever.

Characteristic Radiologic Findings

The radiographic manifestations usually consist of single or multiple areas of consolidation or mass-like lesions. In most cases, thin-section CT shows focal areas of fat density (−30 to −120 Hounsfield units) within the consolidation or masslike lesions. Although the fat may be visible on thick sections (5 to 7 mm), optimal assessment requires thin sections (1 mm).

Less Common Radiologic Manifestations

Occasionally, exogenous lipoid pneumonia may result in unilateral or bilateral ground-glass opacities with superimposed smooth thickening of the interlobular septa (i.e., crazy-paving pattern).

Differential Diagnosis

- Pneumonia
- Carcinoma
- Alveolar proteinosis
- Bronchioloalveolar cell carcinoma

Discussion

The areas of consolidation seen in exogenous lipoid pneumonia are similar to those that may occur in a variety of other conditions, including pneumonia, edema, and hemorrhage. When lipoid pneumonia manifests as a dense focal consolidation with spiculated margins, the appearance resembles that of carcinoma. In most cases, the diagnosis of lipoid pneumonia is suggested by focal areas of fat density on CT. In the remaining cases, the diagnosis often is suspected only at biopsy or bronchoalveolar lavage.

The crazy-paving is relatively nonspecific, and the pattern may be seen in several conditions, including lipoid pneumonia, *Pneumocystis* pneumonia, acute respiratory distress syndrome (ARDS), alveolar proteinosis, and bronchioloalveolar cell carcinoma.

Diagnosis

Lipoid pneumonia

Suggested Readings

Franquet T, Gimenez A, Roson N, et al: Aspiration diseases: Findings, pitfalls, and differential diagnosis. Radiographics 20:673-685, 2000.

Gaerte SC, Meyer CA, Winer-Muram HT, et al: Fat-containing lesions of the chest. Radiographics 22:S61-S78, 2002.

Lee KS, Müller NL, Hale V, et al: Lipoid pneumonia: CT findings. J Comput Assist Tomogr 19:48-51, 1995.

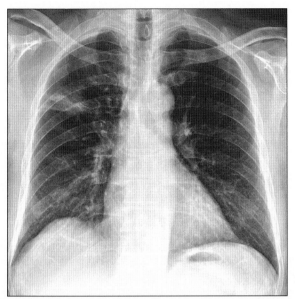

Figure 1. Posteroanterior chest radiograph shows a focal opacity in the right upper lobe. The patient was a 57-year-old man with exogenous lipoid pneumonia due to aspiration of mineral oil.

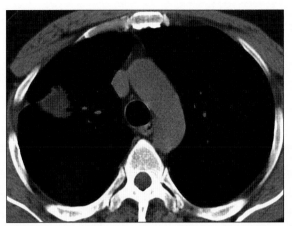

Figure 3. In the same patient, CT (5-mm-thick section) using soft tissue windows shows an inhomogeneous appearance of the spiculated nodule with focal areas of low attenuation, which measured − 30 Hounsfield units, consistent with fat.

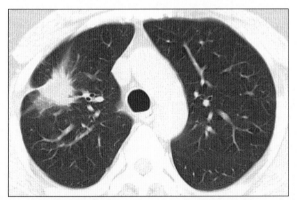

Figure 2. In the same patient, CT (5-mm-thick section) using lung windows shows a spiculated nodule with adjacent ground-glass opacities and a pleural tag.

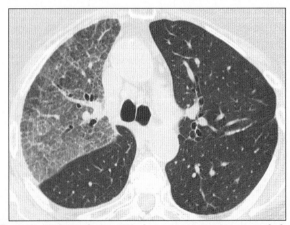

Figure 4. High-resolution CT shows an extensive ground-glass opacity in the right upper lobe with superimposed smooth thickening of the interlobular septa (i.e., crazy-paving pattern). The patient was an 81-year-old woman with exogenous lipoid pneumonia due to aspiration of mineral oil.

Case 148

DEMOGRAPHICS/CLINICAL HISTORY

A 39-year-old woman with progressive shortness of breath over several days and a history of breast cancer and chemotherapy, undergoing radiography and computed tomography (CT).

FINDINGS

Chest radiograph (Fig. 1) shows bilateral, hazy, increased-density areas (i.e., ground-glass opacities) and foci of consolidation in the middle and lower lung zones. High-resolution CT at the level of the middle and lower lobe bronchi (Fig. 2) shows bilateral ground-glass opacities mainly in the central lung regions and peribronchial areas of consolidation. The area of ground-glass opacity in the right lung is marginated by linear consolidation (i.e., reversed halo sign). High-resolution CT at the level of the lung bases (Fig. 3) shows bilateral peribronchial areas of consolidation and patchy ground-glass opacities.

DISCUSSION

Definition/Background

Organizing pneumonia, also known as bronchiolitis obliterans organizing pneumonia (BOOP), is characterized histologically by the presence of buds of organizing granulation tissue in respiratory bronchioles, alveolar ducts, and adjacent alveoli. Organizing pneumonia is an increasingly recognized manifestation of drug reaction. Drugs most commonly associated with an organizing pneumonia reaction pattern include amiodarone, acebutolol, minocycline, nitrofurantoin, bleomycin, cyclophosphamide, methotrexate, carbamazepine mesalamine, hydralazine, and interferon.

Characteristic Clinical Features

Patients have a dry cough and shortness of breath.

Characteristic Radiologic Findings

The most common radiographic manifestation of organizing pneumonia (i.e., BOOP-like reaction) consists of bilateral, patchy areas of consolidation and ground-glass opacities. On CT, the areas of consolidation usually have a predominantly peribronchial or subpleural distribution. Ground-glass opacities often occur in a bilateral, asymmetric, and random distribution.

Less Common Radiologic Manifestations

Imaging may show perilobular opacities, a reversed halo sign, and centrilobular nodules.

Differential Diagnosis

- Pneumonia
- Pulmonary edema
- Pulmonary hemorrhage
- Lymphoma
- Eosinophilic pneumonia

Discussion

The differential diagnosis for organizing pneumonia includes several other conditions that may lead to bilateral consolidation, including bacterial, fungal, and viral pneumonia; pulmonary edema; pulmonary hemorrhage; aspiration; and eosinophilic pneumonia. The diagnosis of organizing pneumonia requires lung biopsy. Criteria for the diagnosis of drug-induced organizing pneumonia include a history of drug exposure, consistent radiologic findings, histologic evidence of organizing pneumonia, and exclusion of other causes, such as pulmonary infection and lymphoma.

Diagnosis

Drug-Induced lung disease: organizing pneumonia pattern

Suggested Readings

Dodd JD, Lee KS, Johkoh T, Müller NL: Drug-associated organizing pneumonia: High-resolution CT findings in 9 patients. J Thorac Imaging 21:22-26, 2006.
Foucher P, Camus P: The Drug-Induced Lung Diseases. Available at http//www.pneumotox.com (accessed July 2009).
Myers JL, Limper AH, Swensen SJ: Drug-induced lung disease: A pragmatic classification incorporating HRCT appearances. Semin Respir Crit Care Med 24:445-453, 2003.
Silva CI, Müller NL: Drug-induced lung diseases: Most common reaction patterns and corresponding high-resolution CT manifestations. Semin Ultrasound CT MR 27:111-116, 2006.

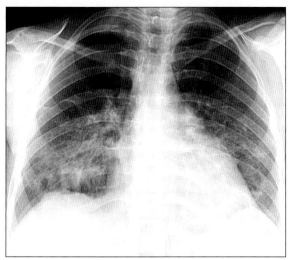

Figure 1. Chest radiograph shows bilateral, hazy, increased-density areas (i.e., ground-glass opacities) and foci of consolidation in the middle and lower lung zones. The patient was a 39-year-old woman with organizing pneumonia resulting from an adverse reaction to trastuzumab, which was used for the treatment of breast cancer.

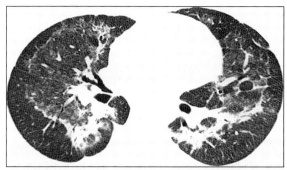

Figure 2. In the same patient, high-resolution CT at the level of the middle and lower lobe bronchi shows bilateral ground-glass opacities mainly in the central lung regions and peribronchial areas of consolidation. The area of ground-glass opacity in the right lung is marginated by linear consolidation (i.e., reversed halo sign).

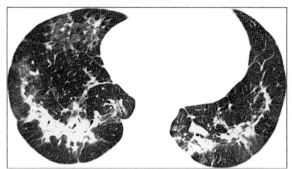

Figure 3. In the same patient, high-resolution CT at the level of the lung bases shows bilateral peribronchial areas of consolidation and patchy ground-glass opacities.

Case 149

DEMOGRAPHICS/CLINICAL HISTORY

A 71-year-old man with progressive shortness of breath over several months and recurrent urinary tract infections, undergoing computed tomography (CT).

FINDINGS

High-resolution CT at the level of the lower lung zones (Fig. 1) shows bilateral ground-glass opacities, mild reticulation, and focal traction bronchiolectasis. Coronal, reformatted, high-resolution CT (Fig. 2) shows involvement of all lung zones and the predominantly peripheral and basal distribution of the ground-glass opacities and mild reticulation.

DISCUSSION

Definition/Background

Nonspecific interstitial pneumonia (NSIP) is characterized histologically by various proportions of interstitial inflammation and fibrosis that are temporally uniform. NSIP is a common reaction pattern associated with drug toxicity. Drugs most commonly associated with an NSIP-like pattern include amiodarone, methotrexate, nitrofurantoin, bleomycin, hydrochlorothiazide, and carmustine.

Characteristic Clinical Features

Patients have a dry cough and progressive shortness of breath.

Characteristic Radiologic Findings

The radiographic manifestations include poorly defined, bilateral, hazy opacities and reticulation. The high-resolution CT findings usually consist of extensive, bilateral ground-glass opacities. With progression to fibrosis, there is superimposed reticulation, traction bronchiectasis, and bronchiolectasis.

Less Common Radiologic Manifestations

Occasionally, focal areas of consolidation may be seen superimposed on the ground-glass opacities due to an associated organizing pneumonia reaction pattern.

Differential Diagnosis

- Hypersensitivity pneumonitis
- *Pneumocystis* pneumonia
- Diffuse pulmonary hemorrhage
- Idiopathic pulmonary findings

Discussion

The differential diagnosis for NSIP includes several conditions that may lead to extensive, bilateral ground-glass opacities with or without associated reticulation, including hypersensitivity pneumonitis, *Pneumocystis* pneumonia (in immunocompromised patients), and diffuse pulmonary hemorrhage. The diagnosis of NSIP requires surgical lung biopsy. Criteria for the diagnosis of drug-induced NSIP include a history of drug exposure, consistent radiologic findings, histologic evidence of NSIP, and exclusion of other causes of NSIP, such as collagen vascular disease and hypersensitivity pneumonitis.

Diagnosis

Drug-induced lung disease: nonspecific interstitial pneumonia pattern

Suggested Readings

Foucher P, Camus P: The Drug-Induced Lung Diseases. Available at http//www.pneumotox.com (accessed July 2009).

Lynch DA, Travis WD, Müller NL, et al: Idiopathic interstitial pneumonias: CT features. Radiology 236:10-21, 2005.

Myers JL, Limper AH, Swensen SJ: Drug-induced lung disease: A pragmatic classification incorporating HRCT appearances. Semin Respir Crit Care Med 24:445-453, 2003.

Silva CI, Müller NL: Drug-induced lung diseases: Most common reaction patterns and corresponding high-resolution CT manifestations. Semin Ultrasound CT MR 27:111-116, 2006.

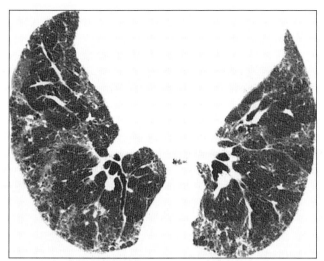

Figure 1. High-resolution CT at the level of the lower lung zones shows bilateral ground-glass opacities, mild reticulation, and focal traction bronchiolectasis. The patient was a 73-year-old man with an NSIP reaction to nitrofurantoin.

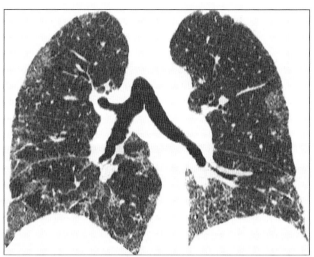

Figure 2. In the same patient, coronal, reformatted, high-resolution CT shows involvement of all lung zones and a predominantly peripheral and basal distribution of the ground-glass opacities and mild reticulation.

Case 150

DEMOGRAPHICS/CLINICAL HISTORY

A 61-year-old man, cough, exertional dyspnea, history of arrhythmias.

FINDINGS

High-resolution CT image at the level of lung bases (Fig. 1) shows focal consolidation and ground-glass opacity in the right middle lobe. Also noted is bilateral emphysema. CT image photographed at soft tissue windows (Fig. 2) demonstrates that the right middle lobe consolidation has attenuation greater than that of the chest wall and cardiac muscle. CT scan through the abdomen (Fig. 3) shows increased attenuation of the liver.

DISCUSSION

Definition/Background

Amiodarone is an iodinated benzofuran derivative used in the treatment of cardiac arrhythmias. Pulmonary toxicity is estimated to occur in approximately 5% of treated patients. Common reaction patterns include diffuse pulmonary damage (DAD), nonspecific interstitial pneumonia (NSIP), and organizing pneumonia (BOOP)-like reaction.

Characteristic Clinical Features

Cough and shortness of breath.

Characteristic Radiologic Findings

The appearance of the parenchymal abnormalities is variable and may consist of bilateral areas of consolidation, bilateral ground-glass opacities, a reticular pattern, or (less commonly) focal round areas of consolidation (Figs. 1 and 2). Because amiodarone contains about 37% iodine by weight, it has a high attenuation value on CT; thus, this procedure allows confident recognition of drug deposition, particularly in the liver and lungs (Figs. 2 and 3). High-attenuation (82–175 Hounsfield units [HU]) of pulmonary abnormalities are seen in approximately 70% of patients who have symptoms of pulmonary toxicity.

Less Common Radiologic Manifestations

Pleural effusions are present in 50% of patients.

Differential Diagnosis

- Pneumonia
- Pulmonary edema
- Pulmonary hemorrhage

Discussion

The radiographic abnormalities resemble those seen in a variety of other conditions, including pneumonia, pulmonary edema, and hemorrhage. The diagnosis of amiodarone lung is usually based on pulmonary parenchymal abnormalities associated with high attenuation, high attenuation of the liver, intake of amiodarone (often more than 400 mg/day), and exclusion of other causes of parenchymal lung abnormalities such as pneumonia, pulmonary edema, and pulmonary hemorrhage.

Diagnosis

Amiodarone lung

Suggested Readings

Camus P, Martin WJ II, Rosenow EC III: Amiodarone pulmonary toxicity. Clin Chest Med 25:65-75, 2004.

Myers JL, Limper AH, Swensen SJ: Drug-induced lung disease: A pragmatic classification incorporating HRCT appearances. Seminars in Respiratory and Critical Care Medicine 24:445-453, 2003.

Silva CI, Müller NL: Drug-induced lung diseases: Most common reaction patterns and corresponding high-resolution CT manifestations. Semin Ultrasound CT MR 27:111-116, 2006.

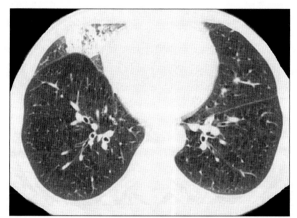

Figure 1. High-resolution CT image at the level of lung bases shows focal consolidation and ground-glass opacity in the right middle lobe. Also noted is bilateral emphysema. The patient was a 61-year-old man with amiodarone pulmonary toxicity.

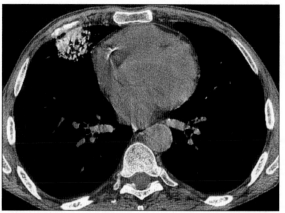

Figure 2. CT image photographed at soft tissue windows demonstrates that the right middle lobe consolidation has attenuation greater than that of the chest wall and cardiac muscle. The patient was a 61-year-old man with amiodarone pulmonary toxicity.

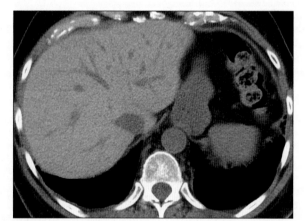

Figure 3. CT image scan through the abdomen shows increased attenuation of the liver. The patient was a 61-year-old man with amiodarone pulmonary toxicity.

Case 151

DEMOGRAPHICS/CLINICAL HISTORY

A 43-year-old woman with cough, exertional dyspnea, and a history of breast cancer, undergoing computed tomography (CT).

FINDINGS

High-resolution CT at the level of the lung apices (Fig. 1) shows peripheral ground-glass opacities and a few linear opacities in the peripheral regions of the left upper lobe. High-resolution CT at the level of the middle lung zones (Fig. 2) shows a focal consolidation in the lingula. The left breast had been surgically removed. Coronal, reformatted CT (Fig. 3) shows peripheral ground-glass opacities in the left upper lobe and consolidation in the lingula.

DISCUSSION

Definition/Background

Radiation pneumonitis is radiation-induced lung injury characterized histologically by the presence of acute and organizing diffuse alveolar damage. It typically occurs 1 to 3 months after completion of radiation therapy and may progress over the next 3 months. Radiation-induced lung disease rarely occurs with fractionated total doses below 20 Gy, occurs in a small percentage of patients who receive doses between 20 and 40 Gy, and is relatively common in patients who receive higher total doses of radiation.

Characteristic Clinical Features

Patients are most commonly asomptomatic but may have cough and dyspnea.

Characteristic Radiologic Findings

Radiation pneumonitis manifests radiographically and on CT as ground-glass opacities or consolidation typically limited to the treatment field.

Less Common Radiologic Manifestations

Uncommonly, radiation pneumonitis may extend beyond the treatment field. Occasionally, radiation therapy can result in patchy, bilateral areas of consolidation due to organizing pneumonia (i.e., BOOP-like reaction) (Fig. 4) or chronic eosinophilic pneumonia.

Differential Diagnosis

- Pneumonia
- Drug reaction
- Organizing pneumonia

Discussion

The main differential diagnosis for patients with a focal area of ground-glass attenuation or consolidation 1 or several months after radiation therapy for a thoracic malignancy is between radiation pneumonitis and pneumonia. The diagnosis of radiation pneumonitis is usually straightforward because it is typically limited to the radiation field. Infection should be considered if the chest radiograph or CT scan shows pulmonary opacities occurring before completion of radiation therapy or outside the radiation treatment fields. Because radiation pneumonitis normally has a more indolent course than an infectious pneumonitis, an abrupt onset can indicate an infection unless there has been recent discontinuation of steroids.

In patients with bilateral areas of consolidation, the main differential diagnosis is between radiation-induced organizing pneumonia or eosinophilic pneumonia and pneumonia or drug-induced lung disease. The clinical and radiologic manifestations of organizing pneumonia and chronic eosinophilic pneumonia after radiation therapy may be similar. Distinction between the two entities is based on the presence of parenchymal and peripheral blood eosinophilia in chronic eosinophilic pneumonia and on typical histologic findings of intraluminal granulation tissue polyps within alveolar ducts and surrounding alveoli associated with chronic inflammation of the surrounding lung parenchyma in organizing pneumonia.

Diagnosis

Radiation-induced pneumonitis

Suggested Readings

Abid SH, Malhotra V, Perry MC: Radiation-induced and chemotherapy-induced pulmonary injury. Curr Opin Oncol 13:242-248, 2001.

Ghafoori P, Marks LB, Vujaskovic Z, Kelsey CR: Radiation-induced lung injury. Assessment, management, and prevention. Oncology (Williston Park) 22:37-47; discussion 52-53, 2008.

Libshitz HI, DuBrow RA, Loyer EM, Charnsangavej C: Radiation change in normal organs: An overview of body imaging. Eur Radiol 6:786-795, 1996.

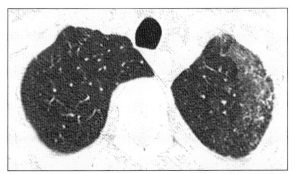

Figure 1. High-resolution CT at the level of the lung apices shows peripheral ground-glass opacities and a few linear opacities in the peripheral regions of the left upper lobe. The patient was a 43-year-old woman with radiation pneumonitis 2 months after radiotherapy for left breast cancer.

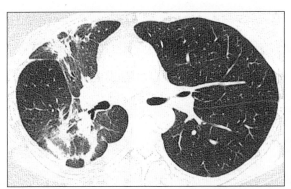

Figure 3. Coronal, reformatted CT shows peripheral ground-glass opacities in the left upper lobe and consolidation in the lingula.

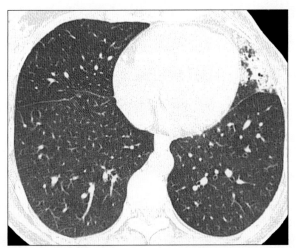

Figure 2. In the same patient, high-resolution CT at the level of the middle lung zones shows a focal consolidation in the lingula. The left breast was surgically removed.

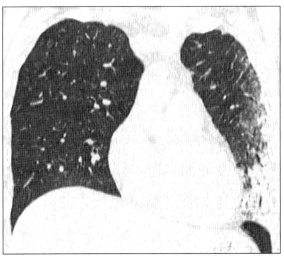

Figure 4. High-resolution CT shows peribronchial areas of consolidation in the right upper and lower lobes and perilobular consolidation in the right lower lobe. Extensive ground-glass opacities can be seen in the right upper and lower lobes. The patient was a 48-year-old woman with organizing pneumonia after radiation therapy for metastatic breast cancer.

Case 152

DEMOGRAPHICS/CLINICAL HISTORY

A 72-year-old woman who is asymptomatic and has a history of pulmonary carcinoma, undergoing computed tomography (CT).

FINDINGS

CT images (5-mm-thick sections) at the level of the lung apices (Fig.1) and main bronchi (Fig. 2) show sharply outlined fibrosis in the medial aspects of the right upper and lower lobes with associated traction bronchiectasis, architectural distortion, and marked volume loss.

DISCUSSION

Definition/Background

Radiation fibrosis is radiation-induced lung injury characterized histologically by the presence of organizing diffuse alveolar damage (DAD) with interstitial fibrosis. Radiation fibrosis typically first becomes apparent approximately 3 months after completion of radiation therapy, progresses gradually over several months, and becomes stable at approximately 1 year after radiation therapy. Radiation fibrosis rarely occurs with fractionated total doses less than 20 Gy, occurs in a small percentage of patients who receive doses between 20 and 40 Gy, and is relatively common in patients who receive higher total doses of radiation.

Characteristic Clinical Features

The patients are usually asymptomatic but may present with cough and dyspnea.

Characteristic Radiologic Findings

Radiation fibrosis manifests on radiographs and CT scans as reticulation, traction bronchiectasis, and volume loss that is typically limited to the treatment field and often superimposed on a background of ground-glass opacities and or dense consolidation.

Less Common Radiologic Manifestations

Patients have pleural thickening.

Differential Diagnosis

- Pneumonia
- Recurrent tumor

Discussion

Infection should be considered if the chest radiograph or CT scan shows pulmonary opacities outside the radiation treatment fields. Local tumor recurrence can be difficult to diagnose during the evolution of radiation-induced lung disease. However, as radiation-induced lung disease stabilizes, alteration in the contour of the fibrosis should raise the suspicion of tumor recurrence. Filling in of bronchi within radiation-induced fibrosis is abnormal and usually results from local recurrence of malignancy or a superimposed infection.

Diagnosis

Radiation-induced fibrosis

Suggested Readings

Abid SH, Malhotra V, Perry MC: Radiation-induced and chemotherapy-induced pulmonary injury. Curr Opin Oncol 13:242-248, 2001.

Ghafoori P, Marks LB, Vujaskovic Z, Kelsey CR: Radiation-induced lung injury. Assessment, management, and prevention. Oncology (Williston Park) 22:37-47; discussion 52-53, 2008.

Libshitz HI, DuBrow RA, Loyer EM, Charnsangavej C: Radiation change in normal organs: An overview of body imaging. Eur Radiol 6:786-795, 1996.

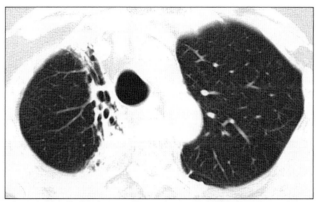

Figure 1. CT image (5-mm-thick sections) at the level of the lung apices shows sharply outlined fibrosis in the medial aspect of the right upper lobe with associated traction bronchiectasis, architectural distortion, and marked volume loss. The patient was a 72-year-old woman with fibrosis after radiotherapy for pulmonary carcinoma.

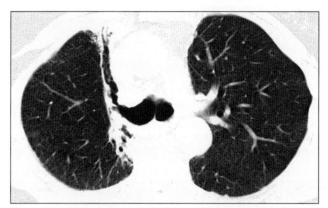

Figure 2. In the same patient, CT (5-mm-thick sections) at the level of the main bronchi show sharply outlined fibrosis in the medial aspects of the right upper and lower lobes with associated traction bronchiectasis, architectural distortion, and marked volume loss.

Case 153

DEMOGRAPHICS/CLINICAL HISTORY

A 29-year-old man, with shortness of breath 2 weeks following double lung transplant.

FINDINGS

High-resolution CT images at the level of the middle (Fig. 1) and lower (Fig. 2) lung zones show thickening of the interlobular septa, mild dependent ground-glass opacities, and small bilateral pleural effusions.

DISCUSSION

Definition/Background

Pulmonary complications of lung and heart-lung transplantation include opportunistic infection, drug-induced disease, rejection, and post-transplant lymphoproliferative disorder. Acute rejection is a common complication of lung and heart-lung transplantation, one or more episodes occurring in 60–75% of lung recipients in the first year after transplantation.

Characteristic Clinical Features

Mild lung rejection is commonly asymptomatic. Manifestations of higher grades of rejection include fever, cough, and dyspnea.

Characteristic Radiologic Findings

The chest radiograph may be normal or may show reticular or air space opacities predominantly in the middle and lower lung zones. High-resolution CT shows findings of interstitial pulmonary edema with septal thickening, interlobar fissure thickening, pleural effusions, and ground-glass opacities (Figs. 1 and 2).

Less Common Radiologic Manifestations

In patients with severe acute rejection, the findings may progress to extensive consolidation.

Differential Diagnosis

- Fluid overload
- Pulmonary vein stenosis
- Pneumonia

Discussion

In patients with bilateral lung transplant, the findings of acute rejection are similar to those of fluid overload or left heart failure. In patients with unilateral transplant, the main differential diagnosis is interstitial edema resulting from pulmonary vein stenosis, an uncommon surgical complication of transplantation. Definitive diagnosis of acute rejection requires transbronchial biopsy.

Diagnosis

Acute lung rejection

Suggested Readings

Kotloff RM, Ahya VN, Crawford SW: Pulmonary complications of solid organ and hematopoietic stem cell transplantation. Am J Respir Crit Care Med 170:22-48, 2004.

Krishnam MS, Suh RD, Tomasian A, Goldin JG, Lai C, Brown K, et al: Postoperative complications of lung transplantation: Radiologic findings along a time continuum. Radiographics 27:957-974, 2007.

Whelan TPM, Hertz MI: Allograft rejection after lung transplantation. Clin Chest Med 26:599-612, 2005.

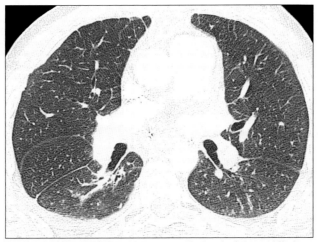

Figure 1. High-resolution CT image at the level of the middle lung zones shows thickening of the interlobular septa, mild dependent ground-glass opacities, and small bilateral pleural effusions. The patient was a 29-year-old man with acute rejection following double lung transplant.

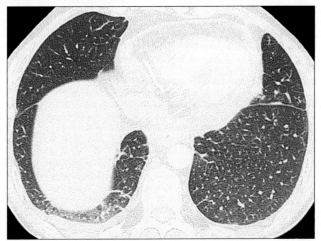

Figure 2. High-resolution CT image at the level of lower lung zones shows thickening of the interlobular septa, mild dependent ground-glass opacities, and small bilateral pleural effusions. The patient was a 29-year-old man with acute rejection following double lung transplant.

Case 154

DEMOGRAPHICS/CLINICAL HISTORY

A 23-year-old man after a motor vehicle accident, undergoing radiography and computed tomography (CT).

FINDINGS

Posteroanterior chest radiograph (Fig. 1) reveals areas of consolidation in the peripheral regions of the right lung. No rib fracture is seen. CT (5-mm-thick sections) (Fig. 2) shows areas of consolidation and ground-glass opacities, mainly in the periphery of the right upper lobe.

DISCUSSION

Definition/Background

Lung contusion represents pulmonary hemorrhage and edema from disruption of the alveolar capillary membrane after blunt chest trauma. It is the most common cause of pulmonary parenchymal opacification in blunt chest trauma and is seen in up to 70% of patients.

Characteristic Clinical Features

Patients usually have no symptoms related to lung contusion. Cough, dyspnea, and hemoptysis may occur in patients with extensive contusion.

Characteristic Radiologic Findings

Pulmonary contusions can manifest as focal, patchy, or diffuse ground-glass opacities or parenchymal consolidations. These opacities typically cross segmental and fissural boundaries and are often found at the site of chest trauma.

Less Common Radiologic Manifestations

Ground-glass opacities and consolidation may result from a contrecoup injury (i.e., parenchymal contusion in which the lungs have been compressed against the denser heart, liver, chest wall, and spine).

Differential Diagnosis

- Aspiration
- Atelectasis
- Pulmonary laceration

Discussion

Pulmonary contusion may be difficult to differentiate from aspiration pneumonitis and atelectasis, and these entities are often present concurrently. Pulmonary contusion may affect any area of the lung, typically crosses anatomic boundaries, and follows a predictable temporal pattern on imaging. Contused lung may not be apparent on initial chest radiography, but it usually is identified within 6 hours after the inciting injury. Conspicuity of pulmonary opacities peaks at 24 to 72 hours and gradually diminishes over 1 week. Aspiration pneumonitis involves mainly the dependent regions, and on CT, it typically is associated with centrilobular nodules and tree-in-bud opacities due to filling of small airways with fluid. This appearance is usually seen acutely, and these opacities coalesce over the next several hours. Aspiration affects the dependent portions of the lungs (i.e., posterior segment of the upper lobes and the superior and posterior segments of the lower lobes in the supine patient). Atelectasis manifests as pulmonary opacities with associated signs of volume loss.

On the initial chest radiograph, pulmonary lacerations are often obscured by the consolidation related to the pulmonary contusion. They can usually be readily recognized on CT.

Diagnosis

Pulmonary contusion

Suggested Readings

Costantino M, Gosselin MV, Primack SL: The ABC's of thoracic trauma imaging. Semin Roentgenol 41:209-225, 2006.

Mirvis SE: Diagnostic imaging of acute thoracic injury. Semin Ultrasound CT MR 25:156-179, 2004.

Sangster GP, González-Beicos A, Carbo AI, et al: Blunt traumatic injuries of the lung parenchyma, pleura, thoracic wall, and intrathoracic airways: Multidetector computer tomography imaging findings. Emerg Radiol 14:297-310, 2007.

Thoongsuwan N, Kanne JP, Stern EJ: Spectrum of blunt chest injuries. J Thorac Imaging 20:89-97, 2005.

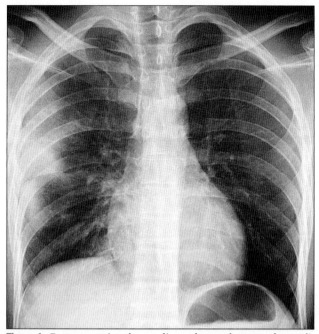

Figure 1. Posteroanterior chest radiograph reveals areas of consolidation in the peripheral regions of the right lung. No rib fracture is seen. The patient was a 23-year-old man with lung contusion due to blunt chest trauma.

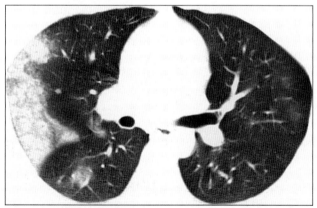

Figure 2. In the same patient, CT (5-mm-thick sections) shows areas of consolidation and ground-glass opacities, mainly in the periphery of the right upper lobe.

Case 155

DEMOGRAPHICS/CLINICAL HISTORY

A 20-year-old woman with progressive shortness of breath 2 years after bilateral lung transplantation, undergoing computed tomography (CT).

FINDINGS

High-resolution CT (Figs. 1 and 2) shows extensive areas of decreased attenuation and vascularity and patchy areas of increased attenuation and vascularity, resulting in a mosaic attenuation pattern. Extensive bronchiectasis can be seen.

DISCUSSION

Definition/Background

Bronchiolitis obliterans is a common complication of lung and heart-lung transplantation, and it remains the single leading cause of morbidity and mortality among these patients. The prevalence of bronchiolitis obliterans after lung transplantation is approximately 20% at 1 year and more than 50% at 3 to 5 years. Bronchiolitis obliterans in these patients is thought to be a manifestation of chronic rejection.

Characteristic Clinical Features

Patients may have a dry cough and progressive shortness of breath 1 or more years after lung or heart-lung transplantation.

Characteristic Radiologic Findings

Chest radiography is of limited value in the diagnosis. High-resolution CT typically shows areas of decreased attenuation and vascularity on inspiratory images and air trapping on expiratory images. Another common finding is bronchiectasis.

Less Common Radiologic Manifestations

Imaging may show pneumothorax or pneumomediastinum.

Differential Diagnosis

- Normal air trapping

Discussion

Air trapping is commonly seen on CT in normal adults, particularly in the dependent lung regions, superior segment of the lower lobe, and tip of the middle lobe and lingula. Air trapping can be considered abnormal when it affects more than 25% of the total volume of the lung and is not limited to the superior segment of the lower lobe or the lingula tip. Another helpful feature in the diagnosis is bronchial dilatation seen on inspiratory CT. The combination of bronchiectasis on inspiratory CT and air trapping on expiratory CT after lung transplantation is seen only in patients with bronchiolitis obliterans.

Diagnosis

Bronchiolitis obliterans after lung transplantation

Suggested Readings

Kotloff RM, Ahya VN, Crawford SW: Pulmonary complications of solid organ and hematopoietic stem cell transplantation. Am J Respir Crit Care 170:22-48, 2004.

Krishnam MS, Suh RD, Tomasian A, et al: Postoperative complications of lung transplantation: Radiologic findings along a time continuum. Radiographics 27:957-974, 2007.

Pipavath SJ, Lynch DA, Cool C, et al: Radiologic and pathologic features of bronchiolitis. AJR Am J Roentgenol 185:354-363, 2005.

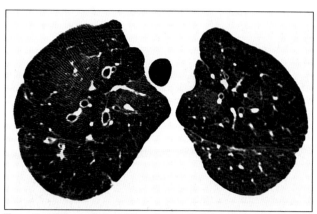

Figure 1. High-resolution CT at the level of the upper lobes shows extensive areas of decreased attenuation and vascularity and patchy areas of increased attenuation and vascularity, resulting in a mosaic attenuation pattern. Notice the bronchiectasis in the right upper lobe. The patient was a 20-year-old woman with severe bronchiolitis obliterans after bilateral lung transplantation.

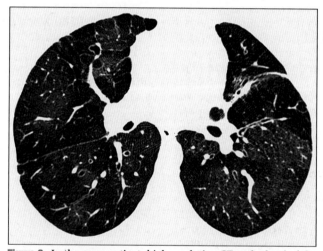

Figure 2. In the same patient, high-resolution CT at the level of the bronchus intermedius shows extensive areas of decreased attenuation and vascularity and patchy areas of increased attenuation and vascularity, resulting in a mosaic attenuation pattern. Mild bilateral bronchiectasis can be seen.

Case 156

DEMOGRAPHICS/CLINICAL HISTORY

A 40-year-old man with shortness of breath after blunt chest trauma, undergoing radiography and computed tomography (CT).

FINDINGS

Anteroposterior chest radiograph (Fig. 1) shows extensive opacification of the left lung. High-resolution CT (Fig. 2) shows a complex cystic lesion with air-fluid levels and ground-glass opacities in the left upper lobe and shows a subtle pneumomediastinum. High-resolution CT at the level of left lower lobe bronchus (Fig. 3) shows mass-like lesion; small, focal lucencies; and ground-glass opacities. Coronal, reformatted CT (Fig. 4) better demonstrates the complex left upper lobe cystic mass, left lower lobe mass, and the extent of ground-glass opacities in the left lung.

DISCUSSION

Definition/Background

Pulmonary laceration is a tear in the lung parenchyma resulting in a traumatic lung cyst, which may be filled with air (i.e., pneumatocele) or blood (i.e., hematoma), or both. It is the most common cause of pulmonary parenchymal opacification in blunt chest trauma and is seen in up to 70% of patients.

Characteristic Clinical Features

Patients usually have no symptoms related to lung laceration, except those of the commonly associated pneumothorax. Cough, dyspnea, and hemoptysis may occur in patients with extensive contusions and lacerations.

Characteristic Radiologic Findings

Pulmonary lacerations manifest as thin-walled cystic spaces (i.e., traumatic pneumatocele) or soft tissue masses (i.e., hematoma), or both. They may be single or multiple and are commonly associated with post-traumatic pneumothorax. Pulmonary lacerations are commonly obscured initially on the chest radiograph by ground-glass opacities and consolidation related to associated lung contusions, but they usually can be seen on CT. As the findings of contusion resolve, pulmonary lacerations become better defined.

Less Common Radiologic Manifestations

Occasionally, traumatic pneumatoceles may increase in size.

Differential Diagnosis

- Pulmonary contusion

Discussion

On the initial chest radiograph, pulmonary lacerations are often obscured by the consolidation related to pulmonary contusion. They can usually be readily recognized on CT.

Diagnosis

Pulmonary laceration

Suggested Readings

Costantino M, Gosselin MV, Primack SL: The ABC's of thoracic trauma imaging. Semin Roentgenol 41:209-225, 2006.

Mirvis SE: Diagnostic imaging of acute thoracic injury. Semin Ultrasound CT MR 25:156-179, 2004.

Sangster GP, González-Beicos A, Carbo AI, et al: Blunt traumatic injuries of the lung parenchyma, pleura, thoracic wall, and intrathoracic airways: Multidetector computer tomography imaging findings. Emerg Radiol 14:297-310, 2007.

Thoongsuwan N, Kanne JP, Stern EJ: Spectrum of blunt chest injuries. J Thorac Imaging 20:89-97, 2005.

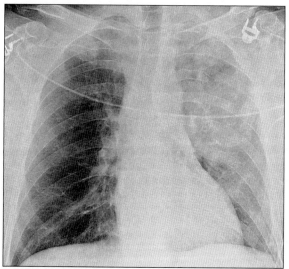

Figure 1. Anteroposterior chest radiograph shows extensive opacification of the left lung. The patient was a 40-year-old man with pulmonary contusion and multiple lacerations due to blunt chest trauma after motor vehicle accident.

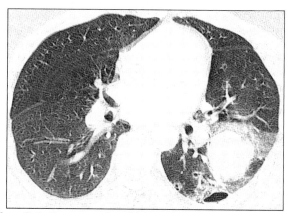

Figure 3. In the same patient, high-resolution CT at the level of left lower lobe bronchus shows masslike lesion; small, focal lucencies; and ground-glass opacities. The image is degraded by respiratory motion artifact.

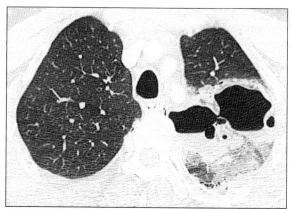

Figure 2. In the same patient, high-resolution CT shows a complex cystic lesion with air-fluid levels and ground-glass opacities in the left upper lobe.

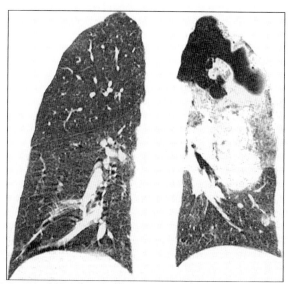

Figure 4. In the same patient, coronal, reformatted CT shows the complex left upper lobe cystic lesion, left lower lobe mass, and the extent of ground-glass opacities in the left lung. The image is degraded by respiratory motion artifact.

Case 157

DEMOGRAPHICS/CLINICAL HISTORY

A 45-year-old man after a motor vehicle accident, undergoing radiography and computed tomography (CT).

FINDINGS

Anteroposterior chest radiograph with the patient supine (Fig. 1) shows widening of the mediastinum, obscuration of the aortic arch, a shift of the trachea and nasogastric tube to the right, and downward deviation of the left main bronchus. Contrast-enhanced CT (Fig. 2) shows a focal irregularity of the proximal descending aorta, mediastinal hematoma, and focal areas of atelectasis. Oblique, sagittal, reformatted CT (Fig. 3) shows a focal irregularity of the proximal descending aorta and para-aortic hematoma.

DISCUSSION

Definition/Background

Traumatic aortic injury is a common and serious complication of blunt chest trauma that usually results from high-speed motor vehicle accidents and occasionally from falls from heights greater than 10 feet (3 m). Ninety percent of injuries occur in the aortic isthmus (i.e., portion of the descending aorta between the origin of the left subclavian artery and the site of attachment of the ligamentum arteriosum); the next most common site is the ascending aorta. Injuries to the ascending aorta are almost invariably fatal because of associated coronary artery compromise, aortic valve rupture, or cardiac tamponade.

Characteristic Clinical Features

Clinical signs of traumatic aortic injury are seldom present. The diagnosis is based on mechanism of injury (e.g., major blunt trauma) and the results of imaging studies.

Characteristic Radiologic Findings

The findings on the chest radiograph are nonspecific and include widening of the mediastinum, loss of aortic arch definition, increased aortic arch density, increased width and density of the descending aorta, rightward deviation of the enteric tube, downward displacement of the left main bronchus, and presence of the left apical cap. The direct signs of aortic injury on CT include an intraluminal clot or a low-density filling defect, focal change in the caliber of the aorta (i.e., pseudocoarctation), focal aortic wall contour abnormality (i.e., pseudoaneurysm), and dissection. The main indirect sign is the presence of mediastinal hematoma adjacent to the aorta.

Less Common Radiologic Manifestations

Imaging may show widening of the right paratracheal stripe, increased right paratracheal density, or rightward deviation of the trachea.

Differential Diagnosis

- Venous bleeding
- Mediastinal fat
- Technical artifact

Discussion

The chest radiograph has a low specificity in the diagnosis of traumatic aortic injury (approximately 15%). Supine imaging, magnification factors, and patient rotation can lead to radiographic mimics of a mediastinal hematoma. The main value of the radiograph is in excluding aortic injury; the negative predictive value of a properly obtained normal chest radiograph is 98%.

Contrast-enhanced multidetector helical CT is the imaging modality of choice in the assessment of patients with blunt chest trauma. Direct signs of aortic injury on CT have a positive predictive value that approaches 100%, and a morphologically normal aorta on CT with no mediastinal hematoma has a 100% negative predictive value for exclusion of aortic injury. However, some patients with equivocal studies (i.e., hematoma only) require aortography or close clinical follow-up.

Diagnosis

Traumatic aortic injury

Suggested Readings

Alkhadhi H, Wildermuth S, Desbiolles L, et al: Vascular emergencies of the thorax after blunt and iatrogenic trauma: Multi-detector row CT and three-dimensional imaging. Radiographics 24:1239-1255, 2004.

Mirvis SE: Thoracic vascular injury. Radiol Clin North Am 44:181-197, vii, 2006.

Mirvis SE, Bidwell JK, Buddemeyer EU, et al: Value of chest radiography in excluding traumatic aortic rupture. Radiology 163:487-493, 1987.

Sammer M, Wang E, Blackmore CC, et al: Indeterminate CT angiography in blunt thoracic trauma: Is CT angiography enough? AJR Am J Roentgenol 189:603-608, 2007.

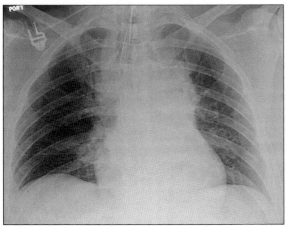

Figure 1. Anteroposterior chest radiograph with the patient supine shows widening of the mediastinum, obscuration of the aortic arch, a shift of the trachea and nasogastric tube to the right, and downward deviation of the left main bronchus. The patient was a 45-year-old man with an aortic tear after a motor vehicle accident.

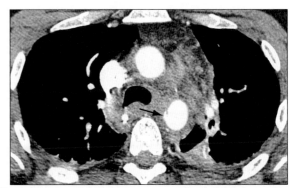

Figure 2. In the same patient, contrast-enhanced CT shows a focal irregularity *(arrow)* of the proximal descending aorta, a mediastinal hematoma, and focal areas of atelectasis.

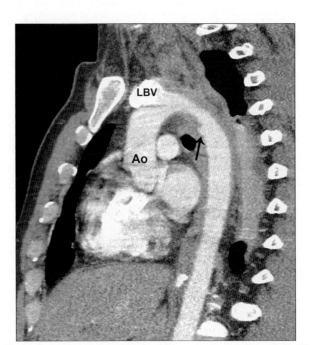

Figure 3. In the same patient, oblique, sagittal, reformatted CT shows a focal irregularity *(arrow)* of the proximal descending aorta (Ao) and a para-aortic hematoma. LBV, left brachiocephalic vein.

Case 158

DEMOGRAPHICS/CLINICAL HISTORY

A 53-year-old woman with shortness of breath after a motor vehicle accident, undergoing radiography.

FINDINGS

Anteroposterior chest radiograph (Fig. 1) reveals left rib fractures, increased opacification of the left hemithorax, and large oval lucency projecting over the left cardiac border and outlined by an irregular curvilinear opacity. In another patient, a posteroanterior chest radiograph (Fig. 2) shows abnormal lucencies above and below the right hemidiaphragm, and a lateral chest radiograph (Fig. 3) shows the abnormal contour of the right hemidiaphragm and adjacent lucencies consistent with bowel.

DISCUSSION

Definition/Background

Traumatic diaphragmatic hernia is herniation of abdominal contents through a tear of the diaphragm. It occurs in up to 8% of patients with major blunt trauma and is most common in young men injured in motor vehicle accidents.

Characteristic Clinical Features

Patients usually have no major symptoms related to the diaphragmatic tear, and clinical findings are obscured by other major trauma. Strangulation of the herniated viscera is typically a late manifestation.

Characteristic Radiologic Findings

Specific findings on the chest radiograph include intrathoracic herniation of a hollow viscus and visualization of the nasogastric tube above the left hemidiaphragm. Suggestive but nonspecific findings include apparent elevation, distortion, or obliteration of the diaphragmatic outline; abnormal lucencies adjacent to the diaphragm; and contralateral shift of the mediastinum.

Less Common Radiologic Manifestations

Air fluid level within the herniated stomach.

Differential Diagnosis

- Hemothorax
- Phrenic nerve palsy
- Eventration of the diaphragm

Discussion

Traumatic hemothorax may obscure traumatic hernias. Elevation of the hemidiaphragm due to phrenic nerve palsy or chronic eventration may mimic a traumatic hernia on the radiograph. In the majority of cases a confident diagnosis can be made on CT.

Diagnosis

Traumatic diaphragmatic hernia, radiographic findings

Suggested Readings

Costantino M, Gosselin MV, Primack SL: The ABC's of thoracic trauma imaging. Semin Roentgenol 41:209-225, 2006.

Scharff JR, Naunheim KS: Traumatic diaphragmatic injuries. Thorac Surg Clin 17:81-85, 2007.

Thoongsuwan N, Kanne JP, Stern EJ: Spectrum of blunt chest injuries. J Thorac Imaging 20:89-97, 2005.

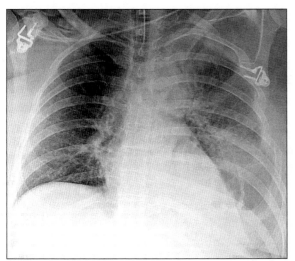

Figure 1. Anteroposterior chest radiograph reveals left rib fractures, increased opacification of the left hemithorax, and large, oval lucency projecting over the left cardiac border and outlined by an irregular curvilinear opacity. The oval lucency was shown to be the herniated stomach. The patient was a 53-year-old woman with traumatic diaphragmatic hernia due to blunt chest trauma.

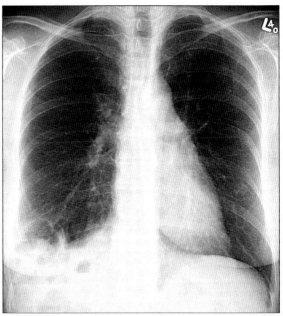

Figure 2. Posteroanterior chest radiograph shows abnormal lucencies above and below right hemidiaphragm. The patient was a 55-year-old woman with herniation of large bowel due to iatrogenic injury of the right hemidiaphragm after partial hepatectomy.

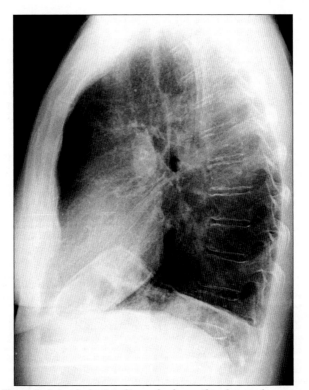

Figure 3. Lateral chest radiograph shows the abnormal contour of right hemidiaphragm and adjacent lucencies consistent with bowel in a 55-year-old woman with herniation of large bowel due to iatrogenic injury of the right hemidiaphragm after partial hepatectomy.

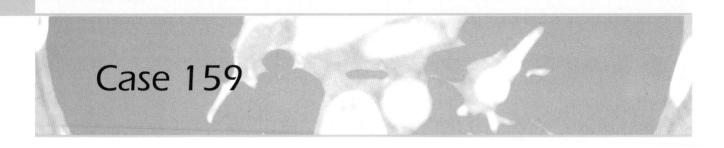

Case 159

DEMOGRAPHICS/CLINICAL HISTORY

A 53-year-old woman with chest pain after a motor vehicle accident, undergoing computed tomography (CT).

FINDINGS

Contrast-enhanced CT (Fig. 1) shows a discontinuity of the left hemidiaphragm, the spleen in close contact with the posterior ribs (i.e., fallen viscera sign), the high position of the stomach and spleen, and a left rib fracture. Coronal, reformatted, multidetector CT (Fig. 2) shows a focal tear of the left hemidiaphragm with herniation of the stomach and omentum. Notice the narrowing of the stomach as it herniates through the diaphragmatic tear (i.e., collar sign). In another patient, contrast-enhanced, multidetector CT (Fig. 3) shows bowel loops and omentum in the right hemithorax, and coronal, reformatted CT (Fig. 4) shows a discontinuity of the right hemidiaphragm and waist-like narrowing of the omentum and large bowel as they herniate through the diaphragm.

DISCUSSION

Definition/Background
Traumatic diaphragmatic hernia is herniation of abdominal contents through a tear of the diaphragm. It occurs in up to 8% of patients with major blunt trauma and is most common in young men injured in motor vehicle accidents.

Characteristic Clinical Features
Patients usually have no major symptoms related to the diaphragmatic tear; the clinical findings are obscured by other major trauma. Strangulation of the herniated viscera is typically a late manifestation.

Characteristic Radiologic Findings
Characteristic findings on CT include visualization of a focal discontinuity of the diaphragm (sensitivity of 75%, specificity of 90%); dependent position of the stomach, spleen, and bowel that has herniated into the thorax (i.e., dependent viscera sign; sensitivity of 55% to 90%); intrathoracic herniation of a hollow viscus or liver (sensitivity of 60%, specificity of 100%); and waist-like constriction of herniated abdominal contents at the level of diaphragmatic rupture (i.e., collar sign; sensitivity of 60%, specificity of 100%) (Fig. 1, Fig. 2, Fig. 3, Fig. 4). A diaphragmatic discontinuity, an intrathoracic herniation, and the collar sign are better seen on multiplanar reformations than on cross-sectional images.

Less Common Radiologic Manifestations
Imaging may show focal thickening of the diaphragm, segmental nonvisualization of the diaphragm, and elevated abdominal organs.

Differential Diagnosis
- Normal variant
- Hemothorax

Discussion
Focal diaphragmatic defects are normal variants that appear and increase in number and severity with age; they are absent in patients younger than 39 years and present in 25% of patients between 40 and 49 years old and in 60% of patients between 70 and 79 years old. Traumatic hemothorax may obscure small diaphragmatic tears on CT.

Diagnosis
Traumatic diaphragmatic hernia, CT findings

Suggested Readings
Costantino M, Gosselin MV, Primack SL: The ABC's of thoracic trauma imaging. Semin Roentgenol 41:209-225, 2006.

Nchimi A, Szapiro D, Ghaye B, et al: Helical CT of blunt diaphragmatic rupture. AJR Am J Roentgenol 184:24-30, 2005.

Thoongsuwan N, Kanne JP, Stern EJ: Spectrum of blunt chest injuries. J Thorac Imaging 20:89-97, 2005.

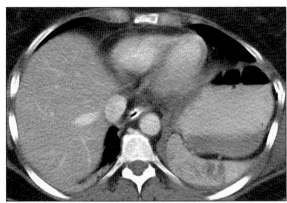

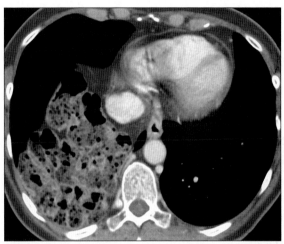

Figure 1. Contrast-enhanced CT shows discontinuity of the left hemidiaphragm, the spleen in close contact with the posterior ribs (i.e., fallen viscera sign), high position of stomach and spleen, and a left rib fracture. The patient was a 53-year-old woman with traumatic tear of the left hemidiaphragm due to a motor vehicle accident.

Figure 3. Contrast-enhanced, multidetector CT shows bowel loops and omentum in the right hemithorax. Notice that the bowel loops are in close contact with the posterior ribs (i.e., dependent viscera sign). The patient was a 55-year-old woman with a diaphragmatic hernia after iatrogenic injury of the right hemidiaphragm during partial hepatectomy for hepatocellular carcinoma.

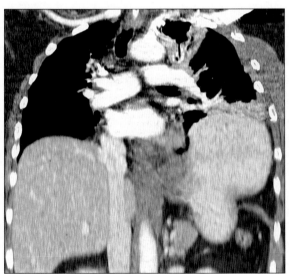

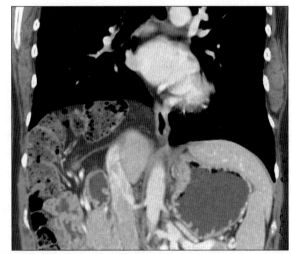

Figure 2. In the same patient, coronal, reformatted, multidetector CT shows a focal tear of the left hemidiaphragm with herniation of the stomach and omentum. Notice the waistlike constriction of the stomach as it herniates through the diaphragmatic tear (i.e., collar sign).

Figure 4. Coronal, reformatted CT shows a discontinuity of the right hemidiaphragm and waist-like narrowing of the omentum and large bowel as they herniate through the diaphragm (i.e., collar sign) in a 55-year-old woman with a diaphragmatic hernia after iatrogenic injury of the right hemidiaphragm during partial hepatectomy for hepatocellular carcinoma.

Case 160

DEMOGRAPHICS/CLINICAL HISTORY

A 68-year-old man with fever 1 week after coronary artery bypass grafting, undergoing computed tomography (CT).

FINDINGS

Contrast-enhanced CT (Fig. 1) shows a retrosternal and anterior mediastinal fluid collection with air bubbles. The scan also shows a loculated, right anterolateral pleural fluid collection that contains areas of high attenuation consistent with residual hemothorax and a small, posterior, right pleural effusion.

DISCUSSION

Mediastinal abscess is a mediastinal inflammatory mass, the central part of which has undergone purulent liquefaction necrosis. It occurs most commonly after median sternotomy, esophageal surgery or perforation, and spread of infection from an adjacent region, usually the lower neck. Mediastinal abscess has a mortality rate of approximately 25%.

Characteristic Clinical Features
Patients have fever, chills, sepsis, retrosternal pain, and pain originating between the scapulas.

Characteristic Radiologic Findings
Imaging shows mediastinal widening due to associated mediastinitis, single or multiple areas of low attenuation consistent with fluid, focal or diffuse ectopic gas bubbles, and commonly, an air-fluid level.

Less Common Radiologic Manifestations
Imaging may show communication with an empyema, fistula formation, sinus tract, or infection in the lower neck.

Differential Diagnosis
- Normal postoperative finding

Discussion
Normal postoperative findings in the first week after median sternotomy include small amounts of air in the operative field, retrosternal soft tissue thickening, localized soft tissue densities due to hematoma, and partial obliteration of the mediastinal fat plane lucency. These findings are difficult to distinguish from mediastinitis or early abscess formation. The diagnosis of mediastinitis and abscess formation requires close correlation of the radiologic and clinical findings.

The anastomosis after transthoracic esophagectomy is usually located around the level of the thoracic inlet. After a gastric pull-up, chest radiography shows a mildly widened mediastinum with intrathoracic air, and CT typically shows a partially collapsed stomach in the right posterior mediastinum anterior to the vertebral body. A fluid-filled collection around the esophagus on CT should raise the possibility of a mediastinal abscess. The radiologic diagnosis of an anastomotic leak is usually made by demonstrating contrast extravasation on contrast-enhanced esophagography.

Diagnosis
Postoperative complication—mediastinal abscess

Suggested Readings
Akman C, Kantarci F, Cetinkaya S: Imaging in mediastinitis: A systematic review based on aetiology. Clin Radiol 59:573-585, 2004.

Giménez A, Franquet T, Erasmus JJ, et al: Thoracic complications of esophageal disorders. Radiographics 22:S247-S258, 2002.

Kim TJ, Lee KH, Kim YH, et al: Postoperative imaging of esophageal cancer: What chest radiologists need to know. Radiographics 27:409-429, 2007.

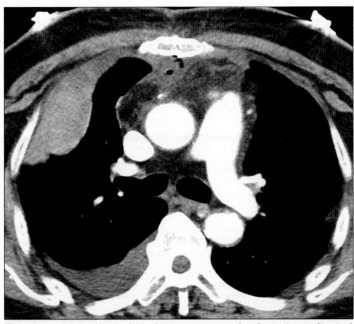

Figure 1. Contrast-enhanced CT shows a retrosternal and anterior mediastinal fluid collection with air bubbles. Notice the a loculated, right anterolateral pleural fluid collection that contains areas of high attenuation consistent with residual hemothorax and a small, posterior, right pleural effusion. The patient was a 68-year-old man with mediastinal abscess and right hemothorax 1 week after coronary artery bypass grafting.

Case 161

DEMOGRAPHICS/CLINICAL HISTORY

A 43-year-old woman with a productive cough 3 months after right lower lobectomy, undergoing radiography and computed tomography (CT).

FINDINGS

Posteroanterior chest radiograph (Fig. 1) shows postoperative changes related to a prior right lower lobectomy, a right pleural effusion, and an air-fluid level. Sequential CT images (Figs. 2 to 4) reveal a communication of the right lower lobe bronchial stump with the pleural space.

DISCUSSION

Definition/Background

Postoperative bronchopleural fistulas may occur after any type of lung resection, but they occur most often after pneumonectomy. Predisposing factors for development of a bronchopleural fistula include preoperative uncontrolled pleuropulmonary infection, preoperative radiation therapy, and trauma.

Characteristic Clinical Features

Patients may have cough, fever, chills, and pleuritic chest pain.

Characteristic Radiologic Findings

Radiographic findings suggesting postoperative bronchopleural fistula include a continuous increase in the amount of air in the pleural space, the appearance of an air-fluid level, a drop in the air-fluid level exceeding 2 cm during the postoperative period, and the reappearance of an air-fluid level in a patient who has undergone pneumonectomy. CT demonstrates air and fluid collections in the pleural space and frequently shows a communication or tract from an airway or the lung parenchyma to the pleural space.

Less Common Radiologic Manifestations

Imaging may show a contralateral shift of the mediastinum.

Diagnosis

Postoperative complication—bronchopleural fistula

Suggested Readings

Chae EJ, Seo JB, Kim SY, et al: Radiographic and CT findings of thoracic complications after pneumonectomy. Radiographics 26:1449-1468.

Kim EA, Lee KS, Shim YM, et al: Radiographic and CT findings in complications following pulmonary resection. Radiographics 22:67-86, 2002.

Ricci ZJ, Haramati LB, Rosenbaum AT, Liebling MS: Role of computed tomography in guiding the management of peripheral bronchopleural fistula. J Thorac Imaging 17:214-218, 2002.

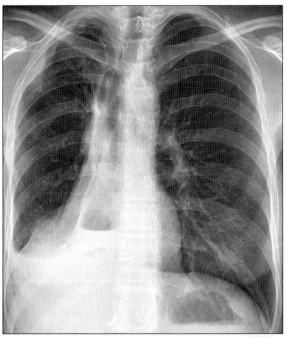

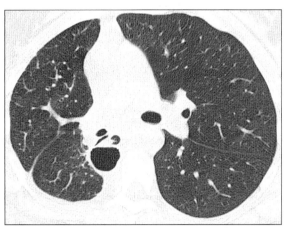

Figure 3. In the same patient, CT at the level of the middle lobe bronchus shows a distal, right lower lobe bronchial stump and a loculated pleural air-fluid level.

Figure 1. Posteroanterior chest radiograph shows postoperative changes related to a prior right lower lobectomy, a right pleural effusion, and an air-fluid level medially. The patient was a 43-year-old woman with bronchopleural fistula 3 months after a right lower lobectomy.

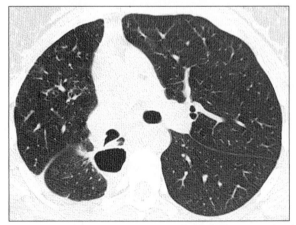

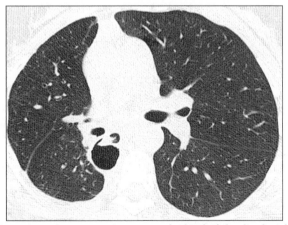

Figure 2. In the same patient, CT at the level of the proximal right middle and lower lobe bronchi shows a right pleural effusion with an air-fluid level medially.

Figure 4. In the same patient, CT at the level of the distal, right lower lobe bronchial stump shows communication of the bronchus with the pleural space.

Case 162

DEMOGRAPHICS/CLINICAL HISTORY

A 76-year-old man with shortness of breath and acute pleuritic left chest pain, undergoing radiography.

FINDINGS

Supine chest radiograph (Fig. 1) shows increased lucency in the region of the left costophrenic sulcus, which is better seen and appears to extend more inferiorly than normal (i.e., deep sulcus sign). Notice the bilateral, perihilar, hazy, increased opacity consistent with pulmonary edema and the various tubes and catheters. In another patient, a supine chest radiograph (Fig. 2) shows increased lucency in the right costophrenic sulcus, subcutaneous emphysema, perihilar consolidation consistent with pulmonary edema, and various tubes and catheters in place.

DISCUSSION

Definition/Background
The deep sulcus sign refers to the very deep radiolucent costophrenic sulcus that results from increased lucency in the lateral costophrenic sulcus extending toward the hypochondrium on the supine chest radiograph of a patient with pneumothorax. Other radiographic findings for supine patients with pneumothorax include increased sharpness of the cardiomediastinal border, increased visualization of the pericardial fat pads, and a visible inferior border of the collapsed lower lobe or the heart.

Characteristic Clinical Features
Patients have ipsilateral pleuritic chest pain and acute dyspnea.

Characteristic Radiologic Findings
Radiographic findings include increased lucency in the lateral costophrenic sulcus extending toward the hypochondrium.

Less Common Radiologic Manifestations
Imaging may show increased sharpness and an angular appearance of the deepened lateral costophrenic angle.

Differential Diagnosis
- Normal lung

Discussion
An apparent deep sulcus sign may also result from technical artifacts and patient rotation.

Diagnosis
Deep sulcus sign in pneumothorax

Suggested Readings
Kong A: The deep sulcus sign. Radiology 228:415-416, 2003.

Qureshi NR, Gleeson FV: Imaging of pleural disease. Clin Chest Med 27:193-213, 2006.

Tschopp JM, Rami-Porta R, Noppen M, Astoul P: Management of spontaneous pneumothorax: State of the art. Eur Respir J 28: 637-650, 2006.

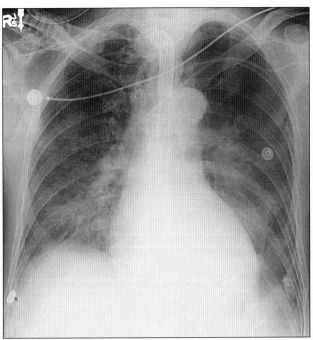

Figure 1. Supine chest radiograph shows increased lucency in the region of the left costophrenic sulcus, which is better seen and appears to extend more inferiorly than normal (i.e., deep sulcus sign). Notice the bilateral, perihilar, hazy, increased opacity consistent with pulmonary edema and the various tubes and catheters in place. The patient was a 76-year-old man with pulmonary edema and a left pneumothorax.

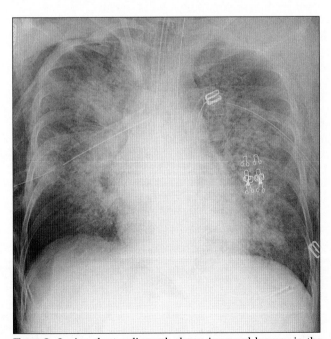

Figure 2. Supine chest radiograph shows increased lucency in the right costophrenic sulcus (i.e., deep sulcus sign), subcutaneous emphysema, perihilar consolidation consistent with pulmonary edema, and various tubes and catheters. The patient was a 33-year-old woman with pulmonary edema and a right pneumothorax after blunt chest trauma.

Case 163

DEMOGRAPHICS/CLINICAL HISTORY

A 16-year-old boy with acute chest pain and shortness of breath, undergoing radiography and computed tomography (CT).

FINDINGS

Chest radiograph (Fig. 1) shows a left pneumothorax and mild irregularity of the left lung apex adjacent to the pleura as it projects over the anterior left first rib. CT (Fig. 2) shows a left pneumothorax and left apical bullae. Coronal, reformatted CT (Fig. 3) shows a left apical bulla and left pneumothorax. The right lung is normal.

DISCUSSION

Definition/Background
Spontaneous pneumothorax refers to the development of pneumothorax in the absence of traumatic injury to the chest or lung, and primary spontaneous pneumothorax refers to spontaneous pneumothorax that occurs in individuals without clinically apparent lung disease. It occurs most often in smokers and in tall, thin, young adults, with a male-to-female ratio of 5:1.

Characteristic Clinical Features
Patients have ipsilateral pleuritic chest pain or acute dyspnea.

Characteristic Radiologic Findings
The characteristic radiographic manifestation of pneumothorax is a thin pleural line (<1 mm thick) parallel to the chest wall, with no lung markings projecting beyond it. CT usually shows localized areas of emphysema mainly at the lung apices or shows isolated blebs (air space of 1 cm or less in diameter) or bullae (air space greater than 1 cm in diameter), even if the patient is a lifelong nonsmoker.

Less Common Radiologic Manifestations
Imaging may show isolated blebs or bullae in the middle or lower lobes.

Differential Diagnosis
- Skin fold

Discussion
On the chest radiograph, the thin, white line of the visceral pleura in pneumothorax can usually be readily distinguished from the black line or interface of a skin fold. Skin folds are straight or only minimally curved, tend not to run parallel to the chest wall, and usually extend beyond the chest cavity.

Diagnosis
Primary spontaneous pneumothorax

Suggested Readings
Baumann MH: Management of spontaneous pneumothorax. Clin Chest Med 27:369-381, 2006.

Qureshi NR, Gleeson FV: Imaging of pleural disease. Clin Chest Med 27:193-213, 2006.

Sahn SA, Heffner JE: Spontaneous pneumothorax. N Engl J Med 342:868-874, 2000.

Tschopp JM, Rami-Porta R, Noppen M, Astoul P: Management of spontaneous pneumothorax: State of the art. Eur Respir J 28: 637-650, 2006.

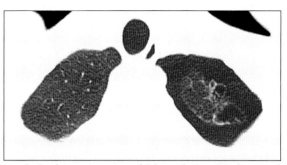

Figure 2. In the same patient, high-resolution CT shows a left pneumothorax and left apical bullae. The right lung apex is normal.

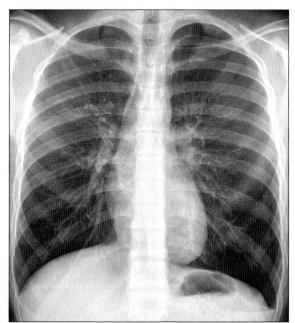

Figure 1. Chest radiograph shows a left pneumothorax and mild irregularity of the left lung apex adjacent to the pleura as it projects over the anterior left first rib. The patient was a 16-year-old boy with recurrent spontaneous pneumothorax.

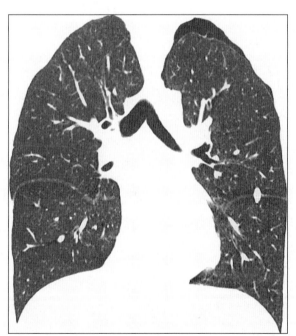

Figure 3. In the same patient, coronal, reformatted CT shows a left apical bulla and left pneumothorax. The right lung is normal.

Case 164

DEMOGRAPHICS/CLINICAL HISTORY

A 50-year-old man with acute-onset shortness of breath, undergoing computed tomography (CT).

FINDINGS

High-resolution CT (Fig. 1) reveals bilateral pneumothorax and numerous bilateral cysts of various shapes and sizes, consistent with pulmonary Langerhans histiocytosis. The scan also shows patchy ground-glass opacities due to hemorrhage, a focal consolidation in the left lower lobe, and a small left pleural effusion.

DISCUSSION

Spontaneous pneumothorax refers to the development of pneumothorax in the absence of traumatic injury to the chest or lung, and secondary spontaneous pneumothorax refers to spontaneous pneumothorax that occurs in individuals with clinically apparent lung disease. Common causes of secondary pneumothorax include chronic obstructive pulmonary disease (COPD), severe pneumonia, *Pneumocystis* pneumonia, interstitial pulmonary fibrosis, and cystic lung diseases such as pulmonary Langerhans cell histiocytosis, lymphangioleiomyomatosis (LAM), and Birt-Hogg-Dubé syndrome.

Characteristic Clinical Features
Patients have ipsilateral pleuritic chest pain or acute dyspnea.

Characteristic Radiologic Findings
The characteristic radiographic manifestation of pneumothorax is a thin pleural line (<1 mm thick) parallel to chest wall, with no lung markings projecting beyond it.

In patients with secondary spontaneous pneumothorax, the radiograph or CT scan shows underlying lung disease, most commonly emphysema. Other common underlying abnormalities include interstitial fibrosis and cystic lung disease.

Less Common Radiologic Manifestations
Extensive bronchiectasis and apical bullae are seen in patients with cystic fibrosis.

Differential Diagnosis
■ Skin fold

Discussion
On the chest radiograph, the thin, white line of the visceral pleura in pneumothorax can usually be readily distinguished from the black line or interface of a skin fold. Skin folds are straight or only minimally curved, tend not to run parallel to the chest wall, and usually extend beyond the chest cavity.

Diagnosis
Secondary spontaneous pneumothorax

Suggested Readings
Baumann MH: Management of spontaneous pneumothorax. Clin Chest Med 27:369-381, 2006.
Qureshi NR, Gleeson FV: Imaging of pleural disease. Clin Chest Med 27:193-213, 2006.
Sahn SA, Heffner JE: Spontaneous pneumothorax. N Engl J Med 342:868-874, 2000.
Tschopp JM, Rami-Porta R, Noppen M, Astoul P: Management of spontaneous pneumothorax: State of the art. Eur Respir J 28:637-650, 2006.

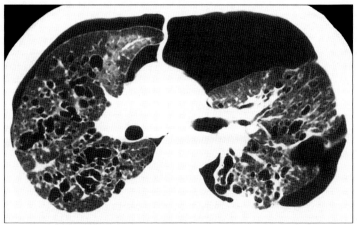

Figure 1. High-resolution CT reveals bilateral pneumothorax and numerous bilateral cysts of various shapes and sizes. Notice the patchy ground-glass opacities due to hemorrhage, focal consolidation in the left lower lobe, and small left pleural effusion. The patient was a 50-year-old man with spontaneous bilateral pneumothorax due to pulmonary Langerhans histiocytosis.

Case 165

DEMOGRAPHICS/CLINICAL HISTORY

A 54-year-old woman with sudden onset of chest pain and a history of multiple skin papules that were shown on biopsy to be fibrofolliculomas, undergoing computed tomography (CT).

FINDINGS

High-resolution CT through the lower lung zones (Figs. 1 and 2) and coronal, reformatted CT (Fig. 3) show sharply marginated, air-containing pulmonary cysts of various sizes with thin walls.

DISCUSSION

Definition/Background

Birt-Hogg-Dubé syndrome is an autosomal dominant disease characterized by benign skin tumors (i.e., fibrofolliculomas) occurring mainly in the face, pulmonary cysts, an increased risk for spontaneous pneumothorax, and an increased risk for development of various renal tumors, including carcinoma. The syndrome should be suspected in patients with characteristic skin lesions or a history of familial pneumothorax.

Characteristic Clinical Features

Patients who present with pneumothorax usually have ipsilateral pleuritic chest pain or acute dyspnea.

Characteristic Radiologic Findings

Radiologic findings include multiple, thin-walled, round or oval cysts of various sizes involving mainly the lower lung zones.

Less Common Radiologic Manifestations

Imaging may show pneumothorax and cysts with an asymmetric distribution.

Differential Diagnosis

- Lymphocytic interstitial pneumonia (LIP)
- Lymphangiomyomatosis
- Pulmonary Langerhans histiocytosis
- Emphysema

Discussion

The cysts in Birt-Hogg-Dubé syndrome usually involve predominantly or exclusively the lung bases, and the lung parenchyma between the cysts is normal. Lung cysts in LIP are almost invariably associated with ground-glass opacities, and LIP occurs almost exclusively in patients with underlying immunologic disorders such as Sjögren syndrome and multicentric Castleman disease. In lymphangiomyomatosis, the cysts are usually small and diffusely distributed throughout the lungs. The cysts in Langerhans histiocytosis are usually associated with lung nodules and typically spare the lung bases.

Diagnosis

Birt-Hogg-Dubé syndrome

Suggested Readings

Ayo DS, Aughenbaugh GL, Yi ES, et al: Cystic lung disease in Birt-Hogg-Dubé syndrome. Chest 132:679-684, 2007.

Souza CA, Finley R, Müller NL: Birt-Hogg-Dubé syndrome: A rare cause of pulmonary cysts. AJR Am J Roentgenol 185:1237-1239, 2005.

Toro JR, Pautler SE, Stewart L, et al: Lung cysts, spontaneous pneumothorax, and genetic associations in 89 families with Birt-Hogg-Dubé syndrome. Am J Respir Crit Care Med 175:1044-1053, 2007.

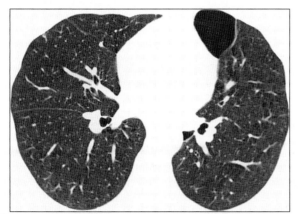

Figure 1. High-resolution CT at level of the inferior pulmonary veins shows a 3.8-cm-diameter, thin-walled cyst in the lingula and a few smaller cysts in the lower lobes. The patient was a 54-year-old woman with Birt-Hogg-Dubé syndrome.

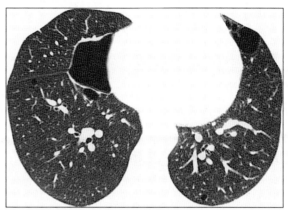

Figure 2. In the same patient, high-resolution CT at level of basal segments of the lower lobes shows multiple bilateral cysts of various sizes.

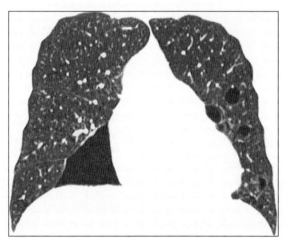

Figure 3. In the same patient, coronal reconstruction CT shows large cystic air space adjacent to the pericardium in the right lower lobe and several smaller cysts in the left lung.

Case 166

DEMOGRAPHICS/CLINICAL HISTORY

A 20-year-old man with pleuritic chest pain, undergoing radiography.

FINDINGS

Posteroanterior chest radiograph (Fig. 1) shows homogeneous opacification of the right lower hemithorax, blunting of the lateral costophrenic sulcus, obscuration of the right hemidiaphragm, and subtle blunting of the posterior left costophrenic recess. Lateral radiograph (Fig. 2) shows blunting of the right and left posterior costophrenic recesses with a concave upper border (i.e., meniscus sign) that is characteristic of pleural fluid.

DISCUSSION

Definition/Background

Pleural effusion is the accumulation of fluid in the pleural space. Pleural effusions may be caused by an imbalance of hydrostatic and oncotic forces (i.e., transudates) or by changes in the pleural surface or local capillary permeability resulting from pleural disease or adjacent lung injury (i.e., exudates).

Characteristic Clinical Features

Patients may be asymptomatic or have ipsilateral pleuritic chest pain and dyspnea.

Characteristic Radiologic Findings

The most characteristic feature is the pleural meniscus (i.e., appearance of fluid as a homogeneous opacity with a concave upper border that is higher laterally than medially). Accumulation in a subpulmonic region causes apparent flattening of the diaphragm without significant blunting of the costophrenic angles; the apex of the pseudodiaphragmatic contour is typically more lateral than the apex of the normal diaphragm. On the supine radiograph, pleural effusion may manifest as increased opacification of a hemithorax; large effusions can cap the apex of the lungs.

Less Common Radiologic Manifestations

Imaging may show large, left pleural effusions that can result in inversion of the hemidiaphragm.

Differential Diagnosis

- Normal pleura
- Pleural thickening

Discussion

Small pleural effusions can be missed on the upright chest radiograph, and even moderate-sized pleural effusions can be overlooked on supine radiographs. The most sensitive radiographic projection for detection of small pleural effusions is the lateral decubitus view. Pleural effusions, particularly when small, can be difficult to differentiate from pleural thickening on the radiograph. The distinction can be made using a radiographic decubitus view, ultrasound, or computed tomography.

Diagnosis

Pleural effusion, radiographic findings

Suggested Readings

Blackmore CC, Black WC, Dallas RV, Crow HC: Pleural fluid volume estimation: A chest radiograph prediction rule. Acad Radiol 3: 103-109, 1996.

Porcel JM, Light RW: Diagnostic approach to pleural effusion in adults. Am Fam Physician 73:1211-1220, 2006.

Qureshi NR, Gleeson FV: Imaging of pleural disease. Clin Chest Med 27:193-213, 2006.

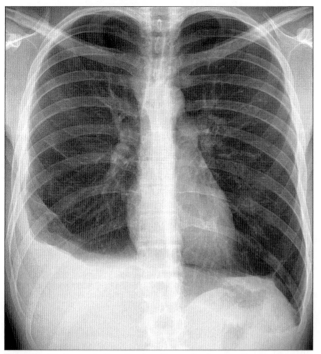

Figure 1. Posteroanterior chest radiograph shows a homogeneous opacification of the right lower hemithorax, blunting of the lateral costophrenic sulcus and obscuration of the right hemidiaphragm. The patient was a 20-year-old man with bilateral pleural effusions.

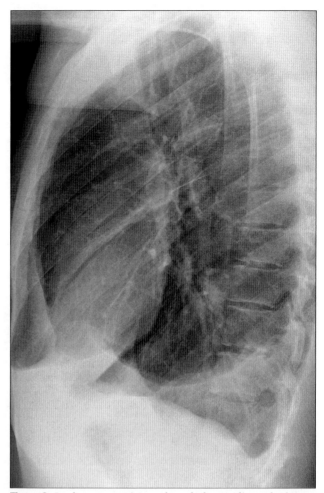

Figure 2. In the same patient, a lateral chest radiograph shows blunting of the right and left posterior costophrenic recesses with a concave upper contour (i.e., meniscus sign) that is characteristic of pleural fluid.

Case 167

DEMOGRAPHICS/CLINICAL HISTORY

A 52-year-old woman with acute shortness of breath, undergoing computed tomography (CT).

FINDINGS

Contrast-enhanced CT at the level of the left atrium (Fig. 1) shows bilateral pleural effusions with a characteristic concave anterior border and low attenuation. Contrast-enhanced CT at the level of the upper abdomen (Fig. 2) shows small, bilateral pleural effusions and ascites. The right pleural effusion is in contact with the bare area of the liver (i.e., bare area sign) and has slightly indistinct margins with the liver, whereas the ascites is anterior to the liver and has a sharply defined interface (i.e., interface sign). In another patient, contrast-enhanced CT (Fig. 3) shows a left pleural effusion and areas of compressive atelectasis in the adjacent lung.

DISCUSSION

Definition/Background
Pleural effusion is the accumulation of fluid in the pleural space. Pleural effusions are common and are estimated to occur in approximately 1 million people each year in the United States. They may result from pleural, parenchymal, or extrapulmonary disease.

Characteristic Clinical Features
Patients may be asymptomatic or present with ipsilateral pleuritic chest pain and dyspnea.

Characteristic Radiologic Findings
On CT, a free-flowing pleural effusion typically results in a sickle-shaped opacity in the most dependent portion of the thorax. Loculated effusions tend to have a lenticular shape, smooth margins, and relatively homogeneous attenuation.

Less Common Radiologic Manifestations
Large, left pleural effusions may result in inversion of the hemidiaphragm.

Differential Diagnosis
- Ascites

Discussion
Differentiation of small pleural effusions from ascites is facilitated by assessment of four signs: diaphragm sign, displaced crus sign, interface sign, and bare area sign. On CT, the fluid in a pleural effusion is outside the diaphragm, whereas the fluid in ascites is inside the diaphragm (i.e., diaphragm sign). The pleural effusion displaces the crus anteriorly and laterally away from spine (i.e., displaced crus sign), forms an indistinct interface with the liver (i.e., interface sign), and can be seen behind bare area of the liver (i.e., bare area sign).

Diagnosis
Pleural effusion, CT findings

Suggested Readings
Müller NL: Imaging of the pleura. Radiology 186:297-309, 1993.
Porcel JM, Light RW: Diagnostic approach to pleural effusion in adults. Am Fam Physician 73:1211-1220, 2006.
Qureshi NR, Gleeson FV: Imaging of pleural disease. Clin Chest Med 27:193-213, 2006.

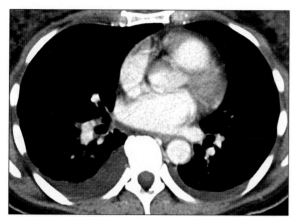

Figure 1. Contrast-enhanced CT at the level of the left atrium shows bilateral pleural effusions with a characteristic concave anterior border and low attenuation. The patient was a 52-year-old woman with bilateral pleural effusions and ascites.

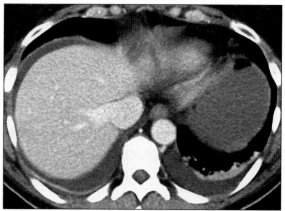

Figure 2. In the same patient, contrast-enhanced CT at the level of the upper abdomen shows small, bilateral pleural effusions and ascites. The right pleural effusion is in contact with the bare area of the liver (i.e., bare area sign) and forms slightly indistinct margins with the liver, whereas the ascites is anterior to the liver and has a sharply defined interface (i.e., interface sign). Notice the compressive atelectasis in the left lower lobe and a fluid-filled stomach.

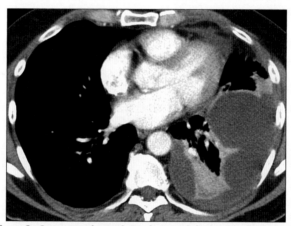

Figure 3. Contrast-enhanced CT shows a left pleural effusion and areas of compressive atelectasis in the adjacent lung. Notice that the pleural effusion has several convex margins consistent of multiple partial or complete loculations. The patient was a 60-year-old man with a loculated, left pleural effusion.

Case 168

DEMOGRAPHICS/CLINICAL HISTORY

A 42-year-old man with pleuritic chest pain and fever, undergoing radiography and computed tomography (CT).

FINDINGS

Posteroanterior chest radiograph (Fig. 1) shows a homogeneous opacification in the lateral aspect of the right hemithorax with a convex border medially, suggesting a large pleural effusion that is at least partially loculated. Medial to the sharply defined border, there is hazy, increased opacification. Contrast-enhanced CT images at the level of the right upper lobe bronchus (Fig. 2) and inferior pulmonary vein (Fig. 3) show a right pleural effusion and thickening and enhancement of the parietal pleura.

DISCUSSION

Definition/Background

Empyema is pus within the pleural space. Common causes include pneumonia, lung abscess, thoracic surgery, and upper abdominal infection. The most common organisms are *Staphylococcus aureus*, *Streptococcus pneumoniae*, and enteric gram-negative bacilli.

Characteristic Clinical Features

Patients typically have fever, chills, and pleuritic chest pain.

Characteristic Radiologic Findings

Radiographic findings include pleural effusion that frequently is loculated. Parietal and visceral pleural enhancement and thickening are seen on contrast-enhanced chest CT. CT shows increased attenuation of the extrapleural fat.

Less Common Radiologic Manifestations

Imaging may show hilar and mediastinal lymphadenopathy and extension of the empyema into the chest wall (i.e., empyema necessitatis).

Differential Diagnosis

- Pleural effusion
- Hemothorax

Discussion

The diagnosis of empyema should be suspected on the basis of CT findings of pleural effusion associated with thickening and enhancement of the pleura and increased attenuation of extrapleural fat. Similar findings may be seen in patients with hemothorax. Definitive diagnosis of empyema requires the presence of pus within the pleural space or positive culture results for organisms from the pleural fluid.

Diagnosis

Empyema

Suggested Readings

Evans AL, Gleeson FV: Radiology in pleural disease: State of the art. Respirology 9:300-312, 2004.

Kearney SE, Davies CW, Davies RJ, Gleeson FV: Computed tomography and ultrasound in parapneumonic effusions and empyema. Clin Radiol 55:542-547, 2000.

Kim EA, Lee KS, Shim YM, et al: Radiographic and CT findings in complications following pulmonary resection. Radiographics 22:67-86, 2002.

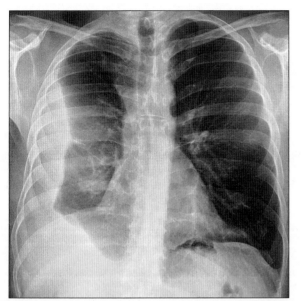

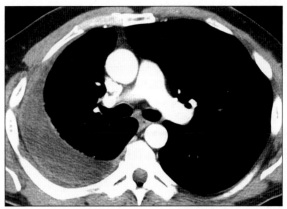

Figure 2. In the same patient, contrast-enhanced CT at the level of the right upper lobe bronchus shows a right pleural effusion and thickening and enhancement of the parietal pleura. Notice the increased density of the right extrapleural space.

Figure 1. Posteroanterior chest radiograph shows a homogeneous opacification of the lateral aspect of the right hemithorax with a convex border medially, suggesting a large pleural effusion that is at least partially loculated. Medial to the sharply defined border, there is hazy, increased opacification. The patient was a 42-year-old man with empyema.

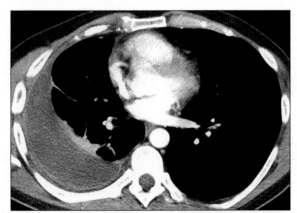

Figure 3. In the same patient, contrast-enhanced CT at the level of the inferior pulmonary vein shows a right pleural effusion and thickening and enhancement of the parietal pleura. Notice the increased density of the right extrapleural space.

Case 169

DEMOGRAPHICS/CLINICAL HISTORY

A 43-year-old man with shortness of breath and left chest pain, undergoing radiography and computed tomography (CT).

FINDINGS

Posteroanterior chest radiograph (Fig. 1) shows opacification of the left lower hemithorax with extension into the lateral and apical regions and a lobulated contour of the left mediastinal interface. Notice the volume loss with an ipsilateral mediastinal shift. Contrast-enhanced CT at the level of the aortopulmonary window (Fig. 2) shows diffuse, nodular, left pleural thickening with involvement of the interlobar fissure and mediastinal pleura. CT at the level of the ventricles (Fig. 3) shows diffuse, left pleural thickening and a loculated, left pleural effusion. In another patient with malignant mesothelioma, CT (Fig. 4) shows circumferential, right pleural thickening with associated volume loss.

DISCUSSION

Definition/Background

Malignant mesothelioma, which usually is caused by asbestos exposure, is a locally aggressive tumor of the pleura that invades the chest wall and surrounding structures. Mesothelioma is classified by three histologic subtypes: epithelial, which is the most common; sarcomatous; and mixed type. It accounts for 20 deaths per 1 million men each year in North America and Europe. The incidence has been increasing over the past few decades, and it has a latency period of 30 to 40 years after asbestos exposure.

Characteristic Clinical Features

Most common first symptoms are dyspnea and chest pain, which often is vague, typically is nonpleuritic, and may be referred to the shoulder.

Characteristic Radiologic Findings

Radiologic findings include unilateral, sheetlike or lobulated pleural thickening encasing the entire lung, with involvement of the mediastinal pleura evident on CT and magnetic resonance imaging (MRI). Unilateral pleural effusion or nodular pleural thickening may be seen. Increased uptake occurs on ^{18}F-fluorodeoxyglucose positron emission tomography (FDG-PET).

Less Common Radiologic Manifestations

CT or MRI may show enlarged pericardiophrenic and internal mammary nodes, ipsilateral volume loss, and evidence of chest wall extension. Pleural plaques are seen in 30% to 40% of patients.

Differential Diagnosis

- Pleural metastases
- Lymphoma
- Diffuse benign pleural thickening
- Benign asbestos-related pleural disease
- Benign pleural effusion

Discussion

Metastatic pleural disease is more common than mesothelioma and may be radiologically indistinguishable from mesothelioma. Features that favor metastases include known primary lung cancer, breast cancer, or lymphoma and systemic metastases.

Diffuse benign pleural thickening of any cause, including prior asbestos exposure, typically results in smooth pleural thickening, seldom involves the mediastinal pleura, and is seldom associated with pleural effusion. Definitive diagnosis of malignant pleural mesothelioma requires thoracoscopic surgery (91% to 98% sensitivity) or image-guided core-needle biopsy.

Diagnosis

Malignant mesothelioma

Suggested Readings

British Thoracic Society Standards of Care Committee: BTS statement on malignant mesothelioma in the UK, 2007. Thorax 62(Suppl 2): ii1-ii19, 2007.

Qureshi NR, Gleeson FV: Imaging of pleural disease. Clin Chest Med 27:193-213, 2006.

Wang ZJ, Reddy GP, Gotway MB, et al: Malignant pleural mesothelioma: Evaluation with CT, MR imaging, and PET. Radiographics 24:105-119, 2004.

Yamamuro M, Gerbaudo VH, Gill RR, et al: Morphologic and functional imaging of malignant pleural mesothelioma. Eur J Radiol 64:356-366, 2007.

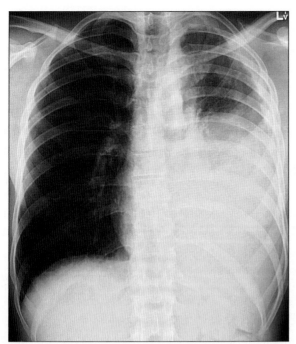

Figure 1. Posteroanterior chest radiograph shows opacification of the left, lower hemithorax with extension into the lateral and apical regions and a lobulated contour of the left mediastinal interface. Notice the volume loss with an ipsilateral mediastinal shift. The patient was a 43-year-old man with malignant mesothelioma.

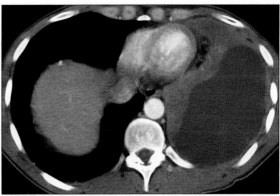

Figure 3. In the same patient, CT at the level of the ventricles shows diffuse, left pleural thickening and a loculated, left pleural effusion.

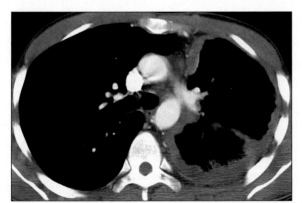

Figure 2. In the same patient, contrast-enhanced CT at the level of the aortopulmonary window demonstrates diffuse, nodular, left pleural thickening with involvement of the interlobar fissure and mediastinal pleura. Notice the volume loss with an ipsilateral mediastinal shift.

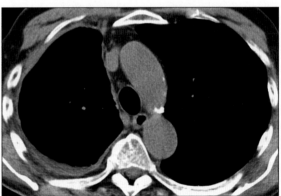

Figure 4. CT shows circumferential, right pleural thickening with associated volume loss. The thickening of the costal pleura is smooth, and that of the mediastinal pleura is nodular. The patient was an 80-year-old man with malignant mesothelioma.

Case 170

DEMOGRAPHICS/CLINICAL HISTORY

A 72-year-old woman with shortness of breath, cough, malaise, and weight loss, undergoing radiography and computed tomography (CT).

FINDINGS

Posteroanterior chest radiograph (Fig. 1) shows a large, right pleural effusion, apical pleural thickening, and increased soft tissue opacity in the right paratracheal region. Contrast-enhanced CT at the level of the trachea (Fig. 2) shows nodular, right pleural thickening with involvement of the mediastinal pleura and enlarged paratracheal and internal mammary lymph nodes. CT at the level of the tracheal carina (Fig. 3) shows a loculated, right pleural effusion and diffuse, right pleural thickening. A pulmonary nodule that is adjacent to the pleura is presumably the primary pulmonary carcinoma.

DISCUSSION

Definition/Background

Pleural metastases account for most malignant tumors of the pleura and approximately 80% percent of all malignant pleural effusions. The most common tumors that metastasize to the pleura are bronchogenic carcinoma, breast cancer, ovarian cancer, gastric carcinoma, and lymphoma.

Characteristic Clinical Features

Patients have dyspnea, pleuritic chest pain, weight loss, and malaise.

Characteristic Radiologic Findings

The most common finding in patients with pleural metastases is pleural effusion. Other common findings include pleural nodules, nodular pleural thickening, and circumferential pleural thickening. Increased radiotracer uptake is seen on ^{18}F-fluorodeoxyglucose positron emission tomography (FDG-PET).

Less Common Radiologic Manifestations

Imaging may show enlarged mediastinal, pericardiophrenic, and internal mammary nodes and extension into adjacent soft tissues.

Differential Diagnosis

- Mesothelioma
- Lymphoma

Discussion

Metastatic pleural disease is more common than mesothelioma and can be radiologically indistinguishable from mesothelioma. Features that favor metastases include a known primary lung cancer, breast cancer, or lymphoma and systemic metastases.

Diagnosis

Pleural metastases

Suggested Readings

Aquino SL: Imaging of metastatic disease to the thorax. Radiol Clin North Am 43:481-495, vii, 2005.

Bonomo L, Feragalli B, Sacco R, et al: Malignant pleural disease. Eur J Radiol 34:98-118, 2000.

English JC, Leslie KO: Pathology of the pleura. Clin Chest Med 27:157-180, 2006.

Qureshi NR, Gleeson FV: Imaging of pleural disease. Clin Chest Med 27:193-213, 2006.

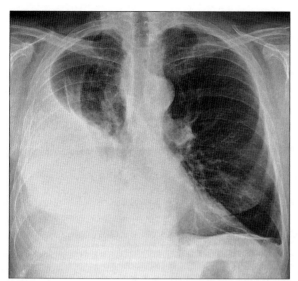

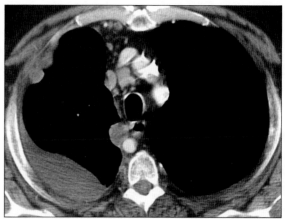

Figure 2. In the same patient, contrast-enhanced CT at the level of the trachea shows nodular, right pleural thickening with involvement of the mediastinal pleura and enlarged paratracheal and internal mammary lymph nodes.

Figure 1. Posteroanterior chest radiograph shows a large, right pleural effusion, apical pleural thickening, and increased soft tissue opacity in the right paratracheal region. The patient was a 72-year-old woman with right pleural metastases from an adenocarcinoma.

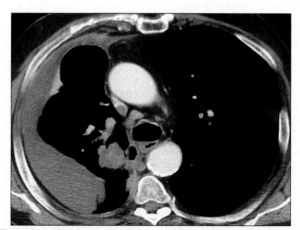

Figure 3. In the same patient, CT at the level of the tracheal carina shows a loculated, right pleural effusion and diffuse, right pleural thickening. A pulmonary nodule that is adjacent to the pleura is presumably the primary pulmonary carcinoma.

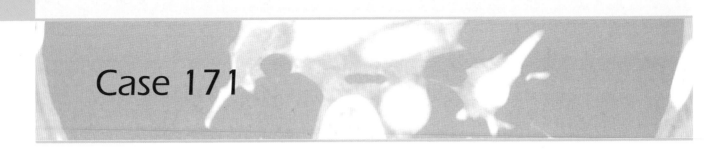

Case 171

DEMOGRAPHICS/CLINICAL HISTORY

A 71-year-old woman who is asymptomatic, undergoing computed tomography (CT).

FINDINGS

CT images using lung (Fig. 1) and soft tissue (Fig. 2) windows show a pleura-based, smoothly marginated nodule in the region of the right major fissure. Sagittal, reformatted CT (Fig. 3) shows that the nodule is located within the major fissure. In another patient with primary fibrous tumor of the pleura, CT (Fig. 4) shows a large, smoothly marginated, homogeneous soft tissue mass in the right lower hemithorax.

DISCUSSION

Definition/Background

Localized fibrous tumor is a relatively uncommon primary neoplasm of the pleura. It has a mesenchymal rather than mesothelial cell origin. It accounts for approximately 5% to 10% of primary tumors of the pleura, has no relation to asbestos exposure, and may be benign or, less commonly, malignant.

Characteristic Clinical Features

Patients may be asymptomatic or present with cough, dyspnea, or chest pain. Approximately 4% of cases are associated with finger clubbing (i.e., hypertrophic osteoarthropathy) and 4% with symptomatic hypoglycemia.

Characteristic Radiologic Findings

Localized fibrous tumor of pleura typically manifests as a single, well-defined, smoothly marginated, pleura-based soft tissue nodule or mass. Small tumors have homogeneous soft tissue attenuation on CT but may have heterogeneous attenuation due to areas of necrosis, hemorrhage, and cystic changes.

Less Common Radiologic Manifestations

Imaging may show foci of calcification, a pedicle, a tumor originating from an interlobar fissure, or a pleural effusion.

Differential Diagnosis

- Pulmonary carcinoma
- Pleural metastasis
- Pleural lipoma
- Neurilemoma

Discussion

The differential diagnosis of a pleura-based mass seen on the chest radiograph is broad and includes peripheral bronchogenic carcinoma, solitary pleural metastasis, pleural lipoma, partial diaphragmatic eventration, and intercostal neurilemoma or neurofibroma. In most cases, the diagnosis of primary fibrous tumor can be suggested on CT. Definitive diagnosis requires core-needle biopsy or surgery.

Diagnosis

Fibrous tumor of the pleura

Suggested Readings

Qureshi NR, Gleeson FV: Imaging of pleural disease. Clin Chest Med 27:193-213, 2006.

Robinson LA: Solitary fibrous tumor of the pleura. Cancer Control 13:264-269, 2006.

Rosado-de-Christenson ML, Abbott GF, McAdams HP, et al: From the archives of the AFIP: Localized fibrous tumor of the pleura. Radiographics 23:759-783, 2003.

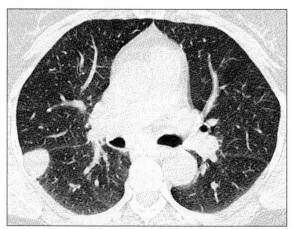

Figure 1. CT using lung windows shows a pleura-based, smoothly marginated nodule in the region of the right major fissure. The patient was a 71-year-old woman with a primary fibrous tumor of the pleura.

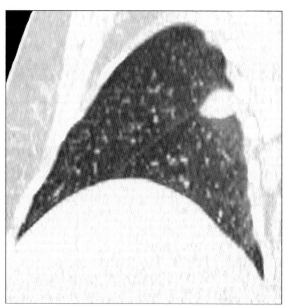

Figure 3. In the same patient, sagittal, reformatted CT shows that the nodule is located within the major fissure.

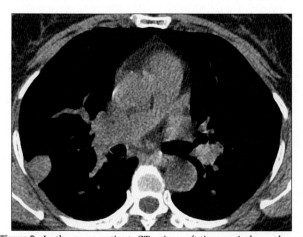

Figure 2. In the same patient, CT using soft tissue windows shows that the nodule has homogeneous soft tissue attenuation.

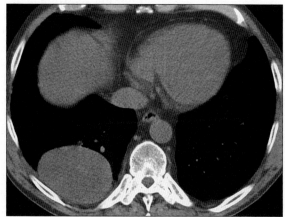

Figure 4. CT shows a large, smoothly marginated, homogeneous soft tissue mass in the right lower hemithorax. The patient was a 70-year-old man with primary fibrous tumor of the pleura.

Case 172

DEMOGRAPHICS/CLINICAL HISTORY

A 55-year-old man who is asymptomatic, undergoing radiography and computed tomography (CT).

FINDINGS

Posteroanterior radiograph (Fig. 1) of the left hemithorax shows a homogeneous opacity with smooth margins, a sharply defined medial edge, and an ill-defined lateral border characteristic of a pleura-based lesion. CT using lung windows (Fig. 2) to view the left hemithorax shows a smoothly marginated lesion forming obtuse angles with the chest wall posteriorly and straight angles anteriorly. CT using soft tissue windows (Fig. 3) shows homogeneous fat attenuation of the pleura-based lesion. In another patient with a pleural lipoma, contrast-enhanced CT (Fig. 4) shows a pleura-based lesion with homogeneous fat attenuation in the right hemithorax.

DISCUSSION

Definition/Background

Pleural and extrapleural lipomas are benign soft tissue neoplasms that likely arise from submesothelial mesenchymal cells. They are the most common pleural soft tissue neoplasm.

Characteristic Clinical Features

Patients are usually asymptomatic.

Characteristic Radiologic Findings

Pleural and extrapleural lipomas typically manifest as a single, well-defined, smoothly marginated, pleura-based soft tissue mass that often has tapering margins and forms obtuse angles with the chest wall. Lipomas have characteristic uniform fat density (-50 to -120 HU) on CT and uniform signal intensity similar to subcutaneous fat on magnetic resonance imaging (MRI).

Less Common Radiologic Manifestations

Imaging may show foci of calcification, a pedicle, a tumor originating from an interlobar fissure, or pleural effusion.

Differential Diagnosis

- Pleural liposarcoma
- Fibrous tumor of the pleura
- Pleural metastasis
- Neurilemoma
- Pulmonary carcinoma

Discussion

The differential diagnosis of a pleura-based mass based on the chest radiographic findings includes fibrous tumor of the pleura, solitary pleural metastasis, intercostal neurilemoma or neurofibroma, and peripheral bronchogenic carcinoma. In most cases, a confident diagnosis of pleural lipoma can be made by demonstrating uniform fat density (-50 to -120 HU) on CT or by showing homogeneous signal intensity similar to that of subcutaneous fat on MRI. When the tumor is heterogeneous and has areas with attenuation values greater than -50 HU, a liposarcoma should be suspected.

Diagnosis

Pleural and extrapleural lipoma

Suggested Readings

McLoud TC: CT and MR in pleural disease. Clin Chest Med 19:261-276, 1998.
Müller NL: Imaging of the pleura. Radiology 186:297-309, 1993.
Qureshi NR, Gleeson FV: Imaging of pleural disease. Clin Chest Med 27:193-213, 2006.

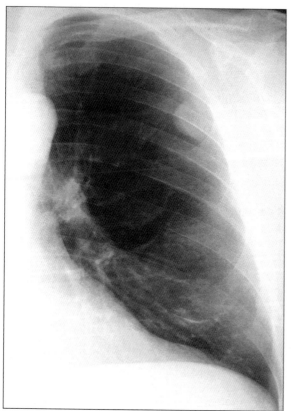

Figure 1. Posteroanterior radiograph of the left hemithorax shows a homogeneous opacity with smooth margins, a sharply defined medial edge, and an ill-defined lateral border characteristic of a pleura-based lesion. The patient was a 55-year-old man with a pleural lipoma.

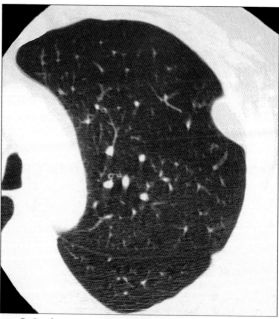

Figure 2. In the same patient, CT using lung windows to view the left hemithorax shows a smoothly marginated lesion forming obtuse angles with the chest wall posteriorly and straight angles anteriorly, consistent with a pleura-based lesion.

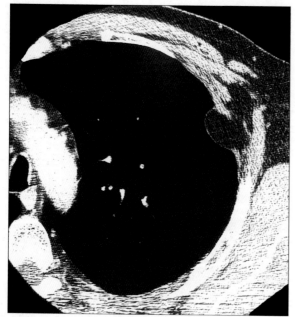

Figure 3. In the same patient, CT using soft tissue windows shows a pleura-based lesion with homogeneous fat attenuation.

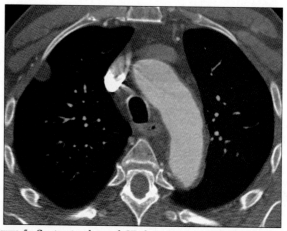

Figure 4. Contrast-enhanced CT shows a pleura-based lesion with homogeneous fat attenuation in the right hemithorax. The patient was a 75-year-old man with a pleural lipoma.

Case 173

DEMOGRAPHICS/CLINICAL HISTORY

A 21-year-old man with acute shortness of breath, undergoing radiography and compared with computed tomography (CT).

FINDINGS

Posteroanterior chest radiograph (Fig. 1) reveals a fine linear shadow parallel to and separated from the left heart border and mediastinum by a band of translucent air. Notice the hyperinflation and bronchial wall thickening. In other patients, chest radiographs show vertical streaks of radiolucency within the upper mediastinum and lower neck (Fig. 2) and mediastinal air along the diaphragm and below the heart (Fig.3), allowing identification of the central portion of the diaphragm in continuity with the lateral portions (i.e., continuous diaphragm sign), and CT (Fig. 4) shows streaks of air within the posterior mediastinum.

DISCUSSION

Definition/Background

Pneumomediastinum is air or other gas in the mediastinal space. The air or gas may reach the mediastinum from ruptured alveoli (e.g., asthma, pneumonia, positive-pressure ventilation), mediastinal airways (e.g., tracheal or bronchial injury due to blunt trauma, endotracheal intubation, bronchoscopy), the esophagus (e.g., Boerhaave's syndrome), the neck (e.g., retropharyngeal abscess), and, occasionally, the abdominal cavity (e.g., perforation of a hollow viscus).

Characteristic Clinical Features

The patients may be asymptomatic or present with chest discomfort, retrosternal pain, dyspnea, or dysphagia.

Characteristic Radiologic Findings

Pneumomediastinum manifests as vertical streaks of radiolucency within the mediastinal shadow. The parietal pleura, peeled off from the mediastinal structures, can be seen as a fine linear shadow that is parallel to and separated from the heart and mediastinum by a band of translucent air.

Less Common Radiologic Manifestations

Radiographic visualization of mediastinal air along the diaphragm and below the heart allows identification of the central portion of the diaphragm in continuity with the lateral portions (i.e., continuous diaphragm sign). A longitudinal or circular gas shadow is visible adjacent to the thoracic aorta and around the pulmonary artery (i.e., ring-around-the-artery sign). The presence of pneumomediastinum and its extent are readily recognized on CT.

Differential Diagnosis

- Pneumopericardium
- Pneumothorax

Discussion

A fine, lucent line along the left heart border, parallel to and separated from the heart and mediastinum, may result from pneumomediastinum or pneumopericardium. The diagnosis depends on the anatomic extent of the air. Pneumopericardium may extend from the diaphragm to just below the aortic arch but does not extend around the aortic arch or into the superior mediastinum. A lateral decubitus view is helpful in differentiating pneumopericardium from pneumomediastinum.

In theory, pneumopericardium should permit visualization of the central portion of the diaphragm (i.e., continuous diaphragm sign), but in clinical practice, pneumopericardium usually is associated with pericardial fluid, which leads to obliteration of the central portion of the diaphragm, at least on radiographs obtained with the patient in an erect position.

Diagnosis

Pneumomediastinum

Suggested Readings

Bejvan SM, Godwin JD: Pneumomediastinum: Old signs and new signs. AJR Am J Roentgenol 166:1041-1048, 1996.
Zylak CM, Standen JR, Barnes GR, Zylak CJ: Pneumomediastinum revisited. Radiographics 20:1043-1057, 2000.

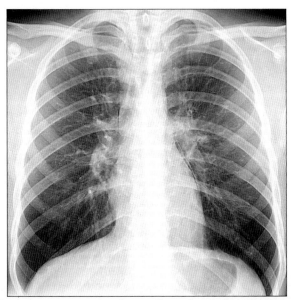

Figure 1. Posteroanterior chest radiograph reveals a fine linear shadow parallel to and separated from the left heart border and mediastinum by a band of translucent air. Notice the hyperinflation and bronchial wall thickening. The patient was a 21-year-old man with acute asthma and pneumomediastinum.

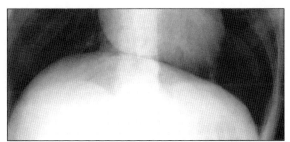

Figure 3. Chest radiograph of the lower chest and upper abdomen shows mediastinal air along the diaphragm and below the heart, allowing identification of the central portion of the diaphragm in continuity with the lateral portions (i.e., continuous diaphragm sign).

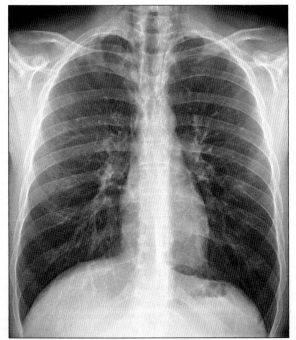

Figure 2. Posteroanterior chest radiograph shows vertical streaks of radiolucency within the upper mediastinum and lower neck. The patient was an 18-year-old boy with pneumomediastinum and subcutaneous emphysema caused by a ruptured esophagus after an episode of excessive vomiting (i.e., Boerhaave syndrome).

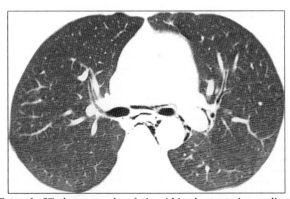

Figure 4. CT shows streaks of air within the posterior mediastinum. The patient was an 16-year-old boy with pneumomediastinum resulting from esophageal perforation caused by a chicken bone.

Case 174

DEMOGRAPHICS/CLINICAL HISTORY

A 25-year-old man with fever and neck and chest pain, undergoing computed tomography (CT).

FINDINGS

Contrast-enhanced CT images at the level of the lower neck (Fig.1), thoracic inlet (Fig. 2), and aortic arch (Fig. 3) show increased soft tissue density with obscuration of the fat planes and several focal areas of low attenuation, some of which have rim enhancement. CT also identifies a small left pleural effusion (Fig. 3).

DISCUSSION

Definition/Background

Mediastinitis is focal or diffuse inflammation of the tissues located in the middle chest cavity (i.e., tissues in the partition between the lungs). The most common cause of acute mediastinitis is perforation or rupture of the esophagus; other causes include perforation or rupture of airways, surgery, and extension of infection from adjacent tissues (e.g., retropharyngeal abscess, paraspinous abscess).

Characteristic Clinical Features

Patients may have sudden onset of retrosternal pain, worsened by breathing or coughing; high fever; chills; tachycardia; and tachypnea. The symptoms may be associated with spontaneous rupture of the esophagus due to a violent vomiting episode (i.e., Boerhaave syndrome).

Characteristic Radiologic Findings

Radiologic findings include widening and poor definition of the margins of the mediastinum. Pneumomediastinum and subcutaneous emphysema may coexist in patients with esophageal or tracheal perforation or rupture. CT shows increased soft tissue density of the mediastinum, obliteration of fat planes, and commonly, localized areas of decreased attenuation with rim enhancement due to abscess formation. CT findings of acute mediastinitis caused by esophageal perforation include esophageal thickening, extraluminal gas, single or multiple mediastinal abscesses, and extraluminal contrast medium.

Less Common Radiologic Manifestations

Mediastinal lymphadenopathy, pleural effusion (Fig. 3), pericardial effusion

Differential Diagnosis

- Mediastinal hemorrhage
- Mediastinal lymphadenopathy
- Mediastinal lipomatosis

Discussion

A widened mediastinum seen on the chest radiograph is a nonspecific finding that may be a normal variant or may be caused by infection, hemorrhage, lymphadenopathy, a mass, or mediastinal lipomatosis. The main role of imaging in the assessment of acute mediastinitis is to confirm mediastinal abnormalities that are consistent with the clinical diagnosis. The radiographic finding of a widened mediastinum in the clinical setting of fever and pleuritic chest pain strongly suggests acute mediastinitis. CT is the imaging modality of choice for the identification of acute mediastinitis and assessment of its extent.

Diagnosis

Acute mediastinitis

Suggested Readings

Akman C, Kantarci F, Cetinkaya S: Imaging in mediastinitis: A systematic review based on aetiology. Clin Radiol 59:573-585, 2004.

Exarhos DN, Malagari K, Tsatalou EG, et al: Acute mediastinitis: Spectrum of computed tomography findings. Eur Radiol 15:1569-1574, 2005.

Gimenez A, Franquet T, Erasmus JJ, et al: Thoracic complications of esophageal disorders. Radiographics 22:S247-S258, 2002.

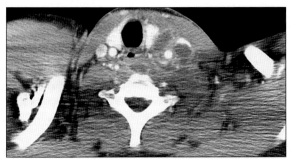

Figure 1. Contrast-enhanced CT shows increased soft tissue density with obscuration of the fat planes in the left lower neck, which is consistent with inflammation, and several focal areas of low attenuation with rim enhancement, which is consistent with abscess formation. The patient was a 25-year-old man with multiple cervical abscesses after wisdom tooth extraction.

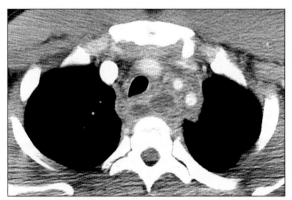

Figure 2. In the same patient, contrast-enhanced CT at the level of the thoracic inlet shows increased soft tissue density with obscuration of the fat planes, which is consistent with mediastinitis, and several focal areas of low attenuation with rim enhancement, which is consistent with abscess formation.

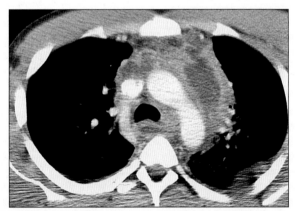

Figure 3. In the same patient, contrast-enhanced CT at the level of the aortic arch shows increased soft tissue density with obscuration of the fat planes, which is consistent with mediastinitis, and several focal areas of low attenuation with rim enhancement, which is consistent with abscess formation. A small, left pleural effusion can be seen.

Case 175

DEMOGRAPHICS/CLINICAL HISTORY

An 82-year-old woman with cough and exertional dyspnea, undergoing computed tomography (CT).

FINDINGS

Contrast-enhanced CT images at the level of the right hilum (Figs. 1 to 3) show increased soft tissue density, narrowing of the distal right interlobar (Fig. 1) and proximal right lower lobe (Figs. 1 and 2) pulmonary arteries, foci of calcification (Fig. 3), and complete obstruction of the right middle lobe artery and bronchus (Fig. 3).

DISCUSSION

Definition/Background

Fibrosing mediastinitis is a rare entity characterized by an excessive focal or diffuse fibrotic reaction of the mediastinal tissues, which can lead to compression of mediastinal structures, particularly vessels and bronchi. Focal fibrosing mediastinitis usually is caused by granulomatous infection, most commonly histoplasmosis or tuberculosis. Diffuse fibrosing mediastinitis may be idiopathic or result from the exposure to certain drugs, such as methysergide.

Characteristic Clinical Features

Clinical manifestations depend on the degree of compression of mediastinal structures. Patients may present with signs and symptoms of obstruction of the superior vena cava, major pulmonary vessels, central airways, or esophagus.

Characteristic Radiologic Findings

Granulomatous mediastinitis due to histoplasmosis or tuberculosis typically results in a localized calcified mass, usually in the right paratracheal region or hilum, with associated narrowing of one or more vessels or airways. Diffuse mediastinitis results in nonspecific widening of the mediastinum, as seen on the radiograph; a diffuse, infiltrative mass of soft tissue attenuation that obliterates normal mediastinal fat planes, as seen on CT; and narrowing of one or more vessels or airways.

Less Common Radiologic Manifestations

Imaging may show collateral circulation in patients with superior vena cava obstruction.

Differential Diagnosis

- Mediastinal hemorrhage
- Mediastinal lymphadenopathy
- Mediastinal lipomatosis
- Lymphoma
- Pulmonary carcinoma

Discussion

A widened mediastinum seen on the chest radiograph is a nonspecific finding that may be a normal variant or be caused by infection, hemorrhage, lymphadenopathy, a mass, or mediastinal lipomatosis. CT is performed almost routinely in the assessment of patients with suspected fibrosing mediastinitis. In the appropriate clinical context, the finding of a localized mediastinal soft tissue mass with calcification is virtually diagnostic of granulomatous fibrosing mediastinitis, and it obviates the need for tissue sampling. If the mass is not calcified or if there is clinical or radiologic evidence of disease progression, biopsy may be required to exclude a neoplasm.

Diagnosis

Fibrosing mediastinitis

Suggested Readings

Akman C, Kantarci F, Cetinkaya S: Imaging in mediastinitis: A systematic review based on aetiology. Clin Radiol 59:573-585, 2004.

Atasoy C, Fitoz S, Erguvan B, Akyar S: Tuberculous fibrosing mediastinitis: CT and MRI findings. J Thorac Imaging 16:191-193, 2001.

Chong S, Kim TS, Kim BT, Cho EY: Fibrosing mediastinitis mimicking malignancy at CT: Negative FDG uptake in integrated FDG PET/CT imaging. Eur Radiol 17:1644-1646, 2007.

Rossi SE, McAdams HP, Rosado-de-Christenson ML, et al: Fibrosing mediastinitis. Radiographics 21:737-757, 2001.

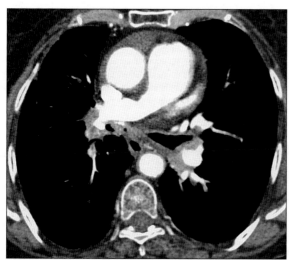

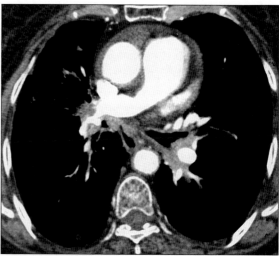

Figure 1. Contrast-enhanced CT at the level of the right pulmonary artery shows increased soft tissue density in the right hilum and narrowing of the distal right interlobar pulmonary artery and bronchus intermedius. The patient was an 82-year-old woman with fibrosing mediastinitis related to prior tuberculosis.

Figure 2. In the same patient, contrast-enhanced CT at the level of the right pulmonary artery immediately caudal to the level in Figure 1 shows increased soft tissue density in the right hilum and narrowing of the distal right interlobar pulmonary artery and bronchus intermedius.

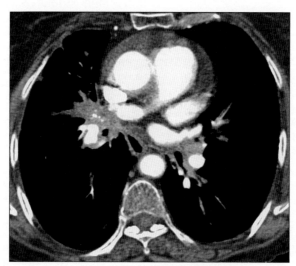

Figure 3. In the same patient, contrast-enhanced CT at the level of the right lower lobe pulmonary artery shows increased soft tissue density and foci of calcification in the right hilum and complete obstruction of the right middle lobe pulmonary artery and bronchus.

Case 176

DEMOGRAPHICS/CLINICAL HISTORY

A 26-year-old man with hyperthyroidism, tachycardia, and muscle weakness, undergoing computed tomography (CT).

FINDINGS

Contrast-enhanced CT (Fig. 1) shows a diffusely enlarged thymus. CT 7 months later (Fig. 2), after treatment of Graves' disease, shows that the size of the thymus is normal.

DISCUSSION

Definition/Background

Thymic hyperplasia is an increase in size and weight of a thymus gland that is otherwise normal. It usually is a rebound phenomenon after atrophy caused by corticosteroids or chemotherapy, and it occurs several months after resolution of the cause of atrophy. Occasionally, it may result from hyperthyroidism.

Characteristic Clinical Features

Patients are asymptomatic.

Characteristic Radiologic Findings

A diffuse increase in the size of the thymus gland is evident on the radiograph or CT scan. Typically, the increase in size develops several months after atrophy of the gland.

Differential Diagnosis

- Normal thymus
- Thymic lymphoid hyperplasia
- Thymoma
- Lymphoma

Discussion

Thymic hyperplasia, also known as rebound hyperplasia, is the most common cause of a diffusely enlarged thymus. It typically is a rebound phenomenon after atrophy caused by corticosteroids or chemotherapy, and it is not associated with any symptoms. Thymic lymphoid hyperplasia refers to the presence of an increased number of lymphoid follicles, and it is most commonly associated with myasthenia gravis (60% to 80% of cases). The thymus in lymphoid hyperplasia usually has a normal size and appearance on CT and magnetic resonance imaging; occasionally lymphoid hyperplasia may result in a diffusely enlarged thymus or a focal mass.

Diagnosis

Thymic hyperplasia

Suggested Readings

Baron RL, Lee JK, Sagel SS, Peterson RR: Computed tomography of the normal thymus. Radiology 142:121-125, 1982.

Bogot NR, Quint LE: Imaging of thymic disorders. Cancer Imaging 5:139-149, 2005.

Kissin CM, Husband JE, Nicholas D, Eversman W: Benign thymic enlargement in adults after chemotherapy: CT demonstration. Radiology 163:67-70, 1987.

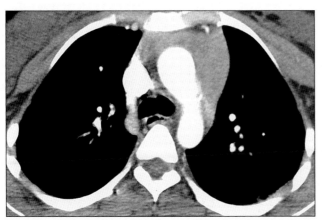

Figure 1. Contrast-enhanced CT shows a diffusely enlarged thymus. The patient was a 26-year-old man with hyperthyroidism due to Graves disease.

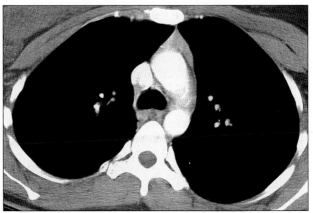

Figure 2. In the same patient 7 months after treatment of Graves disease, CT shows that the size of the thymus is normal.

Case 177

DEMOGRAPHICS/CLINICAL HISTORY

A 33-year-old woman with myasthenia gravis, undergoing computed tomography (CT).

FINDINGS

CT (Fig. 1) shows a normal thymus.

DISCUSSION

Definition/Background

Thymic lymphoid hyperplasia, also know as thymic follicular hyperplasia, refers to an increased number of thymic lymphoid follicles. Lymphoid hyperplasia is seen in 60% to 80% of patients with myasthenia gravis. It may also occur in a number of immunologically mediated disorders, including systemic lupus erythematosus, rheumatoid arthritis, scleroderma, thyrotoxicosis, and Graves disease.

Characteristic Clinical Features

Patients with thymic lymphoid hyperplasia typically present with myasthenia gravis.

Characteristic Radiologic Findings

A normal thymus is usually seen on CT and magnetic resonance imaging (MRI). Occasionally, thymic lymphoid hyperplasia may result in diffuse enlargement of the thymus or a focal mass.

Less Common Radiologic Manifestations

- Diffuse enlargement of thymus
- Focal mass

Differential Diagnosis

- Thymic rebound hyperplasia
- Thymoma

Discussion

The most common cause of a diffusely enlarged thymus is thymic hyperplasia (i.e., rebound hyperplasia). Occasionally, thymic lymphoid hyperplasia may result in a diffusely enlarged thymus. The distinguishing feature is that patients with thymic lymphoid hyperplasia commonly present with myasthenia gravis. Thymic lymphoid hyperplasia manifesting as a focal mass may be clinically and radiologically indistinguishable from thymoma.

Diagnosis

Thymic lymphoid hyperplasia

Suggested Readings

Bogot NR, Quint LE: Imaging of thymic disorders. Cancer Imaging 5:139-149, 2005.

de Kraker M, Kluin J, Renken N, et al: CT and myasthenia gravis: Correlation between mediastinal imaging and histopathological findings. Interact Cardiovasc Thorac Surg 4:267-271, 2005.

Inaoka T, Takahashi K, Mineta M, et al: Thymic hyperplasia and thymus gland tumors: Differentiation with chemical shift MR imaging. Radiology 243:869-876, 2007.

Nicolaou S, Müller NL, Li DKB, Oger JJF: Thymus in myasthenia gravis: Comparison CT and pathologic findings and clinical outcome after thymectomy. Radiology 201:471-474, 1996.

Takahashi K, Inaoka T, Murakami N, et al: Characterization of the normal and hyperplastic thymus on chemical-shift MR imaging. AJR Am J Roentgenol 180:1265-1269, 2003.

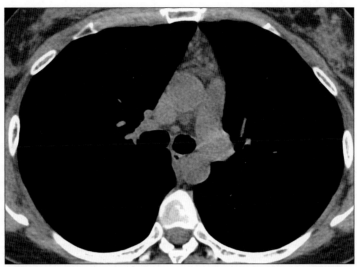

Figure 1. CT shows a normal thymus. The patient was a 33-year-old woman with lymphoid hyperplasia of the thymus and myasthenia gravis.

Case 178

DEMOGRAPHICS/CLINICAL HISTORY

A 58-year-old woman with myasthenia gravis, undergoing radiography and computed tomography (CT).

FINDINGS

Posteroanterior (Fig. 1) and lateral (Fig. 2) chest radiographs show a large, anterior mediastinal mass. Contrast-enhanced CT (Fig. 3) shows a well-defined, anterior mediastinal mass with homogeneous soft tissue attenuation.

DISCUSSION

Definition/Background

Thymomas are thymic epithelial tumors composed of a mixture of thymic epithelial cells and lymphocytes without apparent cellular atypia. Thymomas are seen most commonly in patients who are between 50 and 65 years old.

Characteristic Clinical Features

Patients with thymoma often are asymptomatic, with the tumor found incidentally on the chest radiograph or CT scan. Approximately 40% of patients with thymoma present with myasthenia gravis. Less common paraneoplastic syndromes associated with thymoma include pure red cell aplasia, hypogammaglobulinemia, and stiff person syndrome.

Characteristic Radiologic Findings

The radiographic manifestations of thymoma typically consist of an anterior mediastinal mass situated near the junction of the heart and great vessels. The shape is round or oval, and the margins usually are smooth or lobulated. Tumors usually have homogenous soft tissue attenuation on CT; less commonly and usually in large tumors, hemorrhage, necrosis, or cystic formation leads to focal areas of low attenuation.

Less Common Radiologic Manifestations

Imaging may show punctate, linear, or ring-like calcification in the capsule (or margin) or within the tumor. Radiologic study may reveal irregular tumor margins, tumor invasion of great vascular structures or the chest wall, encasement of mediastinal structures, irregular interface with the adjacent lung, and pleural dissemination (i.e., drop metastases) or pericardial involvement.

Differential Diagnosis

- Thymic lymphoid hyperplasia
- Thymic carcinoma
- Lymphoma
- Germ cell tumor

Discussion

The differential diagnosis for an anterior mediastinal mass includes Hodgkin disease, non-Hodgkin lymphoma, thymic neoplasms, substernal thyroid mass, germ cell tumors, and mediastinal tuberculous lymphadenopathy. Findings that favor Hodgkin disease and lymphoma include lobulation and involvement of multiple lymph node groups. Definitive diagnosis requires biopsy. Thymic lymphoid hyperplasia manifesting as a focal mass may be clinically and radiologically indistinguishable from thymoma. Thymic carcinoma typically manifests as a heterogeneous, anterior mediastinal mass that frequently contains areas of necrosis and commonly invades adjacent structures, whereas thymomas most commonly manifest as smoothly marginated, fairly homogeneous masses. Thymic carcinomas are not associated with myasthenia gravis.

Diagnosis

Thymoma

Suggested Readings

Bogot NR, Quint LE: Imaging of thymic disorders. Cancer Imaging 5:139-149, 2005.

Maher MM, Shepard JAO: Imaging of thymoma. Semin Thorac Cardiovasc Surg 17:12-19, 2005.

Sadohara J, Fujimoto K, Müller NL, et al: Thymic epithelial tumors: Comparison of CT and MR imaging findings of low-risk thymomas, high-risk thymomas, and thymic carcinomas. Eur J Radiol 60:70-79, 2006.

Tomiyama N, Müller NL, Ellis SJ, et al: Invasive and noninvasive thymoma: Distinctive CT features. J Comput Assist Tomogr 25:388-393, 2001.

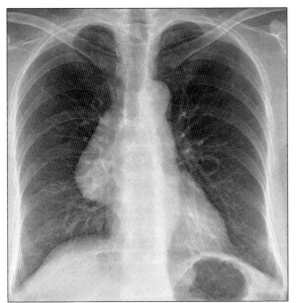

Figure 1. Posteroanterior chest radiograph shows a mediastinal mass projecting over the right hilum. Notice that the hilum is easily seen, indicating that the mass is anterior or posterior to the hilum (i.e., hilum overlay sign). The patient was a 58-year-old woman with thymoma and myasthenia gravis.

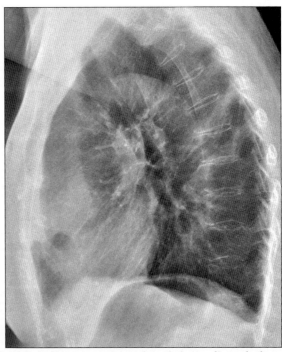

Figure 2. In the same patient, a lateral chest radiograph shows a large anterior mediastinal mass.

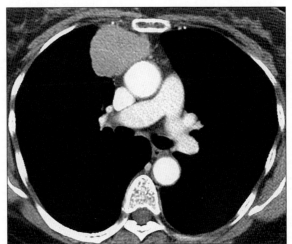

Figure 3. In the same patient, contrast-enhanced CT shows a well-defined, anterior mediastinal mass with homogeneous soft tissue attenuation.

Case 179

DEMOGRAPHICS/CLINICAL HISTORY

A 39-year-old woman with chest pain and fatigue, undergoing radiography and computed tomography (CT).

FINDINGS

Posteroanterior chest radiograph (Fig. 1) shows widening of the mediastinum. Contrast-enhanced CT (Fig. 2) shows an inhomogeneous, anterior mediastinal mass with ill-defined borders and obliteration of the fat planes throughout the anterior mediastinum and soft tissue infiltration between the superior vena cava and aortic arch.

DISCUSSION

Definition/Background
Thymic carcinomas are thymic tumors in which the epithelial cells exhibit the cytologic features of malignancy. The most common type is squamous cell carcinoma. These tumors often lack a capsule and may be adherent to mediastinal structures or be metastatic to mediastinal lymph nodes at the time of resection.

Characteristic Clinical Features
The most common symptoms are chest pain, cough, fatigue, fever, anorexia, and superior vena cava syndrome. Thymic carcinoma is not associated with myasthenia gravis.

Characteristic Radiologic Findings
The characteristic findings consist of a large, anterior mediastinal mass with irregular or lobulated margins and heterogeneous attenuation on CT due to areas of necrosis or cystic changes. The tumor commonly invades adjacent structures and often is associated with mediastinal lymphadenopathy.

Less Common Radiologic Manifestations
Imaging may show foci of calcification within the tumor and metastases to lungs, bone, liver, and brain.

Differential Diagnosis
- Thymoma
- Mediastinal lymphoma
- Germ cell tumors

Discussion
The differential diagnosis for an anterior mediastinal mass includes Hodgkin disease, non-Hodgkin lymphoma, thymic neoplasms, substernal thyroid mass, germ cell tumors, and mediastinal tuberculous lymphadenopathy. Findings that favor Hodgkin disease and lymphoma include lobulation and involvement of multiple lymph node groups. Definitive diagnosis requires biopsy. Thymomas most commonly manifest as smoothly marginated, fairly homogeneous masses without associated lymphadenopathy, whereas thymic carcinoma typically manifests as a heterogeneous, anterior mediastinal mass that frequently contains areas of necrosis, commonly invades adjacent structures, and commonly is associated with mediastinal lymphadenopathy.

Diagnosis
Thymic carcinoma

Suggested Readings
Bogot NR, Quint LE: Imaging of thymic disorders. Cancer Imaging 5:139-149, 2005.
Sadohara J, Fujimoto K, Müller NL, et al: Thymic epithelial tumors: Comparison of CT and MR imaging findings of low-risk thymomas, high-risk thymomas, and thymic carcinomas. Eur J Radiol 60:70-79, 2006.

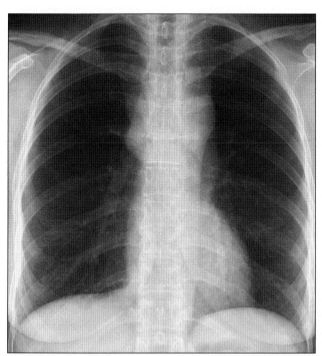

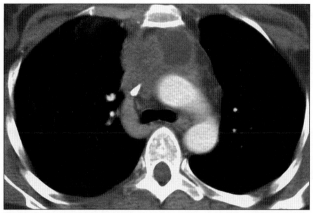

Figure 2. In the same patient, contrast-enhanced CT shows an inhomogeneous, anterior mediastinal mass with ill-defined borders and obliteration of the fat planes throughout the anterior mediastinum and soft tissue infiltration between the superior vena cava and aortic arch.

Figure 1. Posteroanterior chest radiograph shows widening of the mediastinum. The patient was a 39-year-old woman with thymic carcinoma.

Case 180

DEMOGRAPHICS/CLINICAL HISTORY

A 34-year-old woman with chest pain, undergoing computed tomography (CT).

FINDINGS

Contrast-enhanced CT images (Figs. 1 and 2) show an anterior mediastinal mass with inhomogeneous enhancement and areas of low attenuation consistent with necrosis. The mass has ill-defined borders, particularly on the left, and there is obliteration of the fat planes between the mass and the ascending aorta. Notice the enlarged, right, lower paratracheal lymph node (Fig. 1).

DISCUSSION

Definition/Background
Thymic carcinoid tumors are low-grade thymic neuroendocrine carcinomas. There are two types: relatively benign, typical carcinoid tumors and more aggressive, atypical carcinoid tumors. These tumors are considerably less common than thymomas and thymic squamous cell carcinomas.

Characteristic Clinical Features
The patients most commonly present with chest pain, cough, dyspnea, and superior vena cava syndrome. Approximately 20% to 30% of thymic carcinoid tumors in adults are associated with Cushing syndrome due to adrenocorticotropic hormone (ACTH) production. Carcinoid syndrome is rare.

Characteristic Radiologic Findings
The radiologic manifestations range from well-circumscribed to ill-defined, 2- to 20-cm, unencapsulated masses that often contain foci of necrosis and hemorrhage. Invasion of adjacent structures and lymphadenopathy may be seen in approximately 40% to 50% of cases. In patients presenting with Cushing syndrome, the tumors are usually small and may have homogeneous attenuation.

Less Common Radiologic Manifestations
Metastases to lung, liver, and adrenal glands

Differential Diagnosis
- Thymoma
- Thymic carcinoma
- Lymphoma
- Germ cell tumor

Discussion
The differential diagnosis for an anterior mediastinal mass includes Hodgkin disease, non-Hodgkin lymphoma, thymic neoplasms, substernal thyroid mass, germ cell tumors, and mediastinal tuberculous lymphadenopathy. Thymomas most commonly manifest as smoothly marginated, fairly homogeneous masses without associated lymphadenopathy, whereas thymic squamous cell carcinoma typically manifests as a heterogeneous, anterior mediastinal mass that frequently contains areas of necrosis, commonly invades adjacent structures, and is commonly associated with mediastinal lymphadenopathy. Thymic carcinoid tumors may resemble thymomas or, more commonly, thymic squamous cell carcinomas. Findings that favor lymphoma include lobulation and involvement of multiple lymph node group.

Diagnosis
Thymic carcinoid tumor

Suggested Readings
Groves AM, Mohan HK, Wegner EA, et al: Positron emission tomography with FDG to show thymic carcinoid. AJR Am J Roentgenol 182:511-513, 2004.

Quint LE: Imaging of anterior mediastinal masses. Cancer Imaging 7:S56-S62, 2007.

Sadohara J, Fujimoto K, Müller NL, et al: Thymic epithelial tumors: Comparison of CT and MR imaging findings of low-risk thymomas, high-risk thymomas, and thymic carcinomas. Eur J Radiol 60:70-79, 2006.

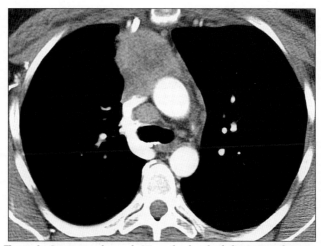

Figure 1. Contrast-enhanced CT at the level of the aortopulmonary window shows an anterior mediastinal mass with inhomogeneous enhancement and areas of low attenuation consistent with necrosis. The mass has ill-defined borders, particularly on the left, and there is obliteration of the fat planes between the mass and the ascending aorta. Notice the right paratracheal lymphadenopathy. The patient was a 34-year-old woman with a thymic carcinoid tumor.

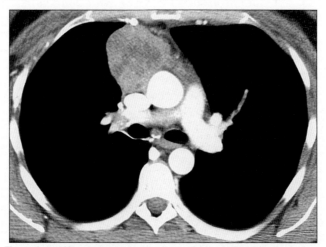

Figure 2. In the same patient, contrast-enhanced CT at the level of the main pulmonary arteries shows an anterior mediastinal mass with inhomogeneous enhancement and areas of low attenuation consistent with necrosis. The mass has ill-defined borders, particularly on the left, and there is obliteration of the fat planes between the mass and the ascending aorta.

Case 181

DEMOGRAPHICS/CLINICAL HISTORY

A 28-year-old man with chest pain, undergoing radiography and computed tomography (CT).

FINDINGS

Posteroanterior (Fig. 1) and lateral (Fig. 2) chest radiographs show a large anterior mediastinal mass. Contrast-enhanced CT (Fig. 3) shows a cystic, anterior mediastinal mass containing areas of soft tissue, fluid, and a focal area of fat density. In another patient with primary mediastinal teratoma, contrast-enhanced CT (Fig. 4) shows a heterogeneous, anterior mediastinal mass containing areas of soft tissue and fat density and several foci of calcification.

DISCUSSION

Definition/Background

Teratoma is a benign germ cell tumor composed of several types of mature and immature somatic tissues derived from two or three germinal layers (i.e., ectoderm, endoderm, and mesoderm). Teratomas account for 50% to 70% of all mediastinal germ cell tumors and approximately 7% to 9% of all mediastinal tumors. The mean age of adults at presentation is 28 years (range, 18 to 60 years).

Characteristic Clinical Features

Mediastinal teratomas are often asymptomatic and incidentally found on a chest radiograph. Symptoms include cough, dyspnea, and chest, back, or shoulder pain.

Characteristic Radiologic Findings

Teratomas usually are seen on the chest radiograph as well-circumscribed, rounded or lobulated, anterior mediastinal masses that are 3 to 25 cm in diameter. The characteristic feature on CT consists of heterogeneous attenuation, most commonly including soft tissue and fluid; foci of fat attenuation are seen in 50% to 70% of cases. Approximately 50% of cases have foci of calcification that may be curvilinear, flocculent, or punctate or that may form part of osseous structures or teeth within the lesion.

Less Common Radiologic Manifestations

The high lipid content of the cystic fluid may result in fat-fluid levels, which are seen in approximately 10% of cases. Intracystic hemorrhage and inflammation or rupture into the pleural or pericardial space may occur.

Differential Diagnosis

- Malignant germ cell tumor
- Thymoma
- Lymphoma
- Thymic carcinoma

Discussion

A mediastinal mass containing fat, calcification, and soft tissue with hairball-like opacities seen on CT strongly suggests a teratoma. Malignant germ cell tumors are seen almost exclusively in males; manifest as large, homogeneous or heterogeneous, anterior mediastinal masses with invasion of adjacent structures; and are usually associated with elevated levels of serum α-fetoprotein (AFP) or β-human chorionic gonadotropin (β-hCG). Thymomas most commonly manifest as smoothly marginated, fairly homogeneous masses; 40% are associated with myasthenia gravis. Primary mediastinal lymphomas may manifest as isolated, typically lobulated, homogeneous or inhomogeneous, anterior mediastinal masses; however, they more commonly are associated with mediastinal lymphadenopathy and other manifestations of systemic lymphoma.

Diagnosis

Mediastinal teratoma

Suggested Readings

Drevelegas A, Palladas P, Scordalaki A: Mediastinal germ cell tumors: A radiologic-pathologic review. Eur Radiol 11:1925-1932, 2001.

Gaerte SC, Meyer CA, Winer-Muram HT, et al: Fat-containing lesions of the chest. Radiographics 22:S61-S78, 2002.

Kim JH, Goo JM, Lee HJ, et al: Cystic tumors in the anterior mediastinum. Radiologic-pathological correlation. J Comput Assist Tomogr 27:714-723, 2003.

Quint LE: Imaging of anterior mediastinal masses. Cancer Imaging 7:S56-S62, 2007.

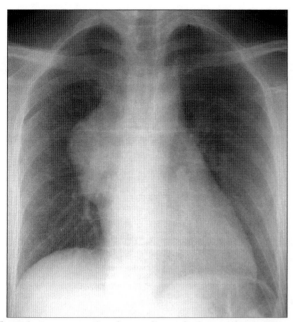

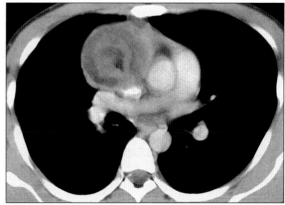

Figure 1. Posteroanterior chest radiograph shows a homogeneous soft tissue density projecting over the right paratracheal region and right hilum and forming obtuse angles with the mediastinum. The patient was a 28-year-old man with primary mediastinal teratoma.

Figure 3. In the same patient, contrast-enhanced CT shows a cystic, anterior mediastinal mass containing areas of soft tissue, fluid, and a focal area of fat density.

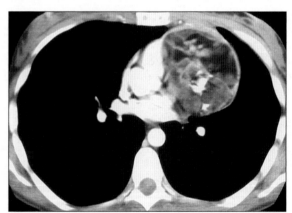

Figure 4. Contrast-enhanced CT shows a heterogeneous, anterior mediastinal mass containing areas of soft tissue and fat density and several foci of calcification. The patient was a 29-year-old woman with primary mediastinal teratoma.

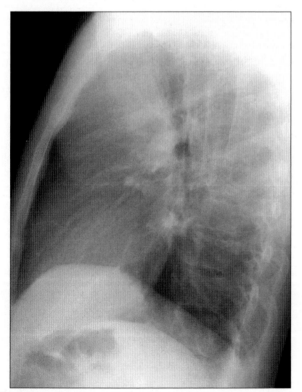

Figure 2. In the same patient, a lateral chest radiograph shows a large anterior mediastinal mass.

Case 182

DEMOGRAPHICS/CLINICAL HISTORY

A 32-year-old man who is asymptomatic and has normal serum α-fetoprotein (AFP) levels, undergoing computed tomography (CT).

FINDINGS

Contrast-enhanced CT shows a small lobulated, anterior mediastinal mass with homogeneous soft tissue attenuation.

DISCUSSION

Definition/Background

Seminoma is a primitive germ cell tumor composed of fairly uniform cells with clear or eosinophilic, glycogen-rich cytoplasm, distinct cell borders, and a round nucleus with one or more nucleoli; they resemble primordial germ cells. Primary mediastinal seminomas account for approximately 8% of extragonadal germ cell tumors and occur almost exclusively in men, who most commonly are between 20 and 40 years old.

Characteristic Clinical Features

Mediastinal seminomas may be asymptomatic or result in symptoms caused by pressure or invasion of mediastinal vessels or the major airways. Common symptoms are chest pain, shortness of breath, and superior vena cava (SVC) syndrome. Approximately one third of patients with seminoma have moderately elevated serum β-human chorionic gonadotropin (β-hCG) levels, but all have normal serum AFP levels.

Characteristic Radiologic Findings

Seminomas typically manifest as large, lobulated, well-marginated, anterior mediastinal masses that typically grow to both sides of the midline. The tumors usually have sharply demarcated borders on CT; however, invasion of adjacent mediastinal structures or the lung can result in irregular margins. The tumor usually shows homogenous soft tissue attenuation, but areas of low attenuation may be present.

Less Common Radiologic Manifestations

Cystic changes and foci of calcification may occur but are uncommon.

Differential Diagnosis

- Teratoma
- Thymoma
- Lymphoma

Discussion

A mediastinal mass containing fat, calcification, and soft tissue with hairball-like opacities seen on CT strongly suggests a teratoma. Thymomas most commonly manifest as smoothly marginated, fairly homogeneous masses; 40% are associated with myasthenia gravis. Primary mediastinal lymphomas may manifest as isolated, typically lobulated, homogeneous or inhomogeneous, anterior mediastinal masses; however, they more commonly are associated with mediastinal lymphadenopathy and other manifestations of systemic lymphoma.

Diagnosis

Mediastinal seminoma

Suggested Readings

Drevelegas A, Palladas P, Scordalaki A: Mediastinal germ cell tumors: A radiologic-pathologic review. Eur Radiol 11:1925-1932, 2001.

Quint LE: Imaging of anterior mediastinal masses. Cancer Imaging 7:S56-S62, 2007.

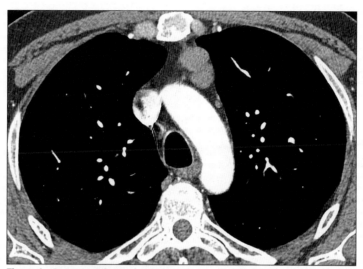

Figure 1. Contrast-enhanced CT shows a small, lobulated, anterior mediastinal mass with homogeneous soft tissue attenuation. The patient was a 32-year-old man with anterior mediastinal seminoma.

Case 183

DEMOGRAPHICS/CLINICAL HISTORY

A 26-year-old man with exertional dyspnea, chest pain, and elevated serum levels of α-fetoprotein (AFP) and β-human chorionic gonadotropin (β-hCG), undergoing computed tomography (CT) and magnetic resonance imaging (MRI).

FINDINGS

CT (Fig. 1) shows a large anterior mediastinal mass with inhomogeneous attenuation and poorly defined margins and reveals bilateral pleural effusions. Axial, T2-weighted MRI (Fig. 2) and coronal, T1-weighted MRI before (Fig. 3) and after (Fig. 4) gadolinium administration show a large anterior mediastinal mass with cystic areas and areas with marked contrast enhancement.

DISCUSSION

Definition/Background

Malignant, nonseminomatous, mediastinal germ cell tumors include embryonal carcinoma, yolk sac tumor, choriocarcinoma, and mixed germ cell tumors. The patients most commonly are between 20 and 40 years old, and virtually all are male.

Characteristic Clinical Features

Patients may have thoracic or shoulder pain and shortness of breath. Most patients have elevated serum levels of AFP or β-hCG, or both.

Characteristic Radiologic Findings

Nonseminomatous, malignant germ cell tumors usually are seen on chest radiographs as large, anterior, mediastinal masses that may have smooth, lobulated, or irregular margins. On CT and MRI, these tumors usually have heterogeneous attenuation and signal intensity due to areas of hemorrhage or necrosis. The fat planes between the tumor and the adjacent structures are usually obliterated, and pleural or pericardial effusions are common.

Less Common Radiologic Manifestations

Imaging may show pulmonary metastases. Direct chest wall invasion, regional lymph node involvement, and distant metastases can occur.

Differential Diagnosis

- Teratoma
- Thymoma
- Lymphoma
- Thymic carcinoma

Discussion

Malignant germ cell tumors are seen almost exclusively in males; manifest as large, homogeneous or heterogeneous, anterior mediastinal masses with invasion of adjacent structures; and are usually associated with elevated serum levels of AFP or β-hCG, or both. A mediastinal mass containing fat, calcification, and soft tissue with hairball-like opacities seen on CT strongly suggests a teratoma. Thymomas most commonly manifest as smoothly marginated, fairly homogeneous masses; 40% are associated with myasthenia gravis. Primary mediastinal lymphomas may manifest as isolated, typically lobulated, homogeneous or inhomogeneous, anterior mediastinal masses; however, they more commonly are associated with mediastinal lymphadenopathy and other manifestations of systemic lymphoma.

Diagnosis

Mediastinal nonseminomatous malignant germ cell tumor

Suggested Readings

Drevelegas A, Palladas P, Scordalaki A: Mediastinal germ cell tumors: A radiologic-pathologic review. Eur Radiol 11:1925-1932, 2001.
Quint LE: Imaging of anterior mediastinal masses. Cancer Imaging 7:S56-S62, 2007.

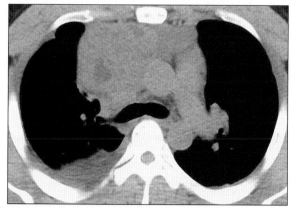

Figure 1. CT shows a large anterior mediastinal mass with inhomogeneous attenuation and poorly defined margins. Notice the bilateral pleural effusions. The patient was a 26-year-old man with malignant, nonseminomatous germ cell tumor.

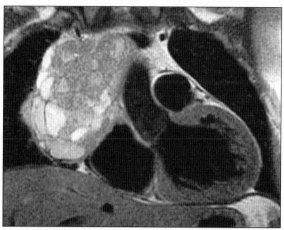

Figure 3. In the same patient, coronal, T1-weighted MRI shows a large, anterior mediastinal mass with inhomogeneous signal characteristics.

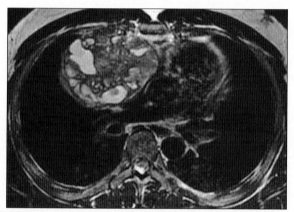

Figure 2. In the same patient, axial, T2-weighted MRI shows a large anterior mediastinal mass with cystic and solid areas.

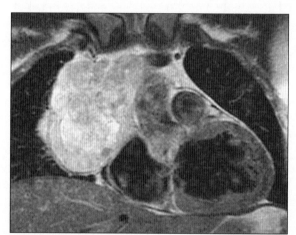

Figure 4. In the same patient, coronal, T1-weighted MRI after intravenous administration of gadolinium shows areas with marked contrast enhancement.

Case 184

DEMOGRAPHICS/CLINICAL HISTORY

A 33-year-old woman with an incidental finding on prior imaging, undergoing computed tomography (CT).

FINDINGS

Cross-sectional CT (Fig. 1) and coronal, reformatted CT (Fig. 2) show a homogeneous, triangular, cystic lesion (attenuation value of 0 HU) in the right cardiophrenic sulcus. In another patient with a pericardial cyst, contrast-enhanced CT (Fig. 3) shows a homogeneous, triangular, cystic lesion adjacent to the left heart border.

DISCUSSION

Definition/Background

Pericardial cysts are outpouchings of the parietal pericardium lined by a single layer of mesothelial cells, and they usually contain clear serous fluid. They are usually congenital but may be acquired after cardiothoracic surgery. They seldom communicate with the pericardial space and usually occur in the cardiophrenic angle, most commonly the right angle.

Characteristic Clinical Features

Most patients are asymptomatic. Symptoms include chest pain and dyspnea.

Characteristic Radiologic Findings

Chest radiograph typically shows a focal opacity in the cardiophrenic angle that obscures the inferior cardiac border. CT shows the characteristic well-circumscribed, unilocular mass with uniform fluid attenuation (0 to 20 HU) that does not enhance after contrast administration. The cysts usually have homogenously low signal intensities on T1-weighted magnetic resonance imaging (MRI) and high signal intensities on T2-weighted MRI.

Less Common Radiologic Manifestations

Rarely, the cyst wall may calcify.

Differential Diagnosis

- Pericardial fat pad
- Morgagni hernia
- Lymphadenopathy
- Lymphangioma
- Bronchogenic cyst

Discussion

A mass in the cardiophrenic angle seen on the chest radiograph must be differentiated from pericardial cyst, prominent pericardial fat pad, Morgagni hernia, and lymphadenopathy. A confident specific diagnosis can usually be made on CT or MRI by demonstrating the typical fluid characteristics of pericardial cysts. The differential diagnosis for cystic lesions in the anterior mediastinum includes thymic cyst, lymphangioma, and bronchogenic cyst. Mediastinal lymphangiomas may be located in the anterior or middle mediastinum, but they commonly extend into the lower neck. Mediastinal bronchogenic cysts typically manifest as a homogenous, water-density lesion in the paratracheal or subcarinal region away from the pericardium, but they sometimes occur in the anterior mediastinum.

Diagnosis

Pericardial cyst

Suggested Readings

Jeung MY, Gasser B, Gangi A, et al: Imaging of cystic masses of the mediastinum. Radiographics 22:S79-S93, 2002.

Kim JH, Goo JM, Lee HJ, et al: Cystic tumors in the anterior mediastinum. Radiologic-pathological correlation. J Comput Assist Tomogr 27:714-723, 2003.

Oyama N, Oyama N, Komuro K, et al: Computed tomography and magnetic resonance imaging of the pericardium: Anatomy and pathology. Magn Reson Med Sci 3:145-152, 2004.

Wang ZJ, Reddy GP, Gotway MB, et al: CT and MR imaging of pericardial disease. Radiographics 23:S167-S180, 2003.

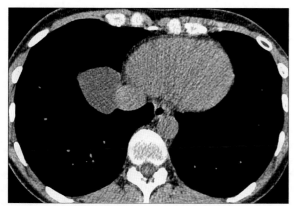

Figure 1. Cross-sectional CT shows a homogeneous, triangular, cystic lesion (attenuation value of 0 HU) adjacent to the inferior vena cava and right pericardium. The patient was a 33-year-old woman with a pericardial cyst.

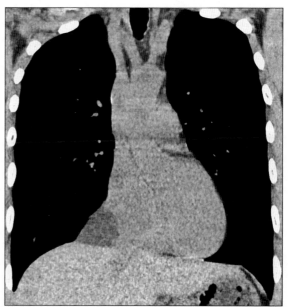

Figure 2. In the same patient, coronal, reformatted CT shows a homogeneous, triangular, cystic lesion (attenuation value of 0 HU) in the right cardiophrenic sulcus.

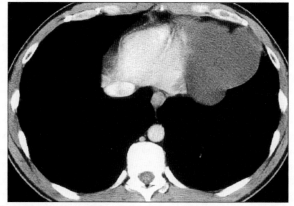

Figure 3. Contrast-enhanced CT shows a homogeneous, triangular, cystic lesion (attenuation value of 0 HU) adjacent to the left heart border. The patient was a 46-year-old man with a pericardial cyst.

Case 185

DEMOGRAPHICS/CLINICAL HISTORY

A 79-year-old man with cough, fatigue, and weight loss, undergoing radiography and computed tomography (CT).

FINDINGS

Posteroanterior chest radiograph (Fig. 1) reveals enlargement and lobulated contour of the right hilum. A focal opacity with increased density projects over the medial aspect of the liver. Lateral radiograph (Fig. 2) shows a right, lower lobe mass projecting over the lower thoracic spine and increased opacity and lobulated contour immediately posterior and inferior to the right hilum. CT image (Fig. 3) shows enlarged right hilar and subcarinal lymph nodes. CT image at the level of lung bases (Fig. 4) shows a right lower lobe mass with focal extrapleural extension.

DISCUSSION

Definition/Background

Lymphadenopathy (i.e., disease of the lymph nodes) is a radiologic term that refers to enlarged lymph nodes. Hilar lymph nodes include the tracheobronchial, peribronchial, and interlobar, lobar, and segmental bronchopulmonary lymph nodes. Similar to mediastinal nodes, hilar lymph nodes are considered to be enlarged when they are more than 10 mm in the short-axis diameter. Unilateral enlargement of the hilar lymph nodes can result from neoplasm (usually pulmonary carcinoma) or infection (usually tuberculosis, histoplasmosis, and bacterial pneumonia).

Characteristic Clinical Features

Patients may be asymptomatic or have symptoms related to the underlying cause, such as cough, weight loss (pulmonary carcinoma), and fever (bacterial pneumonia).

Characteristic Radiologic Findings

Unilateral hilar lymphadenopathy is characterized on the chest radiograph by increased size and opacity of the hilum and a lobulated contour. Enlarged hilar nodes may have homogenous or inhomogeneous attenuation and enhancement on CT

Less Common Radiologic Manifestations

Enlarged nodes may have low-attenuation centers and show rim enhancement, particularly in patients with tuberculosis.

Differential Diagnosis

- Pulmonary carcinoma
- Tuberculosis
- Fungal infection
- Pneumonia
- Lymphoma
- Sarcoidosis

Discussion

Unilateral hilar lymphadenopathy typically results from a neoplasm (e.g., usually pulmonary carcinoma; occasionally lymphoma or metastasis from kidney, breast, or head and neck tumors) or from infection (e.g., tuberculosis, histoplasmosis, coccidioidomycosis, bacterial pneumonia, lung abscess). In tuberculosis, lymph node enlargement is usually seen on the side of lung disease, but contralateral nodes can be involved. Unilateral hilar lymphadenopathy is seen in approximately 5% of patients with sarcoidosis. Contrast-enhanced CT is the best imaging modality for assessing hilar lymphadenopathy and associated findings in adults.

Diagnosis

Unilateral hilar lymphadenopathy

Suggested Readings

Boiselle PM, Patz EF Jr, Vining DJ, et al: Imaging of mediastinal lymph nodes: CT, MR, and FDG PET. Radiographics 18:1061-1069, 1998.

Müller NL, Webb WR: Radiographic imaging of the pulmonary hila. Invest Radiol 20:661-671, 1985.

Sharma A, Fidias P, Hayman LA, et al: Patterns of lymphadenopathy in thoracic malignancies. Radiographics 24:419-434, 2004.

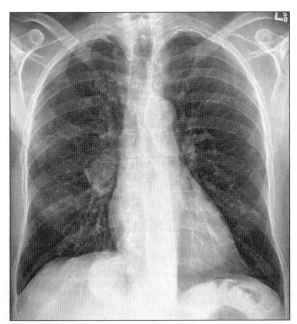

Figure 1. Posteroanterior chest radiograph reveals enlargement and lobulated contour of the right hilum. A focal, increased opacity projects over the medial aspect of the liver. The patient was a 79-year-old man with pulmonary carcinoma and right hilar and subcarinal lymph node metastases.

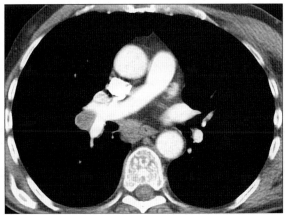

Figure 3. In the same patient, contrast-enhanced CT shows enlarged, right hilar and subcarinal lymph nodes.

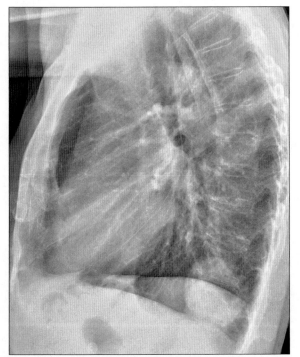

Figure 2. In the same patient, a lateral chest radiograph shows right lower lobe mass projecting over the lower thoracic spine and increased opacity and lobulated contour immediately posterior and inferior to the right hilum.

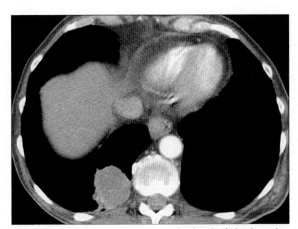

Figure 4. In the same patient, CT at the level of the lung bases shows a right lower lobe mass with focal extrapleural extension.

Case 186

DEMOGRAPHICS/CLINICAL HISTORY

A 31-year-old man with cough and chest pain, undergoing radiography and computed tomography (CT).

FINDINGS

Posteroanterior (Fig.1) and lateral (Fig. 2) chest radiographs show symmetric, bilateral enlargement of the hila, with a lobulated contour characteristic of lymphadenopathy. CT images show enlarged hilar nodes resulting in lobulated contours of the hila (Fig. 3), which may have homogenous (Fig. 4) or inhomogeneous attenuation and enhancement.

DISCUSSION

Definition/Background

Hilar lymph nodes include the tracheobronchial, peribronchial, and interlobar, lobar, and segmental bronchopulmonary lymph nodes. Similar to mediastinal nodes, hilar lymph nodes are considered to be enlarged when they are more than 10 mm in the short-axis diameter. Bilateral enlargement of the hilar lymph nodes is most commonly caused by sarcoidosis. Other causes include Hodgkin and non-Hodgkin lymphoma, leukemia, metastases (e.g., renal cell carcinoma, testicular tumor, breast cancer), cystic fibrosis, silicosis, multicentric Castleman disease, viral pneumonia, tuberculosis, and histoplasmosis.

Characteristic Clinical Features

Patients may be asymptomatic or have symptoms related to the underlying cause, such as fever and night sweats in those with lymphoma.

Characteristic Radiologic Findings

Bilateral hilar lymphadenopathy is characterized on the chest radiograph by increased size and opacity of the hila and a lobulated contour. Enlarged hilar nodes result in lobulated contours of the hila and may have homogenous or inhomogeneous attenuation and enhancement on CT.

Less Common Radiologic Manifestations

Enlarged nodes may have foci of calcification or have characteristic rim calcification (i.e., eggshell calcification), a finding that strongly suggests silicosis.

Differential Diagnosis

- Sarcoidosis
- Lymphoma
- Leukemia
- Metastases
- Silicosis

Discussion

The most common cause of bilateral symmetric hilar lymphadenopathy is sarcoidosis. Other causes include Hodgkin and non-Hodgkin lymphoma, metastases (e.g., renal cell carcinoma, testicular tumor, breast cancer), cystic fibrosis, and silicosis. Common causes of bilateral, asymmetric lymphadenopathy include Hodgkin and non-Hodgkin lymphoma, sarcoidosis, and metastases (e.g., pulmonary carcinoma, renal cell carcinoma, testicular tumor, breast cancer). Less common causes of bilateral hilar lymphadenopathy include leukemia, multicentric Castleman disease, and granulomatous infection (e.g., tuberculosis, histoplasmosis).

Diagnosis

Bilateral hilar lymphadenopathy

Suggested Readings

Boiselle PM, Patz EF Jr, Vining DJ, et al: Imaging of mediastinal lymph nodes: CT, MR, and FDG PET. Radiographics 18:1061-1069, 1998.

Müller NL, Webb WR: Radiographic imaging of the pulmonary hila. Invest Radiol 20:661-671, 1985.

Nunes H, Brillet PY, Valeyre D, et al: Imaging in sarcoidosis. Semin Respir Crit Care Med 28:102-120, 2007.

Sharma A, Fidias P, Hayman LA, et al: Patterns of lymphadenopathy in thoracic malignancies. Radiographics 24:419-434, 2004.

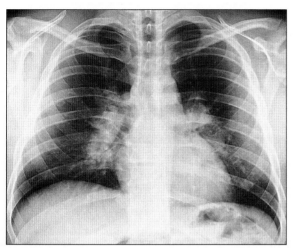

Figure 1. Posteroanterior chest radiograph shows symmetric, bilateral enlargement of the hila, with lobulated contours characteristic of lymphadenopathy. The patient was a 31-year-old man with sarcoidosis.

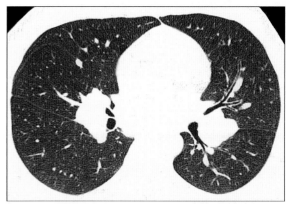

Figure 3. In the same patient, CT using lung windows shows a marked increase in the size and lobulation of the hila.

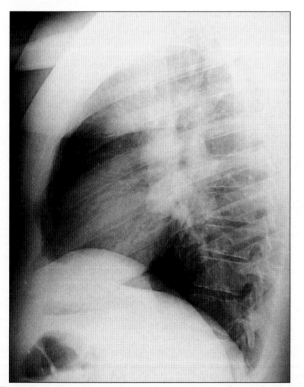

Figure 2. In the same patient, a lateral chest radiograph shows the lobulated contours of the hila and increased opacity in the infrahilar region.

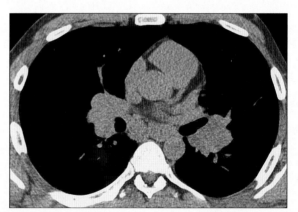

Figure 4. In the same patient, CT using soft tissue windows shows marked bilateral hilar and subcarinal lymphadenopathy.

Case 187

DEMOGRAPHICS/CLINICAL HISTORY

A 71-year-old man who is asymptomatic, undergoing radiography and computed tomography (CT).

FINDINGS

Posteroanterior (Fig. 1) and lateral (Fig. 2) chest radiographs show a homogeneous opacification projecting over the region of the aortic arch, findings consistent with marked dilatation of the aortic arch. Contrast-enhanced CT (Fig. 3) shows a partially thrombosed focal aneurysm of the aortic arch, and volumetric, oblique, sagittal, reformatted CT (Fig. 4) images show a focal aneurysm of the aortic arch.

DISCUSSION

Definition/Background

Aortic aneurysm is an irreversible dilatation of the aorta involving all three wall layers; it may focal or diffuse. The main risk is death from rupture; the risk of rupture within 5 years of detection is approximately 15% for thoracic aneurysms that are less than 6 cm in diameter and 30% for aneurysms equal to or larger than 6 cm. Most aortic aneurysms are caused by atherosclerosis; other causes include cystic medial necrosis (seen in Marfan syndrome and Ehlers-Danlos syndrome), aortitis (infective and inflammatory), and hemodynamic alterations (e.g., aortic stenosis, regurgitation).

Characteristic Clinical Features

Patients often are asymptomatic. The most common presenting symptom of patients with thoracic aortic aneurysms is chest pain, and the most serious complication is death from rupture.

Characteristic Radiologic Findings

On the chest radiograph, aneurysms of the ascending aorta and proximal aortic arch project anteriorly and to the right, and aneurysms of the distal arch and descending aorta project posteriorly and to the left. Any mass-like opacity that is contiguous with any part of the aorta on the radiograph should prompt consideration of an aneurysm. CT and magnetic resonance imaging (MRI) show focal or diffuse dilatation of the aorta and the relation of the aneurysm to adjacent structures.

Less Common Radiologic Manifestations

Imaging may show erosion of the vertebral column, tracheal narrowing, or pleural effusion.

Differential Diagnosis
- Mediastinal mass
- Aortic dissection

Discussion

Focal aortic aneurysms may be indistinguishable from other mediastinal masses on the chest radiograph. Any masslike opacity that appears to be contiguous with any part of the aorta on the radiograph should prompt consideration of an aneurysm. Patients with aneurysmal dilatation of the aorta may also have aortic dissection (i.e., separation of the aortic layers by a stream of blood). The specific diagnosis can be readily made on contrast-enhanced CT and MRI.

Diagnosis

Focal thoracic aortic aneurysm

Suggested Readings

Castañer E, Andreu M, Gallardo X, et al: CT in nontraumatic acute thoracic aortic disease: Typical and atypical features and complications. Radiographics 23:S93-S110, 2003.

Posniak HV, Olson MC, Demos TC, et al: CT of thoracic aortic aneurysms. Radiographics 10:839-855, 1990.

Tatli S, Yucel EK, Lipton MJ: CT and MR imaging of the thoracic aorta: Current techniques and clinical applications. Radiol Clin North Am 42:565-585, vi, 2004.

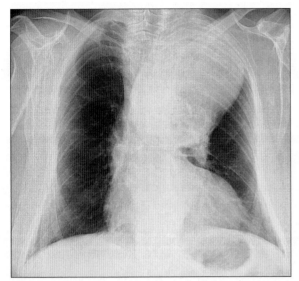

Figure 1. Posteroanterior chest radiograph shows a homogeneous opacification of the left apex that is consistent with a markedly enlarged aortic arch. The patient was a 71-year-old man with a large focal aneurysm of the aortic arch.

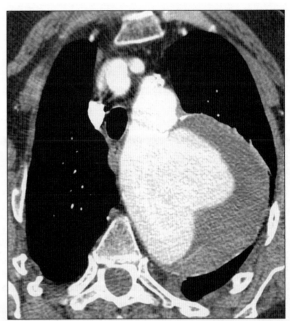

Figure 3. In the same patient, contrast-enhanced CT shows a partially thrombosed focal aneurysm of the aortic arch that is 10.7 cm in diameter.

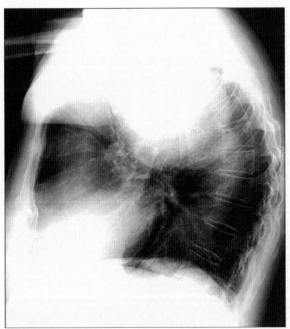

Figure 2. In the same patient, the lateral chest radiograph shows a homogeneous opacity in continuity with the aortic arch and descending aorta and extending to the lung apex.

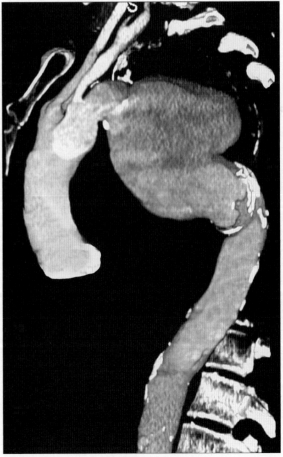

Figure 4. In the same patient, volumetric, oblique, sagittal, reformatted CT shows a focal aneurysm of the aortic arch.

Case 188

DEMOGRAPHICS/CLINICAL HISTORY

A 73-year-old woman with sudden onset of severe chest and back pain, undergoing computed tomography (CT).

FINDINGS

Transverse, contrast-enhanced CT (Figs. 1 and 2) and oblique, sagittal, reformatted CT images (Fig. 3) show an intimal flap involving the entire thoracic aorta.

DISCUSSION

Definition/Background

Aortic dissection is a separation of the layers of the aorta by a stream of blood. The dissection usually occurs between the middle and outer third of the media and results from an intimomedial tear or bleeding of the vasa vasorum into the media. Aortic dissection is classified as type A dissection, which affects the ascending aorta and requires emergency surgical repair to avoid potentially fatal complications, and type B, which starts distal to the left subclavian artery and can usually be treated medically.

Characteristic Clinical Features

Patients may have sudden onset of severe chest pain, pulse deficits, and syncope.

Characteristic Radiologic Findings

The radiographic findings are nonspecific. The diagnostic features on CT angiography and magnetic resonance imaging (MRI) consist of visualization of an intimomedial flap and blood flow within true and false lumens. In most cases, the true lumen can be identified by its continuity with the nondissected portion of the aorta. Another helpful finding is the 'beak sign (i.e., acute angle between the dissection flap and the outer wall at the site of the false lumen).

Less Common Radiologic Manifestations

Imaging may show thrombosis of the false lumen or hemothorax.

Differential Diagnosis

- Primary intramural hematoma of the thoracic aorta

Discussion

Primary intramural hematoma of the aorta, also known as aortic dissection without an intimal flap, represents localized hemorrhage confined to the aortic media. It is characterized on CT and MRI by the absence of a discrete intimomedial flap and the absence of flowing blood within the false lumen.

Diagnosis

Thoracic aortic dissection

Suggested Readings

Castañer E, Andreu M, Gallardo X, et al: CT in nontraumatic acute thoracic aortic disease: Typical and atypical features and complications. Radiographics 23:S93-S110, 2003.

Posniak HV, Olson MC, Demos TC, et al: CT of thoracic aortic aneurysms. Radiographics 10:839-855, 1990.

Tatli S, Yucel EK, Lipton MJ: CT and MR imaging of the thoracic aorta: Current techniques and clinical applications. Radiol Clin North Am 42:565-585, vi, 2004.

Yamada T, Tada S, Harada J: Aortic dissection without intimal rupture: Diagnosis with MR imaging and CT. Radiology 168:347-352, 1988.

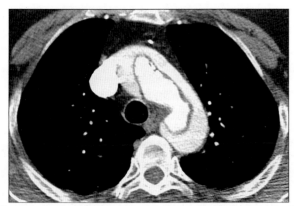

Figure 1. Contrast-enhanced, axial CT at the level of the aortic arch shows a complex intimal flap. The patient was a 73-year-old woman with type A aortic dissection.

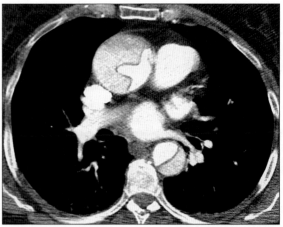

Figure 2. In the same patient, contrast-enhanced, axial CT at the level of the ascending aorta shows an intimal flap in the ascending and descending thoracic aorta.

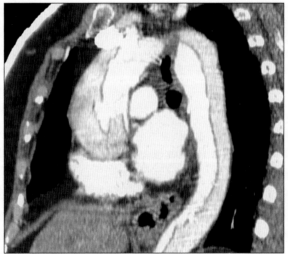

Figure 3. In the same patient, oblique, sagittal, reformatted CT shows an intimal flap involving the entire thoracic aorta.

Case 189

DEMOGRAPHICS/CLINICAL HISTORY

A 52-year-old woman with sudden onset of severe thoracic back pain, undergoing computed tomography (CT).

FINDINGS

Contrast-enhanced CT images at the level of the proximal (Fig. 1) and distal descending thoracic aorta (Fig. 2) show a crescent-shaped area of soft tissue density in the wall of the aorta that forms smooth margins with the lumen. The ascending aorta is normal.

DISCUSSION

Definition/Background

Primary intramural hematoma of the aorta, also known as aortic dissection without an intimal flap, represents localized hemorrhage confined to the aortic media. The clinical manifestations and the treatment are similar to those for aortic dissection. Intramural hematoma is classified as type A, which affects the ascending aorta, and type B, which starts distal to the left subclavian artery.

Characteristic Clinical Features

Patients may have sudden onset of severe chest pain.

Characteristic Radiologic Findings

Non–contrast-enhanced CT typically shows a crescent-shaped area along the wall of the aorta that has higher attenuation than blood. After administration of contrast, the hematoma does not enhance and appears hypodense compared with the enhanced lumen.

Less Common Radiologic Manifestations

Imaging may show pleural effusion or pericardial effusion.

Differential Diagnosis

- Thoracic aortic dissection

Discussion

Thoracic aortic dissection can be readily distinguished from thoracic aortic intramural hematoma on contrast-enhanced CT and magnetic resonance imaging by the presence of an intimomedial flap and flowing blood within the false lumen.

Diagnosis

Primary intramural thoracic aortic hematoma

Suggested Readings

Castañer E, Andreu M, Gallardo X, et al: CT in nontraumatic acute thoracic aortic disease: Typical and atypical features and complications. Radiographics 23:S93-S110, 2003.

Macura KJ, Szarf G, Fishman EK, Bluemke DA: Role of computed tomography and magnetic resonance imaging in assessment of acute aortic syndromes. Semin Ultrasound CT MR 24:232-254, 2003.

Manghat NE, Morgan-Hughes GJ, Roobottom CA: Multi-detector row computed tomography: Imaging in acute aortic syndrome. Clin Radiol 60:1256-1267, 2005.

Sundt TM: Intramural hematoma and penetrating atherosclerotic ulcer of the aorta. Ann Thorac Surg 83:S835-S841, 2007.

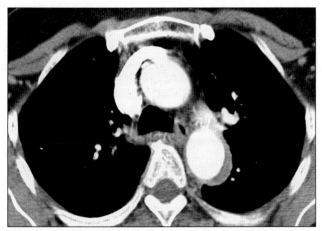

Figure 1. Contrast-enhanced CT at the level of the proximal descending thoracic aorta shows a crescent-shaped area of soft tissue density in the wall of the aorta that forms smooth margins with the lumen. The ascending aorta is normal. The patient was a 52-year-old woman with type B primary aortic intramural hematoma (i.e., aortic dissection without an intimal flap).

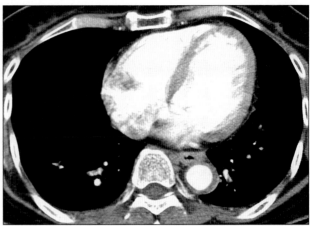

Figure 2. In the same patient, contrast-enhanced CT at the level of the distal descending thoracic aorta shows a crescent-shaped area of soft tissue density in the wall of the aorta that forms smooth margins with the lumen.

Case 190

DEMOGRAPHICS/CLINICAL HISTORY

An 81-year-old woman with acute onset of chest pain, undergoing computed tomography (CT).

FINDINGS

Contrast-enhanced CT (Fig. 1) shows an irregularity of the lumen of the descending aorta, with a focal, irregular outpouching and an intramural hematoma. Notice the small right pleural effusion. Contrast-enhanced CT (Fig. 2) shows a focal, smooth outpouching in the ascending aorta and an extensive intramural hematoma in the ascending and descending thoracic aorta.

DISCUSSION

Definition/Background

Penetrating atherosclerotic aortic ulcer is an ulceration of an atheromatous plaque that extends deeply through the intima and into the aortic media. It is frequently associated with intramural hemorrhage and pseudoaneurysm formation; occasionally, it ruptures. Penetrating aortic ulcer occurs mainly in elderly patients with extensive atherosclerosis of the aorta.

Characteristic Clinical Features

Patients often are asymptomatic, and the ulcer is detected incidentally on CT. Symptoms resemble acute dissection and include sudden onset of chest pain and back pain.

Characteristic Radiologic Findings

Penetrating aortic ulcer manifests on contrast-enhanced CT and magnetic resonance (MR) angiography as an ulcer-like collection of contrast material outside aortic lumen. It can be single or multiple and is usually associated with intramural hemorrhage.

Less Common Radiologic Manifestations

Imaging may show an aortic aneurysm or pseudoaneurysm.

Differential Diagnosis

- Intramural hematoma

Discussion

Penetrating thoracic aortic ulcer can be readily distinguished from intramural hematoma by the presence of an ulcer-like projection of contrast beyond the aortic lumen. Primary aortic intramural hematoma is characterized by an intact intima. Non–contrast-enhanced CT typically shows a crescent-shaped area along the wall of the aorta that has higher attenuation than blood; after administration of contrast, the hematoma does not enhance and appears hypodense compared with the enhanced lumen.

Diagnosis

Thoracic aortic penetrating ulcer

Suggested Readings

Sundt TM: Intramural hematoma and penetrating aortic ulcer. Curr Opin Cardiol 22:504-509, 2007.

Castañer E, Andreu M, Gallardo X, et al: CT in nontraumatic acute thoracic aortic disease: Typical and atypical features and complications. Radiographics 23:S93-S110, 2003.

Macura KJ, Szarf G, Fishman EK, Bluemke DA: Role of computed tomography and magnetic resonance imaging in assessment of acute aortic syndromes. Semin Ultrasound CT MR 24:232-254, 2003.

Quint LE, Williams DM, Francis IR, et al: Ulcerlike lesions of the aorta: Imaging features and natural history. Radiology 218:719-723, 2001.

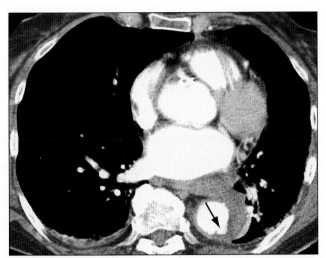

Figure 1. Contrast-enhanced CT shows an irregularity of the lumen of the descending aorta, with a focal irregular outpouching *(arrow)* and an intramural hematoma. Notice the small right pleural effusion. The patient was an 81-year-old woman with a penetrating aortic ulcer and intramural hematoma of the descending thoracic aorta.

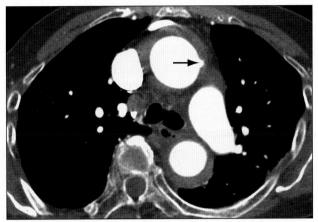

Figure 2. In the same patient, contrast-enhanced CT shows a focal, smooth outpouching *(arrow)* in the ascending aorta and an extensive intramural hematoma in the ascending and descending thoracic aorta.

Case 191

DEMOGRAPHICS/CLINICAL HISTORY

A 79-year-old man with dysphagia and recurrent aspiration, undergoing radiography and computed tomography (CT).

FINDINGS

Posteroanterior (Fig. 1) and lateral (Fig. 2) chest radiographs show a markedly dilated esophagus with an air-fluid level at the level of the right clavicle seen on the posteroanterior view and associated anterior displacement of the trachea evident on the lateral view. Sternal suture wires and vascular clips are from prior coronary artery bypass grafts. CT (Fig. 3) shows contrast material, food residue, and air within a markedly dilated esophagus. Coronal, reformatted CT (Fig. 4) shows marked dilatation of the esophagus.

DISCUSSION

Definition/Background

Achalasia is an esophageal motility disorder characterized by impaired esophageal peristalsis and lack of relaxation of the lower esophageal sphincter, causing marked esophageal dilatation. It is most commonly idiopathic; occasionally, it may result from esophageal carcinoma, vagotomy, diabetic neuropathy, or Chagas disease (particularly in Brazil).

Characteristic Clinical Features

Patients may have dysphagia, regurgitation of food, and chest pain that may increase after eating.

Characteristic Radiologic Findings

Marked dilatation of the esophagus may lead to anterior displacement and bowing of the trachea on the lateral radiograph. Barium esophagogram shows a dilated esophagus, retained fluid and food debris, aperistalsis of the lower esophagus, and inadequate relaxation of the lower esophageal sphincter.

Less Common Radiologic Manifestations

Imaging may show a fluid level within the dilated esophagus, areas of consolidation due to aspiration pneumonia, and lack of a visible gastric air bubble.

Differential Diagnosis

- Esophageal carcinoma
- Esophageal stricture

Discussion

Marked dilatation of the esophagus may be caused by achalasia or distal obstruction by carcinoma, stricture, or extrinsic compression. The diagnosis of achalasia is based on clinical findings, outcome of the barium esophagogram, and esophageal motility testing (i.e., esophageal manometry) results. Endoscopy is necessary to rule out malignancy as the cause of achalasia.

Diagnosis

Achalasia

Suggested Readings

Pohl D, Tutuian R: Achalasia: An overview of diagnosis and treatment. J Gastrointestin Liver Dis 16:297-303, 2007.

Whitten CR, Khan S, Munneke GJ, Grubnic S: A diagnostic approach to mediastinal abnormalities. Radiographics 27:657-671, 2007.

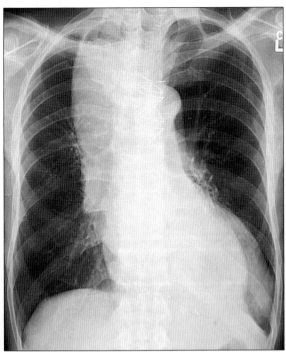

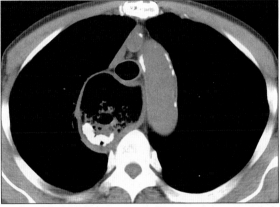

Figure 3. In the same patient, CT shows contrast material, food residue, and air within a markedly dilated esophagus.

Figure 1. Posteroanterior chest radiograph shows a markedly dilated esophagus with an air-fluid level at the level of the right clavicle. Notice the sternal suture wires and vascular clips from prior coronary artery bypass grafts. The patient was a 79-year-old man with achalasia.

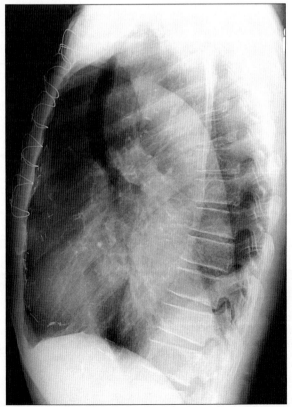

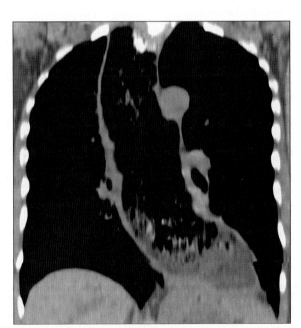

Figure 4. In the same patient, coronal, reformatted CT shows marked dilatation of the esophagus.

Figure 2. In the same patient, the lateral chest radiograph shows a markedly dilated esophagus with associated anterior displacement of the trachea. The sternal suture wires and vascular clips are from prior coronary artery bypass grafts.

Case 192

DEMOGRAPHICS/CLINICAL HISTORY

A 64-year-old woman with dysphagia and weight loss, undergoing computed tomography (CT).

FINDINGS

Contrast-enhanced CT at the level of the aortopulmonary window (Fig. 1) shows paratracheal and paraesophageal lymphadenopathy. CT images at the level of the right pulmonary artery (Fig. 2) and left atrium (Fig. 3) show marked thickening of the esophageal wall and soft tissue infiltration of the adjacent tissues with obscuration of the fat plane between the esophagus and the aorta.

DISCUSSION

Definition/Background

Esophageal carcinomas are of two main types: squamous cell carcinomas, which account for approximately 80% of cases and are associated with cigarette smoking and heavy alcohol consumption, and adenocarcinomas, which account for approximately 20% of cases and are commonly associated with a history of gastroesophageal reflux disease and Barrett esophagus. Esophageal carcinomas usually occur in patients older than 60 years and are associated with a poor prognosis.

Characteristic Clinical Features

Patients may have dysphagia, anorexia, and weight loss.

Characteristic Radiologic Findings

The chest radiograph may show normal anatomy or may show a mass in middle or posterior mediastinum or dilatation of the esophagus. Findings on CT include concentric or eccentric thickening of the esophagus (usually > 5 mm), narrowing of the esophageal lumen, dilatation above the obstructing tumor, a focal intraluminal mass, obscuration of periesophageal fat planes with or without evidence of invasion of adjacent structures, and periesophageal, paratracheal, aortopulmonary window, cervical, and upper abdominal lymphadenopathy.

Less Common Radiologic Manifestations

Imaging may show pulmonary metastases.

Differential Diagnosis

- Esophagitis
- Leiomyoma of the esophagus
- Achalasia

Discussion

Esophageal wall thickening is an early but nonspecific manifestation of esophageal carcinoma. It may also occur with benign processes, such as esophagitis and gastroesophageal reflux. Leiomyoma of the esophagus is a benign tumor that typically manifests on CT as a smoothly marginated mass that usually involves one esophageal wall, and the bulk of the mass often is extrinsic to the esophagus. Diagnosis of esophageal carcinoma and differentiation from other tumors requires biopsy. Dilatation of the esophagus may be caused by achalasia or distal obstruction by carcinoma, stricture, or extrinsic compression. The diagnosis of achalasia is based on clinical findings, outcome of the barium esophagogram, and esophageal motility testing (i.e., esophageal manometry) results. Endoscopy is necessary to rule out malignancy as the cause of achalasia.

Diagnosis

Carcinoma of the esophagus

Suggested Readings

Bruzzi JF, Truong MT, Macapinlac H, et al: Integrated CT-PET imaging of esophageal cancer: Unexpected and unusual distribution of distant organ metastases. Curr Probl Diagn Radiol 36:21-29, 2007.

Gibbs JM, Chandrasekhar CA, Ferguson EC, Oldham SA: Lines and stripes: Where did they go?—From conventional radiography to CT. Radiographics 27:33-48, 2007.

Korst RJ, Altorki NK: Imaging for esophageal tumors. Thorac Surg Clin 14:61-69, 2004.

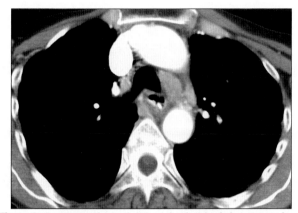

Figure 1. Contrast-enhanced CT at the level of the aortopulmonary window shows paratracheal and paraesophageal lymphadenopathy. The patient was a 64-year-old woman with esophageal carcinoma.

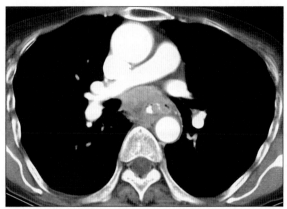

Figure 2. In the same patient, contrast-enhanced CT at the level of the right pulmonary artery shows marked thickening of the esophageal wall and soft tissue infiltration of the adjacent tissues with obscuration of the fat plane between the esophagus and the aorta.

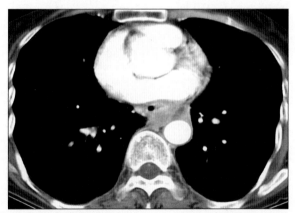

Figure 3. In the same patient, contrast-enhanced CT at the level of the left atrium shows marked thickening of the esophageal wall and soft tissue infiltration of the adjacent tissues with obscuration of the fat plane between the esophagus and the aorta.

Case 193

DEMOGRAPHICS/CLINICAL HISTORY

A 66-year-old man who is asymptomatic, undergoing computed tomography (CT).

FINDINGS

CT (Fig. 1) without intravenous contrast shows a smoothly marginated, low-attenuation (10 HU) lesion adjacent to the esophagus. Contrast-enhanced CT (Fig. 2) shows that the lesion does not increase in density (i.e., attenuation of 10 HU).

DISCUSSION

Definition/Background

Esophageal (foregut) duplication cyst is a congenital cyst lined by esophageal epithelium that contains smooth muscle in its wall and that is intimately attached to the esophagus. Esophageal duplication cysts are less common than bronchogenic cysts.

Characteristic Clinical Features

Patients may be asymptomatic or complain of dysphagia, chest pain, cough, or dyspnea caused by compression of adjacent structures.

Characteristic Radiologic Findings

On the chest radiograph, esophageal duplication cysts appear as smooth, sharply marginated masses located most frequently in the posterior mediastinum and closely associated with the esophagus. The CT findings consist of a rounded or elliptical mass of homogeneous water density or soft tissue density that does not enhance after intravenous administration of contrast and that is adjacent to the esophagus. On magnetic resonance imaging (MRI), esophageal duplication cysts have homogeneous high signal intensity on T2-weighted images, regardless of the nature of the cyst contents, but they have various patterns of signal intensity on T1-weighted images because of the presence of protein or hemorrhage.

Less Common Radiologic Manifestations

Imaging may show esophageal dilatation due to obstruction.

Differential Diagnosis

- Esophageal leiomyoma
- Bronchogenic cyst

Discussion

The radiologic appearance of foregut duplication cysts is identical to that of bronchogenic cysts, except that the latter tend to be closely associated with the airways. Esophageal duplication cysts often can be distinguished from leiomyomas by their location adjacent to the esophagus rather than in the esophageal wall and by fluid density seen on CT (approximately 50% of cases). The distinction can be made in virtually 100% of cases on MRI by the characteristic homogeneous high signal intensity on T2-weighted images.

Diagnosis

Esophageal duplication cyst

Suggested Readings

Jeung MY, Gasser B, Gangi A, et al: Imaging of cystic masses of the mediastinum. Radiographics 22:S79-S93, 2002.
Whitten CR, Khan S, Munneke GJ, Grubnic S: A diagnostic approach to mediastinal abnormalities. Radiographics 27:657-671, 2007.

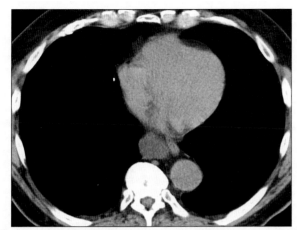

Figure 1. CT without intravenous contrast shows a smoothly marginated, low-attenuation (10 HU) lesion adjacent to the esophagus. The patient was a 66-year-old man with an esophageal (foregut) duplication cyst.

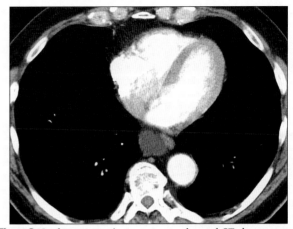

Figure 2. In the same patient, contrast-enhanced CT shows a nonenhancing periesophageal lesion with homogeneous low attenuation (10 HU).

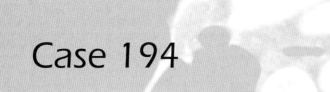

Case 194

DEMOGRAPHICS/CLINICAL HISTORY

A 64-year-old man with an incidental radiographic finding, undergoing computed tomography (CT).

FINDINGS

Contrast-enhanced, axial CT (Fig. 1); coronal CT (Fig. 2); and sagittal, reformatted CT (Fig. 3) show a large mass in the left paravertebral region with enhancing thick walls and a cystic component. Notice the compression and displacement of the aorta. There is no evidence of bony erosion and no enlargement of the neural foramina.

DISCUSSION

Definition/Background

Neurogenic tumors constitute approximately 20% of all resected primary mediastinal neoplasms in adults and 35% in children. Paravertebral nerve sheath tumors include neurilemoma (i.e., schwannoma), neurofibroma, and malignant nerve sheath tumor. More than 90% of peripheral nerve tumors are benign.

Characteristic Clinical Features

Patients often are asymptomatic, but they may present with pain or neurologic symptoms, or both.

Characteristic Radiologic Findings

Neurilemomas and neurofibromas manifest on the chest radiograph as smoothly marginated, rounded or oval masses. Neurilemomas usually have homogeneous attenuation on CT, show homogeneous or heterogeneous enhancement after contrast administration, and may contain cystic areas. They have low to intermediate signal intensity on T1-weighted magnetic resonance imaging (MRI) and areas of intermediate to high signal intensity on T2-weighted sequences. Neurofibromas usually have smooth margins and a round or ellipsoid shape. They have homogeneous attenuation and an early central blush after administration of contrast on CT; homogeneous, low to intermediate signal intensity on T1-weighted MRI; and a target appearance on T2-weighted sequences.

Less Common Radiologic Manifestations

Imaging may show adjacent bone changes, such as erosion, splaying of the ribs, or enlargement of the intervertebral foramen.

Differential Diagnosis

- Malignant nerve sheath tumors

Discussion

Benign nerve sheath tumors (i.e., neurilemoma and neurofibromas) are usually small and have well-defined, smooth margins. Malignant nerve sheath tumors usually are more than 5 cm in diameter, contain areas of low attenuation, and often have irregular or ill-defined margins on CT and MRI. They typically have low-attenuation areas on CT and high-signal-intensity areas on T2-weighted MRI. However, there is considerable overlap of the imaging features of benign and malignant nerve sheath tumors, and definitive diagnosis requires biopsy or surgical resection.

Diagnosis

Paravertebral nerve sheath tumors, neurilemoma or schwannoma

Suggested Readings

Ko SF, Lee TY, Lin JW, et al: Thoracic neurilemomas: An analysis of computed tomography findings in 36 patients. J Thorac Imaging 13:21-26, 1998.

Lee JY, Lee KS, Han J, et al: Spectrum of neurogenic tumors in the thorax: CT and pathologic findings. J Comput Assist Tomogr 23:399-406, 1999.

Tanaka O, Kiryu T, Hirose Y, et al: Neurogenic tumors of the mediastinum and chest wall. MR imaging appearance. J Thorac Imaging 20:316-320, 2005.

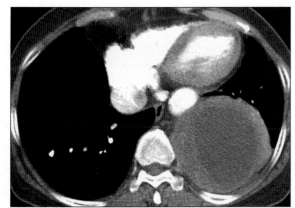

Figure 1. Contrast-enhanced, axial CT shows a large mass in the left paravertebral region with enhancing thick walls and a cystic component. Notice the compression and displacement of the aorta. There is no evidence of bony erosion and no enlargement of neural foramen. The patient was a 64-year-old man with a cystic neurilemoma.

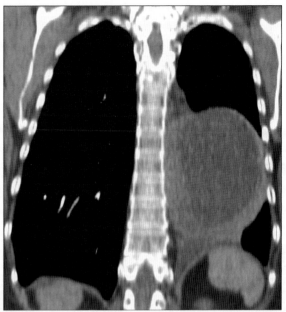

Figure 2. In the same patient, coronal, reformatted CT shows a large mass in the left paravertebral region with enhancing thick walls and a cystic component.

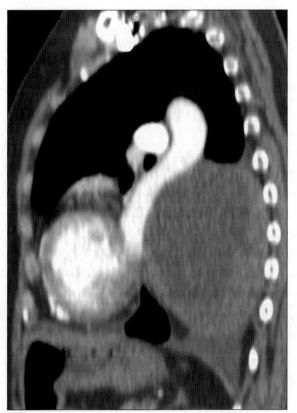

Figure 3. In the same patient, sagittal, reformatted CT shows a large mass with enhancing thick walls and a cystic component displacing the aorta anteriorly.

Case 195

DEMOGRAPHICS/CLINICAL HISTORY

A 64-year-old man with fever and back pain, undergoing computed tomography (CT).

FINDINGS

Contrast-enhanced CT images at the level of T10 (Figs. 1 and 2) show extensive paraspinal soft tissue infiltration with inhomogeneous contrast enhancement and small focal areas of low attenuation. Notice the marked irregularity of the vertebral body and bilateral pleural effusions. Coronal, reformatted CT (Fig. 3) shows marked destruction of the T10 vertebral body and the cephalocaudal extent of the paraspinal soft tissue infiltration.

DISCUSSION

Definition/Background

Paravertebral abscess is a suppurative process involving the paraspinal soft tissues. It may result from direct extension of adjacent infection or from hematogenous dissemination of organisms (most commonly *Staphylococcus aureus* and *Mycobacterium tuberculosis*). Predisposing conditions include intravenous drug use, immunosuppression, spinal surgery, and trauma.

Characteristic Clinical Features

Patients may have fever and back pain.

Characteristic Radiologic Findings

Contrast-enhanced CT findings include a paravertebral, enhancing, inflammatory soft tissue density with obscuration of the fat planes and containing one or more fluid density collections with rim enhancement. The inflammatory tissue is isointense to hypointense on T1-weighted magnetic resonance imaging (MRI), has high signal intensity on T2-weighted MRI, and shows diffuse or peripheral enhancement with gadolinium administration. Features of spondylitis are common and include intervertebral disk or bone destruction seen on CT; end-plate erosion and hyperintense intervertebral disks on T2-weighted MRI; and marrow edema and enhancing disks and marrow on MRI. Increased uptake of indium 111 by white blood cells on the nuclear medicine scan.

Less Common Radiologic Manifestations

Imaging may show intraspinal extension, cord compression, and vertebral collapse with focal kyphosis.

Differential Diagnosis

- Paravertebral neoplasm
- Paravertebral hematoma
- Extramedullary hematopoiesis

Discussion

Paravertebral abscesses usually manifest with fever, and radiologically, they typically are associated with disk or bone destruction and bilateral paraspinal soft tissue and fluid collections, whereas neoplasms are typically unilateral. Paravertebral hematomas follow trauma, may have soft tissue or high attenuation on CT, and are hypointense on T1- and T2- weighted MRI in the acute stage and hyperintense in the late stage. Paravertebral extramedullary hematopoiesis is uncommon and seen only in patients with severe chronic hemolytic anemia (e.g., thalassemia).

Diagnosis

Paravertebral abscess

Suggested Readings

Balériaux DL, Neugroschl C: Spinal and spinal cord infection. Eur Radiol 14(Suppl 3):E72-E83, 2004.

Forrester DM: Infectious spondylitis. Semin Ultrasound CT MR 25: 461-473, 2004.

James SL, Davies AM: Imaging of infectious spinal disorders in children and adults. Eur J Radiol 58:27-40, 2006.

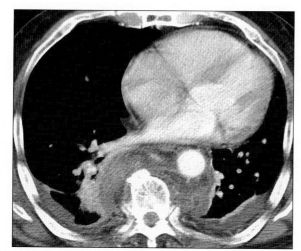

Figure 1. Contrast-enhanced CT at the level of T10 shows extensive paraspinal soft tissue infiltration with inhomogeneous contrast enhancement and small focal areas of low attenuation. Bilateral pleural effusions and compressive atelectasis of the adjacent areas of the lower lobes also can be seen. The patient was a 64-year-old man with paraspinal abscess.

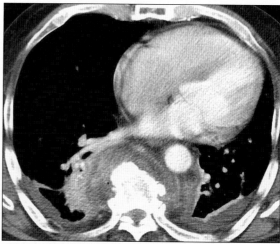

Figure 2. In the same patient, contrast-enhanced CT at the level of T10 and slightly caudal to the view in Figure 1 shows extensive paraspinal soft tissue infiltration with inhomogeneous contrast enhancement and small focal areas of low attenuation. Notice the marked irregularity of the vertebral body and small, bilateral pleural effusions.

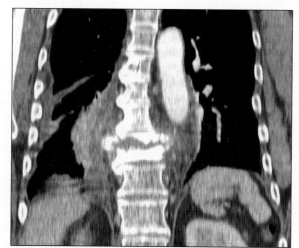

Figure 3. In the same patient, coronal, reformatted CT shows marked destruction of the T10 vertebral body and the cephalocaudal extent of the paraspinal soft tissue infiltration.

Case 196

DEMOGRAPHICS/CLINICAL HISTORY

A 67-year-old man with an incidental finding on radiography, undergoing radiography and CT.

FINDINGS

The posteroanterior chest radiograph (Fig. 1) shows a focal bulge of the left hemidiaphragm with a double contour and slightly increased opacity in the region of the left costophrenic sulcus. The lateral radiograph (Fig. 2) shows an apparent mass in the posterior costophrenic sulcus.

DISCUSSION

Definition/Background

Bochdalek hernias are hernias between the lateral (costal) and the posterior (crural) components of the diaphragm. They are seen on CT in about 10% of adults, are typically small, and unlike the infantile form are almost always asymptomatic. Their incidence increases with age, suggesting that they are acquired. They are rare in patients younger than 40 years but are seen in approximately 5% of patients between 40 and 49 years old, 15% of patients between 50 and 69 years old, and 35% of older patients.

Characteristic Clinical Features

Patients are usually asymptomatic. Occasionally, patients may complain of epigastric or lower sternal pressure and discomfort and sometimes describe cardiorespiratory and gastrointestinal symptoms.

Characteristic Radiologic Findings

Bochdalek hernia can manifest on the chest radiograph as a focal bulge in the hemidiaphragm or as a mass adjacent to the posteromedial aspect of either hemidiaphragm. The diagnosis is readily made on CT (Fig. 3), which typically shows a defect between the costal and crural components of the diaphragm and herniation of omental fat.

Less Common Radiologic Manifestations

Occasionally, adult Bochdalek hernias may contain abdominal viscera, most commonly the kidney.

Differential Diagnosis

- Pulmonary tumor
- Mediastinal mass
- Paravertebral mass
- Congenital Bochdalek hernia
- Traumatic diaphragmatic hernia

Discussion

Although the diagnosis can often be suspected on the radiograph by the typical location and by the lower than soft tissue density of the mass because of its fat content, the appearance can mimic that of pulmonary, mediastinal, or paravertebral masses. Bochdalek hernias seen in adults are almost always acquired and totally distinct from congenital Bochdalek hernias seen in newborns and young infants, which represent herniation through a persistent embryonic pleuroperitoneal hiatus and are typically large and associated with high morbidity and mortality rates.

Diagnosis

Bochdalek hernia in adults

Suggested Readings

Caskey CI, Zerhouni EA, Fishman EK, Rahmouni AD: Aging of the diaphragm: A CT study. Radiology 171:385-389, 1989.

Eren S, Ciris F: Diaphragmatic hernia: Diagnostic approaches with review of the literature. Eur J Radiol 54:448-459, 2005.

Mullins ME, Stein J, Saini SS, et al: Prevalence of incidental Bochdalek's hernia in a large adult population. AJR Am J Roentgenol 177:363-366, 2001.

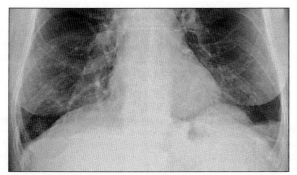

Figure 1. Posteroanterior chest radiograph shows a focal bulge of the left hemidiaphragm with a double contour and slightly increased opacity in the region of the left costophrenic sulcus. The patient was a 76-year-old man with an incidental left Bochdalek hernia identified on the chest radiograph and bilateral Bochdalek hernias seen on CT.

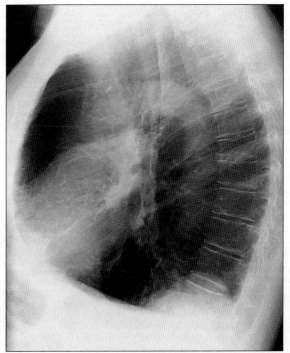

Figure 2. In the same patient, the lateral chest radiograph shows an apparent mass in the posterior costophrenic sulcus.

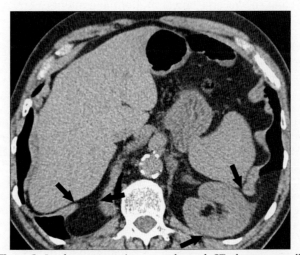

Figure 3. In the same patient, unenhanced CT shows a small defect in the right hemidiaphragm *(arrows)* with herniation of abdominal fat and a large defect in the left hemidiaphragm *(arrows)* with herniation of abdominal fat and kidney, accounting for the abnormalities seen on corresponding radiographs. Notice the herniation of abdominal fat into the region of the left costophrenic sulcus, which accounts for the focal opacity seen on corresponding radiographs.

Case 197

DEMOGRAPHICS/CLINICAL HISTORY

A 37-year-old man with epigastric pain, undergoing radiography and compared with computed tomography (CT).

FINDINGS

Posteroanterior (Fig. 1) and lateral (Fig. 2) chest radiographs show increased soft tissue and air lucencies in the region of the right cardiophrenic angle and in the retrosternal space. The lateral view (Fig. 2) shows continuity of these lucencies with similar findings in the upper abdomen. In another patient with a Morgagni hernia, CT shows large bowel loops and fat in the right cardiophrenic angle and compressing the heart (Fig. 3) and shows large bowel loops and omental fat herniating into the chest through a defect in the diaphragm (Fig. 4).

DISCUSSION

Definition/Background

Morgagni hernias are anterior hernias through the sternocostal hiatus of the diaphragm; approximately 90% of cases occur on the right side. Although the defects are developmental in origin, hernias are more common in adults than children and are often associated with obesity or other situations involving increased intra-abdominal pressure, such as severe effort or trauma. The content of the hernial sac may include, in order of decreasing frequency, the omentum, colon, stomach, liver, and small intestine.

Characteristic Clinical Features

Patients are usually asymptomatic. Occasionally, patients may complain of epigastric or lower sternal pressure and discomfort and sometimes describe cardiorespiratory and gastrointestinal symptoms.

Characteristic Radiologic Findings

Morgagni hernia typically manifests as a smooth, well-defined opacity in the right cardiophrenic angle. In most patients, the shadow is of homogeneous density; less commonly, lucencies due to bowel gas may be seen. CT and magnetic resonance imaging (MRI) are diagnostic, demonstrating herniation of abdominal contents between the costal and sternal attachments of the diaphragm. Most contain only omentum; occasionally, they may be large and contain portions of the liver or large bowel.

Less Common Radiologic Manifestations

Imaging may show an inhomogeneous opacity in the right cardiophrenic angle as a result of an air-containing loop of bowel or the predominantly fatty nature of the hernial contents.

Differential Diagnosis

- Prominent pericardial fat pad
- Pericardial cyst
- Lymphadenopathy

Discussion

The main differential diagnosis for a mass in the cardiophrenic angle on the chest radiograph includes Morgagni hernia, pericardial cyst, prominent pericardial fat pad, and lymphadenopathy. A confident diagnosis of Morgagni hernia can be readily made on CT or MRI.

Diagnosis

Morgagni hernia

Suggested Readings

Eren S, Ciris F: Diaphragmatic hernia: Diagnostic approaches with review of the literature. Eur J Radiol 54:448-459, 2005.

Horton JD, Hofmann LJ, Hetz SP: Presentation and management of Morgagni hernias in adults: A review of 298 cases. Surg Endosc 22:1413-1420, 2008.

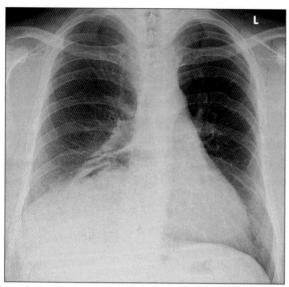

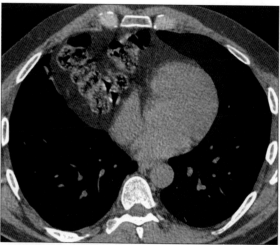

Figure 1. Posteroanterior chest radiograph reveals increased soft tissue and air lucencies in the region of the right cardiophrenic angle, with obscuration of the right heart border and hemidiaphragm. The mild deformity of the left posterior 7th rib is a healed fracture. The patient was a 37-year-old man with Morgagni hernia related to prior trauma.

Figure 3. Unenhanced CT shows large bowel loops and fat in the right cardiophrenic angle that are compressing the heart. The patient was a 54-year-old man with Morgagni hernia.

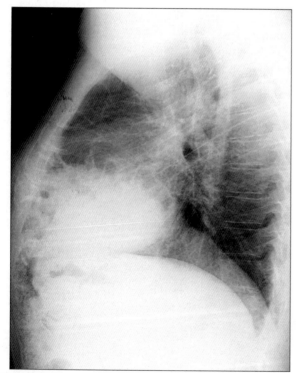

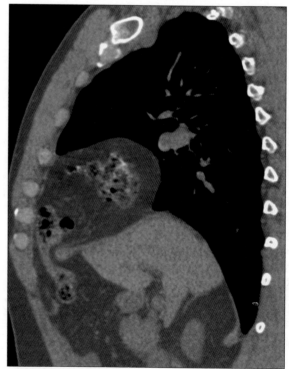

Figure 2. In the same patient, the lateral chest radiograph shows increased soft tissue and air lucencies in the retrosternal space and in continuity with similar findings in the upper abdomen, characteristic of bowel loops.

Figure 4. Sagittal, reformatted CT shows large bowel loops and omental fat herniating into the chest through a defect in the diaphragm in a 54-year-old man with Morgagni hernia.

Case 198

DEMOGRAPHICS/CLINICAL HISTORY

An 86-year-old man with an incidental radiographic finding, undergoing radiography and computed tomography (CT).

FINDINGS

Posteroanterior (Fig. 1) and lateral (Fig. 2) chest radiographs show a large, retrocardiac, air-containing structure with a fluid level. CT performed after oral and intravenous contrast administration shows retrocardiac position of stomach (Fig. 3), and CT at the level of the upper abdomen shows a large diaphragmatic defect with herniation of omental fat and vessels (Fig. 4).

DISCUSSION

Definition/Background

The prevalence of esophageal hiatus hernias increases with age. The abnormality is evident on CT in approximately 5% of individuals younger than 40 years, 30% of those between 40 and 59 years, and 65% of those between 60 and 79 years.

Characteristic Clinical Features

Most patients do not have symptoms. For a few patients, symptoms include epigastric or lower sternal pressure and discomfort, and they sometimes have recurrent aspiration.

Characteristic Radiologic Findings

Hiatus hernia typically manifests radiographically as a retrocardiac mass, usually containing air or an air-fluid level. The diagnosis can be readily made on CT.

Esophageal hernias usually result from widening of the esophageal hiatus, allowing the stomach and the omentum to protrude into the chest. The esophageal hiatus is an opening just to the left of the midline and is marginated by the right and left crura. It is normally elliptical and is 15 mm wide or less (i.e., distance between the medial margins of the crura).

Less Common Radiologic Manifestations

In cases in which most of the stomach has herniated through the hiatus, the stomach may undergo volvulus, resulting in the presence of a large mass containing a double air-fluid level; incarceration the hernial contents is common, and strangulation may occur. Although the stomach is the most common component of the hernial contents, other structures, such as a portion of the transverse colon, omentum, liver, or pancreas, may be seen.

Differential Diagnosis

- Mediastinal mass

Discussion

Hiatus hernia manifesting radiographically as an air-containing, retrocardiac mass can be readily diagnosed on the radiograph. Hiatus hernias not containing air resemble other esophageal or paraesophageal masses. The diagnosis can be readily confirmed on CT or esophagography.

Diagnosis

Hiatus hernia

Suggested Readings

Caskey CI, Zerhouni EA, Fishman EK, Rahmouni AD: Aging of the diaphragm: A CT study. Radiology 171:385-389, 1989.

Eren S, Ciris F: Diaphragmatic hernia: Diagnostic approaches with review of the literature. Eur J Radiol 54:448-459, 2005.

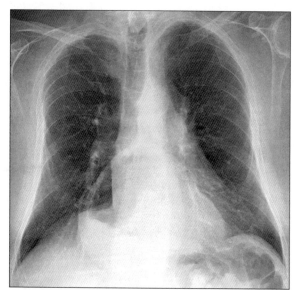

Figure 1. Posteroanterior chest radiograph shows a large, air-containing structure projecting over the cardiopericardial silhouette. The patient was an 86-year-old man with a hiatus hernia.

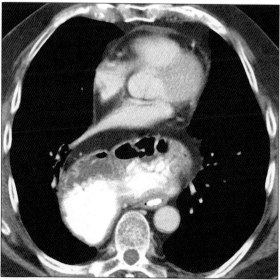

Figure 3. In the same patient, CT performed after oral and intravenous contrast administration shows the retrocardiac position of stomach.

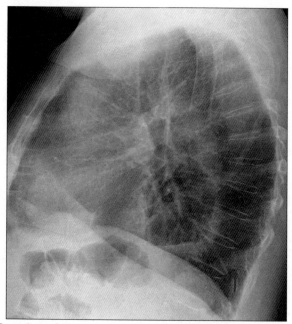

Figure 2. In the same patient, the lateral chest radiograph shows a large, retrocardiac, air-containing structure with a fluid level.

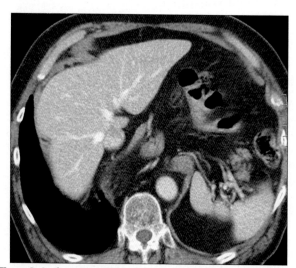

Figure 4. In the same patient, CT at the level of the upper abdomen shows a large diaphragmatic defect with herniation of omental fat and vessels.

Case 199

DEMOGRAPHICS/CLINICAL HISTORY

A 59-year-old man with an incidental finding, undergoing computed tomography (CT) and magnetic resonance imaging (MRI).

FINDINGS

Unenhanced CT (Fig. 1) at the level of the undersurface of the right 6th rib shows a homogenous soft tissue opacity adjacent to and parallel to the rib. There is no associated bone erosion. The lesion is isointense on T1-weighted MRI (Fig. 2) and has areas of signal intensity similar to cerebrospinal fluid on T2-weighted MRI image (Fig. 3).

DISCUSSION

Definition/Background

Neurilemoma (i.e. schwannoma) is a benign, encapsulated nerve sheath tumor composed of neoplastic Schwann cells. They are usually found in the paravertebral region. Occasionally, they may be located along the vagus or phrenic nerve or along a rib.

Characteristic Clinical Features

Most patients are asymptomatic.

Characteristic Radiologic Findings

The radiograph may show normal anatomy or an extrapleural or paraspinal soft tissue mass. The tumor may be associated with rib erosion or widening of the spinal canal. CT shows a well-demarcated, round or oval mass with homogeneous attenuation that may be equal to or less than that of soft tissue on unenhanced scans and shows homogeneous or heterogeneous enhancement after administration of contrast. Neurilemomas typically have low to intermediate signal intensity on T1-weighted MRI and may have areas of intermediate to high signal intensity on T2-weighted sequences.

Less Common Radiologic Manifestations

CT may show cystic areas in large tumors.

Differential Diagnosis

■ Malignant nerve sheath tumor

Discussion

Neurilemomas are radiologically indistinguishable from neurofibromas. Benign nerve sheath tumors (i.e., neurilemoma and neurofibromas) are usually small and have well-defined, smooth margins. Malignant nerve sheath tumors usually are more than 5 cm in diameter, contain areas of low attenuation, and often have irregular or ill-defined margins on CT and MRI. They typically have low-attenuation areas on CT and high-signal-intensity areas on T2-weighted MRI. Definitive diagnosis requires biopsy or surgical resection.

Diagnosis

Intercostal neurilemoma

Suggested Readings

Ko SF, Lee TY, Lin JW, et al: Thoracic neurilemomas: An analysis of computed tomography findings in 36 patients. J Thorac Imaging 13:21-26, 1998.

Lee JY, Lee KS, Han J, et al: Spectrum of neurogenic tumors in the thorax: CT and pathologic findings. J Comput Assist Tomogr 23:399-406, 1999.

Tanaka O, Kiryu T, Hirose Y, et al: Neurogenic tumors of the mediastinum and chest wall. MR imaging appearance. J Thorac Imaging 20:316-320, 2005.

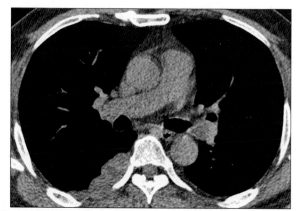

Figure 1. Unenhanced CT at the level of the undersurface of the right 6th rib shows a homogenous soft tissue opacity with a lobulated contour adjacent to and parallel to the rib. The patient was a 59-year-old man with an intercostal nerve neurilemoma.

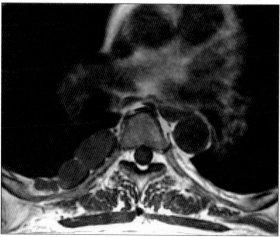

Figure 2. In the same patient, T1-weighted MRI at the level of the undersurface of the right 6th rib shows a lobulated lesion parallel to the rib and having signal intensity that is isointense with muscle.

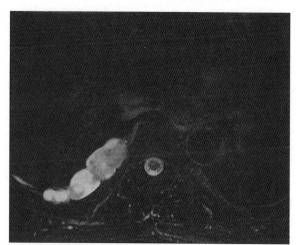

Figure 3. In the same patient, T2-weighted MRI shows areas of intermediate and high signal intensity.

Case 200

DEMOGRAPHICS/CLINICAL HISTORY

A 24-year-old woman with rotoscoliosis and a chest wall deformity, undergoing radiography and computed tomography (CT).

FINDINGS

The posteroanterior chest radiograph (Fig. 1) shows rotoscoliosis, increased soft tissue opacity projecting over the region of the right heart border, obscuration of the right heart border, and displacement of the heart to the left. The lateral radiograph (Fig. 2) shows depression of the lower portion of the sternum, which projects over the anterior aspect of the heart shadow. CT (Fig. 3) at the level of the lower sternum shows the caved-in appearance of the anterior chest wall, with compression and displacement of the heart to the left.

DISCUSSION

Definition/Background

Pectus excavatum (i.e., funnel chest) is a congenital chest wall deformity characterized by a caved-in appearance of the anterior chest wall due to abnormal growth of the sternum and several adjacent ribs. The condition is usually present at birth but typically worsens during rapid bone growth in the early teenage years. Pectus excavatum may occur as the only abnormality or occur with other syndromes; approximately 20% of patients have associated scoliosis.

Characteristic Clinical Features

Most patients do not have symptoms. A few patients have symptoms that include chest pain and, occasionally, shortness of breath.

Characteristic Radiologic Findings

Depression and deformity of the lower portion of the sternum is best seen on a lateral radiograph, CT, or magnetic resonance imaging (MRI). The manifestations on the posteroanterior radiograph include obscuration of the right heart border, displacement of the heart to the left, and spurious cardiomegaly. Patients have a pectus index (Haller index) value greater than 3.25; it is derived from dividing the transverse diameter of the chest by the anteroposterior diameter seen on CT and is often used as a criterion for surgical candidacy.

Less Common Radiologic Manifestations

More vertical than normal orientation of the anterior ribs.

Differential Diagnosis

- Right middle lobe consolidation
- Right middle lobe atelectasis
- Cardiophrenic angle mass

Discussion

Obscuration of the right heart border on the chest radiograph usually is caused by a right middle lobe consolidation or atelectasis. The diagnosis of pectus excavatum can be readily made on the lateral radiographic findings.

Diagnosis

Pectus excavatum

Suggested Readings

Fefferman NR, Pinkney LP: Imaging evaluation of chest wall disorders in children. Radiol Clin North Am 43:355-370, 2005.

Goretsky MJ, Kelly RE Jr, Croitoru D, Nuss D: Chest wall anomalies: Pectus excavatum and pectus carinatum. Adolesc Med Clin 15:455-471, 2004.

Haller JA Jr, Kramer SS, Lietman SA: Use of CT scans in selection of patients for pectus excavatum surgery: A preliminary report. J Pediatr Surg 22:904-906, 1987.

Jeung MY, Gangi A, Gasser B, et al: Imaging of chest wall disorders. Radiographics 19:617-637, 1999.

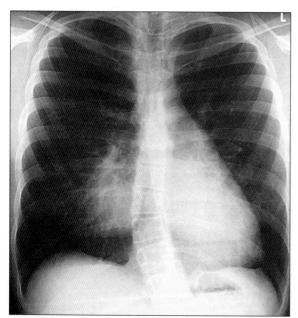

Figure 1. Posteroanterior chest radiograph shows rotoscoliosis, increased soft tissue opacity projecting over the region of the right heart border, obscuration of the right heart border, and displacement of the heart to the left. The patient was a 24-year-old woman with rotoscoliosis and pectus excavatum.

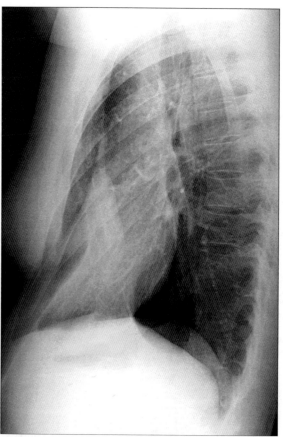

Figure 2. In the same patient, the lateral radiograph shows depression of the lower portion of the sternum, which projects over the anterior aspect of the heart shadow.

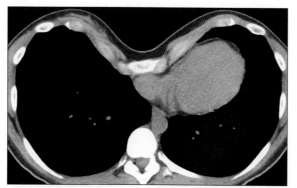

Figure 3. In the same patient, CT at the level of the lower sternum shows the caved-in appearance of the anterior chest wall, with compression and displacement of the heart to the left. The pectus index was 4.77.

Index of Cases

Index

Page numbers followed by f indicate figures.